500
HIGH-FIBER
RECIPES

500
HIGH-FIBER
RECIPES

Fight Diabetes, High Cholesterol, High Blood
Pressure, and Irritable Bowel Syndrome with
Delicious Meals That Fill You Up and
Help You Shed Pounds!

DICK LOGUE

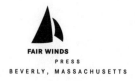

FAIR WINDS
PRESS
BEVERLY, MASSACHUSETTS

Text © 2009 Dick Logue

First published in the USA in 2009 by
Fair Winds Press, a member of
Quayside Publishing Group
100 Cummings Center
Suite 406-L
Beverly, MA 01915-6101
www.fairwindspress.com

13 12 11 10 09   1 2 3 4 5

ISBN-13: 978-1-59233-408-7
ISBN-10: 1-59233-408-3

Library of Congress Cataloging-in-Publication Data

Logue, Dick.
    500 high fiber recipes : fight diabetes, high cholesterol, high blood pressure, irritable bowel syndrome, and cancer with delicious meals that fill you up-and help you shed pounds! / Dick Logue.
        p. cm.
    Includes bibliographical references and index.
    ISBN-13: 978-1-59233-408-7 (alk. paper)
    ISBN-10: 1-59233-408-3 (alk. paper)
    1. High-fiber diet–Recipes.   I. Title.   II. Title: Five hundred high fiber recipes.
    RM237.6.L64 2009
    641.5'63–dc22

                                                                    2009027491

Cover and book design by Fair Winds Press

Printed and bound in Canada

The information in this book is for educational purposes only. It is not intended to replace the advice of a physician or medical practitioner. Please see your health care provider before beginning any new health program.

Dedication

In loving memory of my mother, Laura Wright Logue, who got me started cooking, and I'm sure is still watching over my efforts.

Table of Contents

What's All This about High Fiber?

Recently there has been a lot of talk on the news and in other sources about the benefits of increasing the amount of fiber in your diet. Perhaps you've seen or heard some of these reports, and that is why you are looking at this book. If so, you probably have a number of questions. I'm going to try to address some of those questions here.

We'll look at things like the following:

- Why all the talk about increasing fiber? Is this just another diet craze?
- What are some of the benefits of a high-fiber diet?
- Aren't there concerns about and drawbacks to eating a high-fiber diet?
- How much fiber should we be eating every day?
- How did I end up writing a book of high-fiber recipes?

After we've looked at these questions, chapter 1 will go into detail about how to increase the amount of fiber you eat. We'll look at what the best high-fiber foods are; how you can make some simple substitutions when you go shopping to greatly increase the fiber in your diet; and some surprising foods that contain fiber (like chocolate!).

The rest of the book contains 500 recipes that will help you think about ways to get more fiber in your diet. I'm not going to give you some meal plan to stick to. The ones I've seen in other books are not the kind of thing that most people would follow anyway. And they generally only contain a day's or at the most a week's worth of meals. What I am going to do is give you *lots* of recipes, literally everything from soup to nuts (both of which are usually good high-fiber choices). These aren't the kind of recipes that will make you think you are on some strictly regimented diet. They are the kind that you can pick and choose from to add fiber to your diet, while still providing yourself and your family food that tastes good and is like the kinds of things you've always eaten.

Why All This Talk about High-Fiber Diets?

The first question many people are going to have is probably "Why am I hearing so much about high-fiber diets lately?" First of all, fiber is not a new topic. Dr. John Kellogg, who founded the company that was to become Kellogg's cereal, was a big proponent of fiber in the late 1800s. And Charles Post invented Grape-Nuts, still a popular high-fiber cereal, in 1897. However, fiber has had a bit of an up-and-down history. During the middle of the 20th century it was common to consider fiber a relatively unimportant part of a diet, and it was typically removed from items like white flour.

It is true, however, that talk about fiber has increased in recent years. Part of this is due to the increased awareness of healthy eating over the past 30 or 40 years. Vegetarian cooking tends to be higher in fiber than diets containing meat. And heart-healthy cooking, which is where I got started in creating healthier versions of recipes, also generally includes higher fiber, for reason that we'll discuss. A number of recent medical studies have also confirmed the medical benefits of high-fiber diets for a number of different conditions. Here are a few:

- A study published in the May 11, 2000, issue of the *New England Journal of Medicine* reported that patients with diabetes who maintained very high fiber in their daily diet lowered their glucose levels by 10 percent.
- A 1976 study by the Veterans Administration Medical Center, Lexington, Kentucky, showed that fiber is useful in treating diabetes, high blood pressure, and obesity and in reducing cholesterol levels.
- Two studies published in the *Lancet* showed that people with high-fiber diets suffered from fewer incidents of colon polyps and colon cancer.

So there are a lot of good reasons to add more fiber to your diet, even if you aren't currently being treated for a medical condition that requires it. In the next section we'll look at some of those reasons in more detail.

Why Increase the Amount of Fiber in Your Diet?

So what are the benefits of a high-fiber diet? Let's take a look at some of the more common ones.

Lose Weight

Let's start with this one since it's on a lot of people's minds. If you do a search online, you'll find any number of people pushing high-fiber eating as a way to lose weight. And it does work. We'll get into more details in the next section, but the short explanation is that by eating more fiber, you'll feel more full and want to eat fewer calories. And the bottom line in losing weight is to burn more calories than you eat.

Reduce the Rick of Certain Cancers

A major benefit for everyone is the role that fiber has been shown to have in reducing cancer. I already mentioned the studies that showed people who eat a high-fiber diet have less colon cancer. It appears there are a number of benefits to colon health from fiber. First, it helps to push stools through the colon more quickly, which contributes to overall colon health. Water-soluble fiber also encourages the growth of beneficial bacteria in the colon. And finally, it helps to bind potential carcinogens and excrete them from the body. The bottom line is that the people who eat a high-fiber diet have been shown to have a 40 percent reduction in the risk of colon cancer.

But colon cancer isn't the only cancer that fiber can reduce. Studies done in England have revealed not only that women who eat a high-fiber diet are less likely to develop breast cancer, but also that women who already had breast cancer had a longer life expectancy on a high-fiber diet. And finally, studies have shown a significant reduction in uterine cancer in women who ate a high-fiber diet.

Help the Heart and Circulatory System

Fiber has also had positive effects in fighting heart disease, the number-one killer of both men and women in the United States. Primarily, getting to and staying at a desirable weight reduces one of the biggest risk factors for heart disease. But fiber also contributes in other more active ways. First of all, it helps to reduce cholesterol levels. It does this in several ways. One is by encouraging the production of propionic acid in the intestines, which inhibits the production of cholesterol. Secondly, it removes bile acids from the intestines. In order to make more bile acids, the liver requires cholesterol, which it removes from the bloodstream. The bottom line . . . high-fiber diets have reduced the bad kind of cholesterol, LDL, by 10 to 15 percent.

Help Control Blood Pressure

Another way that fiber contributes to heart and overall health is by reducing high blood pressure. High-fiber diets have been shown to reduce blood pressure by three to seven points, enough to reduce the risk of heart disease by up to 9 percent. Cholesterol reduction contributes to lower blood pressure. Fiber also tends to widen the arteries, reducing the risk of blockage.

Strengthen the Immune System

Fiber can help to keep you healthy by strengthening your immune system. Other diets rely on drastic reductions of food intake. This often has the effect of reducing the number and health of white blood cells. A high-fiber diet, on the other hand, has the opposite effect, strengthening the white blood cells. It also promotes health by increasing beneficial bacteria in the intestines.

Help Fight Diabetes

Finally, a high-fiber diet can reduce your risk of developing type 2 diabetes. Reducing your weight is again a positive thing for reducing the risk of diabetes; but it also helps in other ways. It slows the absorption of sugar into the bloodstream. Research has found that a high-fiber meal can reduce blood sugar levels by as much as 28 percent. It also has been proven to improve insulin sensitivity, which better enables the body to process sugar.

How Does Fiber Work in the Body?

Fiber provides its benefits through a complex series of actions in the body. Without getting into a lot a medical details (which I don't really understand anyway), let's look at a few of them.

High-fiber foods require you to work a little more. In general, they are going to require more chewing. This is good, as it encourages you to eat more slowly. Since it takes a while for the body to determine that it is full, this happens earlier in the meal process, causing you to eat less.

In the stomach, high-fiber food also contributes to that full feeling. Fiber absorbs water, making the stomach feel more full. It also tends to stay in the stomach longer, meaning that you won't feel hungry as soon.

In the intestines, fiber triggers the production of chemicals that again tell the brain that you are full. An additional benefit is that fiber is not absorbed, so it represents calories that will not be stored in the body.

Fiber's ability to reduce the blood sugar level means that you will feel less hungry and feel fewer cravings for high-calorie foods.

How Much Fiber Should I Eat?

So how much fiber is enough? The American Dietetic Association recommends between 20 and 35 grams. However, the average intake in the United States is only 12 to 15 grams. The recommended amount for children under 18 is determined by adding five to a child's age. For example, a 7-year-old child would need 12 grams of fiber a day. The National Academy of Sciences' Institute of Medicine gives the following daily recommendations for adults:

- Men 50 and younger—38 grams
- Men 51 and older—30 grams
- Women 50 and younger—25 grams
- Women 51 and older—21 grams

There's good news and bad news there. The bad news is that unless you are consciously watching your fiber intake, you probably aren't getting nearly the recommended amounts. The good news is that if you do watch what you eat, it isn't as difficult as you think to reach them.

What About the Potential Problems I've Heard About?

Okay, to get right to the point, what do you think about when you think high fiber? Beans. And what do you think of when you think of beans? Gas.

It's true that high-fiber foods can produce gas. It's especially true if you suddenly start eating lots of high-fiber foods. So there are a few things you should consider as you start adding fiber to your diet.

- Start slowly and build up. If you've been eating 10 grams of fiber a day, don't suddenly jump to 35 grams. Add fiber a little at a time, perhaps starting with breakfast, then lunch, and then dinner.

- Drink more water. Fiber absorbs water in the digestive tract. So you'll want to make sure you drink plenty. Some experts recommend doubling your water intake until you know how your body is going to handle the fiber increase.
- If beans or other foods cause gas problems, take an enzyme product such as Beano. It actually works to reduce the amount of gas by helping you break down the starches that cause the gas when they are digested in the intestines.
- If certain raw foods cause gas, cook them, which makes them easier to digest.

How This Book Came About

Perhaps the best way to start telling you who I am is by telling you who I'm not. I'm not a doctor. I'm not a dietitian. I'm not a professional chef. What I *am* is an ordinary person just like you who has some special dietary needs. What I am going to do is give you 500 recipes I have made for myself and my family, which I think will help you increase the amount of fiber in your diet and your family's. Many of them are the things people cook in their own kitchens all the time but modified to make them healthier without losing the flavor.

I've enjoyed cooking most of my life. I guess I started seriously about the time my mother went back to work when I was 12 or so. In those days it was simple stuff like burgers and hot dogs and spaghetti. But the interest stayed. After I married my wife, we got pretty involved in some food-related stuff . . . growing vegetables in our garden, making bread and other baked goods, and canning and jelly making . . . that kind of thing. She always said that my "mad chemist" cooking was an outgrowth of the time I spent in college as a chemistry major, and she might be right.

Some of you may already know me from my Low Sodium Cooking website and newsletter or from my *500 Low-Sodium Recipes* book. I started thinking about low-sodium cooking after being diagnosed with congestive heart failure in 1999. One of the first and biggest things I had to deal with was the doctor's insistence that I follow a low-sodium diet—1200 mg a day or less. At first, like many people, I found it easiest to just avoid the things that had a lot of sodium in them. But I was bored. And I was convinced that there had to be a way to create low-sodium versions of the foods I missed. So I learned all kinds of *new* cooking things. I researched where to get low-sodium substitutes for the things that I couldn't have anymore, bought cookbooks, and basically redid my whole diet.

Along the way I learned some things. And I decided to try to share this information with others who might be in the same position. I started a website, www.lowsodiumcooking.com, to share recipes and information. I sent out an e-mail newsletter with recipes that now has more than 17,000 subscribers. And I wrote my first book.

Along the way, I discovered that there were other areas of the diet besides sodium that contribute to heart health. I began to incorporate these into my diet also. Some of those are detailed in my second book, *500 Low-Cholesterol Recipes*. But I also began to read more and more about the importance of increasing the fiber in your diet, not just for heart health, but also for all the reasons listed earlier in this chapter. So our diet changed again, this time to increase the amount of fiber. And this book is a result of that change.

How Is the Nutritional Information Calculated?

The nutritional information included with these recipes was calculated using the AccuChef program. It calculates the values using the latest US Department of Agriculture standard reference nutritional database. I've been using this program since I first started trying to figure out how much sodium was in the recipes I've created. It's inexpensive, easy to use, and has a number of really handy features. For instance, if I go in and change the nutrition figures for an ingredient, it remembers those figures whenever I use that ingredient. AccuChef is available online from www.accuchef.com. They offer a free-trial version if you want to try it out, and the full version costs less than $20 US.

Of course, that implies that these figures are estimates. Every brand of tomatoes or any other product is a little different in nutritional content. These figures were calculated using products that I buy here in southern Maryland. If you use a different brand, your nutrition figures may be different. Use the nutritional analysis as a guideline in determining whether a recipe is right for your diet.

1

How Do I Add More Fiber to My Diet?

Now that we've looked at why adding more fiber to our diet is a good idea, let's take a quick look at the *how*. It isn't really as difficult as you might think. We'll look at a few simple things you can do when you go to the grocery store and then some specific recommendations for different groups of foods that are high in fiber.

The first thing to do is to be aware of the fiber content of foods. Become a label reader. If you are just starting out, take an extra hour at the store reading nutrition labels and looking at the fiber content. There really are a lot of foods out there with fiber in them. Unlike when I first started on a low-sodium diet, you don't have to make nearly everything from scratch. All you need to do is make smart choices. And the things you pick don't all have to have huge amounts to help you get to your goal. Sure, a serving of beans might have 15 grams, but no one wants to eat beans every day. But you can get that same 15 grams from two or three servings of vegetables or any of a number of combinations.

Just as an example, here are a couple of low-fiber or high-fiber choices:

- Puffed rice cereal—0 grams; shredded wheat—5 grams
- White bread (such as Wonder)—0 grams; light wheat bread (such as Wonder)—5 grams
- Regular pasta (such as Barilla)—2 grams; whole wheat pasta (such as Barilla)—6 grams
- White flour—0 grams; whole wheat pastry flour—3 grams

The great news about these choices is that you'll find the higher-fiber choice also tastes better, has more flavor, and leaves you feeling more satisfied.

Even the kind of ice cream you choose can make a difference. Ben and Jerry's Super Fudge Chunk has 2 grams of fiber!

And of course, you should be looking to add more foods from the following groups to your diet.

Legumes

Beans and other legumes are the poster child for high-fiber foods. A single serving can provide 15 grams or more of fiber. They also have been proven effective at keeping you from feeling hungry the longest and have been linked to reduced risk of heart disease, diabetes, and certain kinds of cancer.

Of course, as I said, you probably won't eat beans every day, but you should strive for two or three servings a week. And there are lots of ways to incorporate legumes into your diet. This book contains 70 recipes that feature just legumes and a number more where they are included as an ingredient along with other high-fiber foods.

Here are a few suggestions for including more legumes in your diet:

- Use legumes as snacks. There are a number of recipes here for bean dips, spreads, and other snack items. True, most of them only contain 2 or 3 grams of fiber, but combined with a high-fiber dipper like fresh vegetables or whole wheat pita chips, they can contribute quickly to your daily fiber goal.
- Add them into other recipes. Beans and chickpeas make a great addition to many soups, salads, and dishes like rice or grain side dishes. You'll find lots of those kind of recipes here in the chapters featuring combinations.
- Think of different ways to use them in dishes. True, you can make chili or baked beans, but there are also things like burritos, split pea soup, and marinated bean salads.

Here are examples of the amount of fiber in a serving of a few common legumes:

- Navy beans—19 grams
- Split peas—16 grams
- Lentils—16 grams
- Black beans—15 grams

- Lima beans—13 grams
- Kidney beans—11 grams
- Black-eyed peas—9 grams

Whole Grains

Whole grains are a great source of fiber and one that's easy to include in your diet. You should eat two or three servings of whole grains a day. Whole grains contribute to that full feeling that keeps you from overeating and have been shown to slow the absorption of sugar into the blood. They also contain many other minerals and nutrients that are removed from processed grains.

Here are some ways to increase the amount of whole grains in your diet:

- Use whole grain bread instead of white bread. This is a simple choice to make and an easy one. Today's grocery stores offer an incredible variety of whole grain breads to choose from.
- Choose whole grain pastas and rice. This is a change that we've made in our diet fairly recently. I never really paid much attention to whole grain pasta, but now I find that I much prefer the flavor to the bland regular pasta. And I generally avoided brown rice because it took longer to cook, even though I preferred the flavor of it also. But now there are quick-cooking and microwaveable varieties of brown rice that make it as easy as white rice.
- Choose high-fiber cereals. A number of studies show that starting the day with a bowl of high-fiber cereal is one of the things that is most positively linked with weight loss.
- Consider alternative grains. Rather than just pasta or rice or potatoes, think about main dishes and side dishes that contain barley, bulgur, kasha, and other grains. You'll find a number of recipes in this book that contain them.

Here is the amount of fiber in a cup of several kinds of whole grains:

- Whole wheat flour—18 grams
- Barley—13 grams
- Whole grain pasta—4 grams or more, depending on the brand
- Oats—4 grams
- Brown rice—3 grams

Fruits and Vegetables

Fruits and vegetables offer a number of health benefits, and increased fiber is just one of them. The five-serving-a-day goal has been well established and publicized. That may seem like a lot, but when you start counting, you'll find that it is not really that difficult to reach. They are a great food value when you are trying to lose weight, since they provide needed bulk while generally being low in calories.

In order to get the most fiber benefit from your fruits and vegetables, here are a few tips:

- Eat whole fruits and vegetables as much as possible. The skin contains many nutrients, as well as fiber. And the seeds in items like fresh tomatoes add fiber that's missing in many processed tomato products.
- Choose fresh fruits and vegetables over frozen or canned if necessary, choose and frozen over canned. The more an item is processed, the more likely it is to have had the healthful nutrients and fiber removed and undesirable things like salt added.
- Don't just think of salads. True, salads are a low-calorie, healthy addition to your diet. But they may not pack the fiber punch that other vegetable servings do. Lettuce, for example, is not one of the better sources of fiber, generally containing less than 1 gram per serving.

The following is the amount of fiber in a 1-cup serving of some common fruits and vegetables:

- Prunes—12 grams
- Avocado—10 grams
- Green peas—9 grams
- Raspberries—8 grams
- Pumpkin and winter squash—6 or 7 grams
- Collard greens—5 grams
- Potato, medium—5 grams
- Pear, medium—5 grams
- Apple, large—5 grams
- Corn—4 grams
- Green beans—4 grams
- Asparagus—4 grams
- Bell pepper—3 grams
- Strawberries—3 grams

- Banana—3 grams
- Cabbage—3 grams
- Eggplant—2 grams
- Broccoli—2 grams
- Peaches—2 grams
- Pineapple—2 grams

Nuts and Seeds

Nuts and seeds provide a surprising amount of fiber in a small serving. You should plan on several servings a week.

Here are some suggestions for including more nuts and seeds in your diet:

- Use them as snacks. Unlike snack items like chips, nuts provide a significant nutritional benefit. We've included a number of recipes for snack mixes and other ways to incorporate more nuts into your diet.
- Use them as toppings and additions. Nuts and seeds can be added to salads, used to top baked goods, and sprinkled over vegetables and casseroles.

The following shows the amount of fiber in an ounce of various nuts and seeds.

- Almonds—3 grams
- Pistachios—3 grams
- Peanut butter, chunky, 3 tablespoons—2 grams
- Sunflower seeds—2 grams
- Peanuts—2 grams
- Sesame seeds, 1 tablespoon—1 gram

Other Fiber Sources

There are several other rather surprising sources of fiber. These aren't where you'll get the majority of your fiber, but if you can pick up a few grams while indulging in something you like, why not?

- Coffee—Coffee contains between 1 gram per serving for filtered coffee and up to almost 2 grams for instant coffee.

- Chocolate—An ounce of chocolate candy contains almost 2 grams of fiber.
- Spices—A teaspoon of spice may contain up to a gram of fiber. In addition, some spices like fennel, cayenne, cumin, and turmeric have been shown to improve digestion and reduce gas and bloating.

A Few Final Thoughts

Hopefully the information in this chapter has gotten you thinking about some of the ways that you can increase the amount of fiber in your diet. The rest of this book contains 500 recipes to help you do just that. As I said earlier, there is no strict meal plan or counting of grams here, just a lot of recipes that may contain as little as a gram of fiber or as much as 20 grams. It's up to you to pick and choose, depending on your tastes, and decide which of these recipes will be best for you.

The book is organized by type of food and the source of fiber. We have sections on appetizers and snack foods, breakfast, main dishes, side dishes, bread, and desserts. Those sections have chapters with recipes containing legumes, grains, fruits and vegetables, nuts, and combinations of those items. Not all sections contain all the categories; there just aren't that many main dishes where nuts are the main source of fiber. But I felt this organization would let you focus on the types of recipes you're looking for.

One final question that many people ask when they start to try to add fiber to their diet is whether they should be taking a fiber supplement. These have been heavily marketed on television, and it seems like an easy fix. However, most experts recommend against it. In the first place, most supplements don't really add that much fiber to your diet. Typically they contain 3 to 5 grams, the amount that you could get from a banana or a slice of whole grain bread. However, the fruit or the bread also contains a number of other nutrients that the supplement doesn't. In the long run, you'll be better off making smart diet choices and eating as much food as possible in its natural state.

2

Appetizers, Snacks, and Party Foods:
Legumes

We'll start our trip with appetizers and snack foods and begin that journey with legumes. The first thing that probably comes to mind is bean dip. We have five different bean dips, and you'll also find dips and spreads using less common legumes such as black-eyed peas and chick peas. There are also a number of other items like salsa, nachos, stuffed eggs and one of my new personal favorites, roasted chickpeas.

Cheddar Bean Dip

This simple to make hot bean-and-cheese dip is great with tortilla chips or crispy wedges of pita bread and is sure to be a hit.

½ cup (115 g) mayonnaise

2 cups (342 g) cooked pinto beans, drained and mashed

1 cup (115 g) shredded Cheddar cheese

4 ounces (115 g) chopped green chiles

¼ teaspoon Tabasco sauce

Stir all ingredients until well mixed. Spoon into a small ovenproof dish. Bake at 350°F (180°C, gas mark 4) for 30 minutes or until bubbly.

Yield: 12 servings

Each with: 32 g water; 153 calories (64% from fat, 14% from protein, 22% from carb); 5 g protein; 11 g total fat; 3 g saturated fat; 3 g monounsaturated fat; 4 g polyunsaturated fat; 8 g carb; 3 g fiber; 0 g sugar; 102 mg phosphorus; 97 mg calcium; 1 mg iron; 159 mg sodium; 149 mg potassium; 149 IU vitamin A; 36 mg vitamin E; 3 mg vitamin C; 15 mg cholesterol

Cowboy Bean Dip

This variation on the usual layered dip is with black beans.

15 ounces (420 g) black beans

¼ cup (40 g) finely chopped olives

2 tablespoons (28 ml) lime juice

¼ teaspoon ground cumin

½ teaspoon finely chopped garlic

⅛ teaspoon black pepper

8 ounces (225 g) cream cheese, softened

¼ cup (25 g) sliced scallions

(continued on page 24)

Drain and rinse the beans. Drain the chopped olives. Mix all the ingredients except cream cheese and scallions. Cover and refrigerate at least 2 hours. Spread cream cheese on serving plate. Spoon bean mixture evenly over cream cheese. Sprinkle with scallions.

Yield: 12 servings

Each with: 48 g water; 127 calories (54% from fat, 15% from protein, 31% from carb); 5 g protein; 8 g total fat; 4 g saturated fat; 3 g monounsaturated fat; 0 g polyunsaturated fat; 10 g carb; 4 g fiber; 0 g sugar; 72 mg phosphorus; 36 mg calcium; 1 mg iron; 139 mg sodium; 164 mg potassium; 318 IU vitamin A; 68 mg vitamin E; 2 mg vitamin C; 21 mg cholesterol

Horseradish Bean Dip

Horseradish adds zip to this dip. It is good on toasted pita bread triangles or tortilla chips.

¼ cup (60 g) mayonnaise

¼ cup (60 ml) low-sodium ketchup

¼ cup (60 g) pickle relish

½ cup (80 g) chopped onion

1 tablespoon horseradish

1 tablespoon dry mustard

1 tablespoon (15 ml) Worcestershire sauce

1½ cups (150 g) cooked kidney beans, drained and mashed

Mix mayonnaise and ketchup. Mix in other ingredients adding kidney beans last. Refrigerate.

Yield: 24 servings

Each with: 15 g water; 39 calories (42% from fat, 12% from protein, 46% from carb); 1 g protein; 2 g total fat; 0 g saturated fat; 0 g monounsaturated fat; 1 g polyunsaturated fat; 5 g carb; 1 g fiber; 1 g sugar; 19 mg phosphorus; 10 mg calcium; 0 mg iron; 50 mg sodium; 71 mg potassium; 38 IU vitamin A; 2 mg vitamin E; 2 mg vitamin C; 1 mg cholesterol

Red Bean Dip

This is a great bean-and-cheese dip that not only tastes better than commercial ones but is healthier too.

2 tablespoons (28 ml) olive oil

½ teaspoon crushed garlic

1 cup (160 g) finely chopped onion

1 jalapeño, finely chopped

1 teaspoon chili powder

2 cups (100 g) cooked kidney beans

½ cup (58 g) shredded Cheddar cheese

Heat oil in a skillet. Add garlic, onion, jalapeño, and chili powder and cook gently 4 minutes. Drain kidney beans, reserving juice. Process beans in a blender or food processor to a puree. Add to onion mixture and stir in 2 tablespoons of reserved bean liquid; mix well. Stir in cheese. Cook gently about 2 minutes, stirring until cheese melts. If mixture becomes too thick, add a little more reserved bean liquid. Spoon into serving dish and serve warm with tortilla chips.

Yield: 12 servings

Each with: 19 g water; 151 calories (26% from fat, 23% from protein, 52% from carb); 9 g protein; 4 g total fat; 2 g saturated fat; 1 g monounsaturated fat; 1 g polyunsaturated fat; 20 g carb; 8 g fiber; 1 g sugar; 158 mg phosphorus; 87 mg calcium; 3 mg iron; 44 mg sodium; 463 mg potassium; 126 IU vitamin A; 14 mg vitamin E; 3 mg vitamin C; 6 mg cholesterol

White Bean Dip

This is tasty appetizer that is good either warm or cold.

1 cup (208 g) dry navy beans

½ cup (80 g) chopped onion

¾ teaspoon minced garlic

1 tablespoon (15 ml) Dijon mustard

¼ cup (25 g) chopped scallions

2 tablespoons (28 ml) lime juice

1 teaspoon tarragon

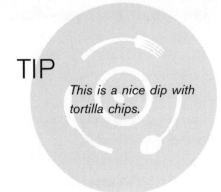

TIP

This is a nice dip with tortilla chips.

Bring beans to a boil for 1 minute and remove from heat to soak for 1 hour. Rinse well. Add onion and cook beans until tender, about 1 hour. Drain beans and rinse well. In a food processor place mustard, scallions, lime juice, and tarragon. Pulse to combine. Add beans and blend until smooth.

Yield: 8 servings

Each with: 40 g water; 45 calories (5% from fat, 24% from protein, 72% from carb); 3 g protein; 0 g total fat; 0 g saturated fat; 0 g monounsaturated fat; 0 g polyunsaturated fat; 8 g carb; 2 g fiber; 1 g sugar; 51 mg phosphorus; 23 mg calcium; 1 mg iron; 169 mg sodium; 128 mg potassium; 38 IU vitamin A; 0 mg vitamin E; 3 mg vitamin C; 0 mg cholesterol

Hummus

A traditional Middle Eastern dip made with chickpeas, this is a simple version that doesn't include the usual tahini sesame butter. But don't make the mistake of thinking that it is short on flavor because it's not. Toasted pita triangles are the perfect dippers for this.

2 cups (328 g) cooked chickpeas, drained

1 teaspoon cumin

½ teaspoon minced garlic

¼ teaspoon cayenne pepper

3 tablespoons (45 ml) lemon juice

1 teaspoon smoked paprika

⅓ cup (78 ml) olive oil

Thoroughly process all ingredients in a blender. Add additional cumin and cayenne pepper to taste. Sprinkle with paprika; drizzle olive oil on top.

Yield: 16 servings

Each with: 15 g water; 75 calories (59% from fat, 10% from protein, 31% from carb); 2 g protein; 5 g total fat; 1 g saturated fat; 3 g monounsaturated fat; 1 g polyunsaturated fat; 6 g carb; 2 g fiber; 1 g sugar; 36 mg phosphorus; 12 mg calcium; 1 mg iron; 2 mg sodium; 70 mg potassium; 95 IU vitamin A; 0 mg vitamin E; 2 mg vitamin C; 0 mg cholesterol

Black-Eyed Pea Pâté

This is especially good with one of the pita chips recipes, but it is also great with vegetable dippers or tortilla chips.

8 ounces (225 g) cream cheese, softened

16 ounces (455 g) black-eyed peas, drained

½ cup (80 g) onion, quartered

½ teaspoon minced garlic

½ cup (130 g) salsa

(continued on page 28)

1 teaspoon Tabasco sauce

3 tablespoons (45 ml) Worcestershire sauce

2 packets unflavored gelatin

2 tablespoons (30 ml) cold water

¼ cup minced fresh parsley

Put cream cheese, peas, onion, garlic, salsa, Tabasco, and Worcestershire sauce in food processor with knife blade. Process until smooth. Sprinkle gelatin over cold water in small saucepan; let stand 1 minute. Cook over low heat, stirring until dissolved. Add gelatin mixture to pea mixture. Spin again until well blended. Spoon into glass casserole dish. Cover and chill until firm. Unmold and sprinkle with parsley.

Yield: 20 servings

Each with: 34 g water; 107 calories (34% from fat, 13% from protein, 53% from carb); 4 g protein; 4 g total fat; 3 g saturated fat; 1 g monounsaturated fat; 0 g polyunsaturated fat; 15 g carb; 2 g fiber; 9 g sugar; 58 mg phosphorus; 18 mg calcium; 1 mg iron; 113 mg sodium; 147 mg potassium; 258 IU vitamin A; 41 mg vitamin E; 6 mg vitamin C; 12 mg cholesterol

Split Pea Spread

This unusual spread is made with split peas and is good on toasted wedges of pita bread.

1 cup (196 g) cooked split peas

2 tablespoons (27 g) cottage cheese

2 tablespoons grated Parmesan cheese

2 tablespoons (28 ml) olive oil

¼ teaspoon dried basil

½ teaspoon crushed garlic

After cooked split peas have cooled, mash them up. Mix in other ingredients and refrigerate.

Yield: 6 servings

Each with: 26 g water; 90 calories (51% from fat, 18% from protein, 31% from carb); 4 g protein; 5 g total fat; 1 g saturated fat; 3 g monounsaturated fat; 1 g polyunsaturated fat; 7 g carb; 3 g fiber; 1 g sugar; 51 mg phosphorus; 30 mg calcium; 0 mg iron; 33 mg sodium; 124 mg potassium; 15 IU vitamin A; 3 mg vitamin E; 0 mg vitamin C; 2 mg cholesterol

Texas Caviar

Being tasty and just a little spicy, this dip is typical of the Texas/Louisiana area.

2 cups (342 g) cooked black-eyed peas, drained

1 cup (100 g) chopped scallions

1 cup (160 g) chopped onion

1 cup (150 g) chopped green bell pepper

¼ cup (34 g) chopped jalapeño pepper

2 ounces (55 g) chopped pimento

8 ounces (225 ml) Italian dressing

Mix all ingredients together and chill.

Yield: 20 servings

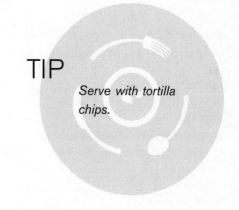

TIP

Serve with tortilla chips.

Each with: 40 g water; 63 calories (47% from fat, 11% from protein, 42% from carb); 2 g protein; 3 g total fat; 1 g saturated fat; 1 g monounsaturated fat; 2 g polyunsaturated fat; 7 g carb; 2 g fiber; 2 g sugar; 28 mg phosphorus; 11 mg calcium; 1 mg iron; 190 mg sodium; 115 mg potassium; 179 IU vitamin A; 0 mg vitamin E; 11 mg vitamin C; 0 mg cholesterol

Shortcut Black Bean Salsa

Combine canned beans and canned salsa with some extra spices for a quick dip that's more than the sum of its parts.

1 cup (172 g) cooked black beans, drained

12 ounces (340 g) salsa

¼ cup chopped fresh cilantro

¼ teaspoon cumin

2 tablespoons (28 ml) lime juice

Roughly chop beans in food processor. Do not puree them. Stir in remaining ingredients. Serve immediately or refrigerate overnight. Serve with corn chips or raw vegetables.

Yield: 20 servings

Each with: 23 g water; 17 calories (4% from fat, 23% from protein, 73% from carb); 1 g protein; 0 g total fat; 0 g saturated fat; 0 g monounsaturated fat; 0 g polyunsaturated fat; 3 g carb; 1 g fiber; 1 g sugar; 18 mg phosphorus; 8 mg calcium; 0 mg iron; 40 mg sodium; 86 mg potassium; 87 IU vitamin A; 0 mg vitamin E; 1 mg vitamin C; 0 mg cholesterol

Chickpea-Stuffed Eggs

Definately a healthier alternative to the usual deviled eggs, these have no cholesterol but contain 2 grams of fiber.

7 eggs, hard boiled and peeled

1 cup (164 g) cooked chickpeas, drained

2 tablespoons (30 g) plain fat-free yogurt

1 teaspoon Dijon mustard

½ teaspoon minced garlic

Slice eggs in half and discard yolks. In food processor, combine all other ingredients. Spoon mixture into egg cavities.

Yield: 7 servings

Each with: 58 g water; 61 calories (7% from fat, 37% from protein, 56% from carb); 6 g protein; 0 g total fat; 0 g saturated fat; 0 g monounsaturated fat; 0 g polyunsaturated fat; 8 g carb; 2 g fiber; 1 g sugar; 44 mg phosphorus; 23 mg calcium; 1 mg iron; 169 mg sodium; 126 mg potassium; 9 IU vitamin A; 0 mg vitamin E; 1 mg vitamin C; 0 mg cholesterol

Skillet Nachos

This is great as an appetizer, served right from the skillet. But it is also good as a meal, wrapped up in a tortilla.

1 pound (455 g) ground beef

1 cup (160 g) chopped onion

2 cups (520 g) salsa

2 cups (344 g) cooked black beans, drained

1 teaspoon chili powder

1 cup (180 g) chopped tomato

1 avocado, seeded and diced

½ cup (50 g) sliced black olives

1 cup (115 g) shredded Cheddar cheese

1 cup (230 g) sour cream

In a 12-inch (30 cm) skillet, brown beef with onion; drain. Add salsa, beans, and chili powder; bring to a boil. Reduce heat and simmer uncovered 5 minutes. Stir in tomato, avocado, and olives; remove from heat. Sprinkle with cheese. Spoon sour cream onto center of meat mixture. Serve with tortilla chips and/or flour tortillas.

Yield: 6 servings

Each with: 276 g water; 486 calories (41% from fat, 30% from protein, 29% from carb); 28 g protein; 17 g total fat; 7 g saturated fat; 7 g monounsaturated fat; 1 g polyunsaturated fat; 27 g carb; 9 g fiber; 5 g sugar; 392 mg phosphorus; 267 mg calcium; 4 mg iron; 360 mg sodium; 970 mg potassium; 1035 IU vitamin A; 97 mg vitamin E; 9 mg vitamin C; 91 mg cholesterol

Roasted Chickpeas

This is a healthy, tasty snack that is high in fiber and very low in fat. Vary the seasonings according to your taste.

4 cups (656 g) cooked chickpeas

¼ teaspoon cayenne pepper

1 teaspoon garlic powder

1 teaspoon cumin

1 teaspoon paprika

Preheat oven to 400°F (200°C, gas mark 6). In a mesh strainer, gently rinse beans. Drain on paper towels and gently roll them dry. Line a baking sheet with aluminum foil and spread chickpeas evenly across sheet. Bake chickpeas, checking at 10-minute intervals. When chickpeas are dried and crunchy, about 30 to 40 minutes, remove from oven and spray with an olive oil cooking spray. Place spices in a plastic bowl with a tight-fitting lid or resealable plastic bag. Add chickpeas and shake to coat. For best results, store in an airtight container in the refrigerator.

Yield: 12 servings

Each with: 33 g water; 92 calories (14% from fat, 21% from protein, 65% from carb); 5 g protein; 1 g total fat; 0 g saturated fat; 0 g monounsaturated fat; 1 g polyunsaturated fat; 15 g carb; 4 g fiber; 3 g sugar; 94 mg phosphorus; 29 mg calcium; 2 mg iron; 4 mg sodium; 170 mg potassium; 133 IU vitamin A; 0 mg vitamin E; 1 mg vitamin C; 0 mg cholesterol

3

Appetizers, Snacks, and Party Foods:
Grains

Whole grain snack and party foods can be a quick way to add a few extra grams of fiber to your daily total. Our whole wheat pita chips contain 2 grams of fiber and are a lot healthier than chips as a dipping option. We also have crackers, snack mixes, and a couple of tortilla roll-ups that you can slice and serve for snacking.

Cheese Crisps

These little snacks taste great either warm from the oven or cold. However, there usually aren't any left to eat cold when we make them.

1 cup (120 g) grated Cheddar cheese
¼ cup (55 g) unsalted butter
½ cup (60 g) whole wheat flour

In large bowl, combine the cheese and butter. Add the flour and mix thoroughly. Roll into small balls. Place the balls on an baking sheet sprayed with nonstick vegetable oil spray and flatten. Bake at 400°F (200°C, gas mark 6) for 5 to 8 minutes. Do not let the edges get browned.

Yield: 12 servings

Each with: 5 g water; 95 calories (70% from fat, 14% from protein, 16% from carb); 3 g protein; 8 g total fat; 5 g saturated fat; 2 g monounsaturated fat; 0 g polyunsaturated fat; 4 g carb; 1 g fiber; 0 g sugar; 75 mg phosphorus; 82 mg calcium; 0 mg iron; 69 mg sodium; 32 mg potassium; 229 IU vitamin A; 60 mg vitamin E; 0 mg vitamin C; 22 mg cholesterol

Wheat Germ Crackers

These tasty little crackers are good without anything, but they also make a healthy dipper for any of the dips and spreads in chapters 3 through 6.

3 cups (240 g) quick-cooking oats
2 cups (240 g) whole wheat pastry flour
1 cup (112 g) wheat germ
3 tablespoons (39 g) sugar
1 cup (235 ml) water
¾ cup (175 ml) canola oil

Mix dry ingredients together. Add water and oil; stir until blended. Roll out on inverted baking sheet. Score and prick with fork. Bake at 325°F (170°C, gas mark 3) for 30 minutes or until brown. This is enough for 2 baking sheets, approximately 10 × 15 inches (25 × 37 cm) or 11 × 16 inches (27 × 40 cm).

Yield: 60 servings

Each with: 5 g water; 63 calories (46% from fat, 11% from protein, 44% from carb); 2 g protein; 3 g total fat; 0 g saturated fat; 2 g monounsaturated fat; 1 g polyunsaturated fat; 7 g carb; 1 g fiber; 1 g sugar; 55 mg phosphorus; 4 mg calcium; 0 mg iron; 1 mg sodium; 48 mg potassium; 2 IU vitamin A; 0 mg vitamin E; 0 mg vitamin C; 0 mg cholesterol

Pita Chips

These are simple and easy. Make your own low-fat, high-fiber chips for snacking or dipping in about 5 minutes.

2 whole wheat pitas

Cut pita into triangles and then separate. Place on foil-covered baking sheet. Spray with nonstick vegetable oil spray; season if desired. Bake in 375°F (190°C, gas mark 5) oven until crisp, about 5 minutes. Remove and cool.

Yield: 4 servings

Each with: 10 g water; 85 calories (8% from fat, 14% from protein, 78% from carb); 3 g protein; 1 g total fat; 0 g saturated fat; 0 g monounsaturated fat; 0 g polyunsaturated fat; 18 g carb; 2 g fiber; 0 g sugar; 58 mg phosphorus; 5 mg calcium; 1 mg iron; 170 mg sodium; 54 mg potassium; 0 IU vitamin A; 0 mg vitamin E; 0 mg vitamin C; 0 mg cholesterol

Parmesan-Garlic Pita Toasts

Use these flavorful pita crisps for any of the spreads or dips in the book. Or just nibble on them for a healthier-than-usual snack option.

3 tablespoons (42 g) unsalted butter

1 teaspoon minced garlic

½ teaspoon black pepper, fresh ground

¼ cup (25 g) grated Parmesan cheese

2 whole wheat pitas, cut into 8 triangles each

Melt butter; cook garlic in butter over low heat, stirring occasionally, for 5 minutes. Brush mixture lightly on rough side of pita triangles. Arrange butter side up in 1 layer on baking sheet. Sprinkle pepper and Parmesan cheese on top. Bake in oven preheated to 350°F (180°C, gas mark 4) for 12 to 15 minutes, until crisp and light brown. Cool on racks and store in airtight container in a dry place.

Yield: 8 servings

Each with: 7 g water; 95 calories (51% from fat, 12% from protein, 37% from carb); 3 g protein; 6 g total fat; 3 g saturated fat; 1 g monounsaturated fat; 0 g polyunsaturated fat; 9 g carb; 1 g fiber; 0 g sugar; 54 mg phosphorus; 40 mg calcium; 1 mg iron; 134 mg sodium; 35 mg potassium; 147 IU vitamin A; 39 mg vitamin E; 0 mg vitamin C; 14 mg cholesterol

Spicy Pita Dippers

Pepper and cumin give these pita triangles a southwestern flavor that goes particularly well with bean dips.

½ cup (112 g) unsalted butter, melted

2 teaspoons lemon pepper

2 teaspoons ground cumin

6 whole wheat pitas, cut into triangles

To make dippers, preheat the broiler. Combine the melted butter, lemon pepper, and cumin in a bowl. Dip the pita pieces quickly in the mixture and then place on a baking sheet. Broil 2 to 4 minutes, until crisp. Cool on a rack.

Yield: 12 servings

Each with: 12 g water; 155 calories (48% from fat, 8% from protein, 44% from carb); 3 g protein; 9 g total fat; 5 g saturated fat; 2 g monounsaturated fat; 1 g polyunsaturated fat; 18 g carb; 2 g fiber; 0 g sugar; 62 mg phosphorus; 12 mg calcium; 1 mg iron; 172 mg sodium; 67 mg potassium; 242 IU vitamin A; 63 mg vitamin E; 0 mg vitamin C; 20 mg cholesterol

Whole Wheat Honey Mustard Pretzels

This was one of those extended work-in-progress things as I tried different combinations to get the taste I wanted. The breakthrough was finding the large hard pretzels in a honey wheat with sesame seeds variety from Harry's Premium Snacks at a gourmet food store not too far away. They are great tasting alone, but they also made a great base for this recipe.

¼ cup (55 g) unsalted butter

2 tablespoons (40 g) honey

¼ cup (60 ml) honey mustard

½ teaspoon onion powder

¼ teaspoon Tabasco sauce

8 ounces (225 g) whole wheat pretzels, broken up

Melt butter in microwave. Stir in honey, honey mustard, and spices. Pour over pretzels and stir to coat evenly. Bake at 300°F (150°C, gas mark 2) for 30 minutes, stirring every 10 minutes. Cool on waxed paper. Store in an airtight container.

Yield: 10 servings

Each with: 8 g water; 137 calories (32% from fat, 7% from protein, 60% from carb); 3 g protein; 5 g total fat; 3 g saturated fat; 1 g monounsaturated fat; 0 g polyunsaturated fat; 22 g carb; 2 g fiber; 4 g sugar; 32 mg phosphorus; 9 mg calcium; 1 mg iron; 83 mg sodium; 110 mg potassium; 236 IU vitamin A; 38 mg vitamin E; 1 mg vitamin C; 12 mg cholesterol

Ranch-Style Pretzels

These are flavorful pretzel snacks with the taste of ranch dressing.

12 ounces (340 g) whole wheat pretzels, broken

1 packet Hidden Valley Ranch or other ranch dressing mix

1 cup (235 ml) olive oil

1 teaspoon lemon pepper

1 teaspoon dill weed

1 teaspoon garlic powder

Mix all ingredients in large bowl and toss to coat. Spread on baking sheet. Don't preheat oven. Bake at 300°F (150°C, gas mark 2) for 20 minutes, 10 minutes on one side and then turn and bake another 10 minutes.

Yield: 24 servings

Each with: 1 g water; 132 calories (61% from fat, 5% from protein, 34% from carb); 2 g protein; 9 g total fat; 1 g saturated fat; 7 g monounsaturated fat; 1 g polyunsaturated fat; 12 g carb; 1 g fiber; 0 g sugar; 19 mg phosphorus; 5 mg calcium; 0 mg iron; 29 mg sodium; 65 mg potassium; 3 IU vitamin A; 0 mg vitamin E; 0 mg vitamin C; 0 mg cholesterol

Cajun Party Mix

Because it's a little spicier than some party mixes, this one will definitely let you know that you are eating it.

12 ounces (340 g) almonds

6 cups (180 g) Crispix or other hexagonal multigrain cereal

1 cup (45 g) goldfish-shaped or other small crackers

¼ cup (55 g) unsalted butter

1 tablespoon (15 ml) Worcestershire sauce

½ teaspoon paprika

½ teaspoon thyme

¼ teaspoon black pepper

¼ teaspoon Tabasco sauce

Preheat oven to 250°F (120°C, gas mark ½). In a large shallow roasting pan, combine almonds, cereal, and goldfish crackers. Melt butter and stir in seasonings. Pour over mixture and toss to coat. Bake 1 hour, stirring every 20 minutes. Spread on paper towel to cool. Store in an airtight container.

Yield: 36 servings

Each with: 1 g water; 86 calories (61% from fat, 11% from protein, 28% from carb); 2 g protein; 6 g total fat; 1 g saturated fat; 3 g monounsaturated fat; 1 g polyunsaturated fat; 6 g carb; 1 g fiber; 1 g sugar; 51 mg phosphorus; 22 mg calcium; 2 mg iron; 45 mg sodium; 76 mg potassium; 212 IU vitamin A; 55 mg vitamin E; 2 mg vitamin C; 3 mg cholesterol

Curried Snack Mix

This is a savory version of the old favorite Chex mix, with curry powder dominating.

2 cups (60 g) round toasted oat cereal, such as Cheerios

2 cups (60 g) square wheat cereal, such as Wheat Chex

2 cups (50 g) square rice cereal, such as Rice Chex

2 cups (90 g) pretzel sticks

1½ cups bite-size shredded wheat cereal

1½ teaspoons onion powder

1 teaspoon garlic powder

½ tablespoon curry powder

1 teaspoon ground celery seeds

1½ tablespoons (22 ml) Worcestershire sauce

1 teaspoon Tabasco sauce

(continued on page 40)

Combine first 5 ingredients in large roasting pan. Spray thoroughly with nonstick vegetable oil spray. Combine remaining ingredients. Pour over cereal mixture, tossing to coat. Bake at 250°F (120°C, gas mark ½) for 2 hours, stirring and spraying with butter-flavored nonstick cooking spray every 15 minutes. Cool and store in an airtight container.

Yield: 25 servings

Each with: 1 g water; 48 calories (6% from fat, 10% from protein, 83% from carb); 1 g protein; 0 g total fat; 0 g saturated fat; 0 g monounsaturated fat; 0 g polyunsaturated fat; 11 g carb; 1 g fiber; 1 g sugar; 39 mg phosphorus; 27 mg calcium; 4 mg iron; 79 mg sodium; 68 mg potassium; 117 IU vitamin A; 34 mg vitamin E; 3 mg vitamin C; 0 mg cholesterol

S'more Snack Mix

This is a great idea. Everyone likes S'mores, so why not a snack mix that gives you that flavor whenever you want it? And all you have to do is mix it up.

2 cups (80 g) honey grahams cereal, such as Golden Grahams

1 cup (50 g) miniature marshmallows

1 cup (145 g) peanuts

½ cup (87.5 g) chocolate chips

½ cup (75 g) raisins

Combine all ingredients and mix thoroughly.

Yield: 20 servings

Each with: 3 g water; 68 calories (29% from fat, 6% from protein, 65% from carb); 1 g protein; 2 g total fat; 1 g saturated fat; 1 g monounsaturated fat; 0 g polyunsaturated fat; 11 g carb; 1 g fiber; 8 g sugar; 24 mg phosphorus; 12 mg calcium; 1 mg iron; 51 mg sodium; 58 mg potassium; 86 IU vitamin A; 26 mg vitamin E; 1 mg vitamin C; 1 mg cholesterol

Caramel Corn

This is an easier version than most for caramel corn, not requiring candy thermometers and all that. But the taste is just as good.

½ cup (112 g) unsalted butter

1 cup (225 g) brown sugar

¼ cup (60 ml) corn syrup

½ teaspoon baking soda

4 quarts (128 g) popped popcorn

2 cups (290 g) peanuts

Cook butter, brown sugar, and syrup 1½ minutes; stir and cook an additional 2 to 3 minutes until at a rolling boil. Take off heat and add soda. Stir well. Pour mixture over popped corn and nuts in grocery sack and shake. Microwave 1 minute and shake; 1 minute and shake; 30 seconds and shake; and 30 seconds and shake. Pour into pan, cool, and eat.

Yield: 18 servings

Each with: 5 g water; 184 calories (52% from fat, 4% from protein, 45% from carb); 2 g protein; 11 g total fat; 4 g saturated fat; 3 g monounsaturated fat; 3 g polyunsaturated fat; 21 g carb; 1 g fiber; 13 g sugar; 38 mg phosphorus; 17 mg calcium; 0 mg iron; 164 mg sodium; 74 mg potassium; 173 IU vitamin A; 42 mg vitamin E; 0 mg vitamin C; 14 mg cholesterol

Rocky Road Popcorn Bars

This is an easy microwave recipe for tasty popcorn-and-peanut bars.

¼ cup (55 g) unsalted butter

2 tablespoons (28 g) shortening

12 ounces (340 g) chocolate chips

5 cups (250 g) miniature marshmallows

¾ cup (109 g) peanuts

6 cups (48 g) popped popcorn

(continued on page 42)

Spray a 9 × 12 × 2-inch (23 × 30 × 5 cm) microwave-safe dish with nonstick vegetable oil spray. Set aside. Measure and mix butter, shortening, and chocolate chips in bowl. Microwave uncovered on high (100%) until chips are softened and mixture becomes smooth when stirred—about 2½ minutes. Stir in marshmallows. Microwave uncovered until they are almost melted—15 to 20 seconds. Stir in peanuts and popcorn until evenly covered with mixture. When cool, press in pan with spoon. Refrigerate until firm—about 1 hour. Cut into squares.

Yield: 10 servings

Each with: 8 g water; 378 calories (49% from fat, 4% from protein, 46% from carb); 4 g protein; 21 g total fat; 9 g saturated fat; 8 g monounsaturated fat; 3 g polyunsaturated fat; 45 g carb; 2 g fiber; 32 g sugar; 97 mg phosphorus; 69 mg calcium; 1 mg iron; 153 mg sodium; 150 mg potassium; 211 IU vitamin A; 54 mg vitamin E; 0 mg vitamin C; 20 mg cholesterol

Mexican Pinwheels

These make a great snack or lunch. You can also slice them about ¾ inch (2 cm) thick and serve as an appetizer.

1 avocado, chopped

3 ounces (85 g) cream cheese, softened

6 whole wheat tortillas, 6 inch (15 cm)

4 ounces (113 g) shredded Monterey Jack cheese

1 ounce (28 g) leaf lettuce

½ cup (17 g) alfalfa sprouts

½ cup (130 g) salsa

Combine avocado and cream cheese; blend dip. Spread each tortilla evenly with avocado mixture to within ½ inch (1 cm) of edge. Arrange cheese, lettuce, and sprouts over avocado mixture. Spoon on salsa. Roll up each tortilla. Cut in half and secure with toothpicks. Serve immediately or wrap in plastic wrap and refrigerate.

Yield: 6 servings

Each with: 67 g water; 259 calories (57% from fat, 14% from protein, 30% from carb); 9 g protein; 17 g total fat; 8 g saturated fat; 6 g monounsaturated fat; 1 g polyunsaturated fat; 19 g carb; 3 g fiber; 1 g sugar; 158 mg phosphorus; 203 mg calcium; 2 mg iron; 388 mg sodium; 269 mg potassium; 787 IU vitamin A; 87 mg vitamin E; 3 mg vitamin C; 32 mg cholesterol

Tortilla Roll-Ups

These tasty little tortilla snacks have just enough heat to be interesting.

8 whole wheat tortillas

8 ounces (225 g) cream cheese, softened

4 ounces (115 g) black olives, chopped

4 ounces (115 g) diced green chiles

¼ teaspoon Tabasco sauce

Cream together cream cheese, olives, chiles, and Tabasco sauce. Spread approximately 2 tablespoons onto a tortilla, roll jelly-roll fashion, roll in plastic wrap, and chill. Before serving cut into ⅜-inch-wide (1-cm) pieces.

Yield: 16 servings

Each with: 25 g water; 105 calories (59% from fat, 9% from protein, 32% from carb); 2 g protein; 7 g total fat; 3 g saturated fat; 3 g monounsaturated fat; 0 g polyunsaturated fat; 9 g carb; 2 g fiber; 0 g sugar; 34 mg phosphorus; 37 mg calcium; 1 mg iron; 200 mg sodium; 41 mg potassium; 221 IU vitamin A; 51 mg vitamin E; 0 mg vitamin C; 16 mg cholesterol

4

Appetizers, Snacks, and Party Foods:
Vegetables and Fruits

Fruits and vegetables make great snacks just as they are. Eating an apple or some carrot sticks provides all kinds of good nutritional benefits, fiber being just one of them. But we also have some recipes here for other ways to incorporate fruits and veggies into your snacking, including dips and some great vegetable and fruit nibbles.

Artichoke Dip

This is the kind of appetizer you can serve to anyone, without any questions about what kind of diet you are on. It also is good just for the family when you want something to nibble on.

1 cup (225 g) low-fat mayonnaise

½ cup (50 g) grated Parmesan cheese

¼ teaspoon Worcestershire sauce

¼ teaspoon garlic powder

1 can artichoke hearts, chopped

TIP *Spread warm on crackers. Recipe can be doubled.*

Mix all ingredients but artichoke hearts until well blended. Add chopped hearts and mix. Bake at 350°F (180°C, gas mark 4) until lightly browned.

Yield: 8 servings

Each with: 44 g water; 141 calories (74% from fat, 10% from protein, 16% from carb); 4 g protein; 12 g total fat; 3 g saturated fat; 1 g monounsaturated fat; 0 g polyunsaturated fat; 6 g carb; 1 g fiber; 2 g sugar; 82 mg phosphorus; 77 mg calcium; 0 mg iron; 352 mg sodium; 105 mg potassium; 132 IU vitamin A; 7 mg vitamin E; 2 mg vitamin C; 16 mg cholesterol

Spinach Dip

Try this with one of our pita dippers.

8 ounces (225 g) cream cheese, softened

2 cups (300 g) grated Monterey Jack cheese

10 ounces (280 g) frozen spinach, thawed and squeezed dry

½ cup (90 g) finely chopped peeled tomato

¾ cup (120 g) chopped onion

⅓ cup (71 ml) half and half

1 tablespoon finely chopped jalapeño pepper

For the dip, beat together the cheeses, spinach, tomato, onion, half-and-half, and jalapeños in a mixing bowl until very smooth. Spread in a buttered dish and bake at 400°F (200°C, gas mark 6) for 20 to 25 minutes until bubbly. Serve hot, warm, or at room temperature with dippers.

Yield: 10 servings

Each with: 73 g water; 204 calories (73% from fat, 19% from protein, 8% from carb); 10 g protein; 17 g total fat; 11 g saturated fat; 5 g monounsaturated fat; 1 g polyunsaturated fat; 4 g carb; 1 g fiber; 1 g sugar; 168 mg phosphorus; 270 mg calcium; 1 mg iron; 241 mg sodium; 180 mg potassium; 4007 IU vitamin A; 140 mg vitamin E; 4 mg vitamin C; 51 mg cholesterol

Carrot Cheese Ball

Carrots provide the color and crunch for this different type of appetizer.

1½ cups (165 g) shredded carrot

8 ounces (225 g) cream cheese, softened

2 cups (225 g) shredded Cheddar cheese

½ teaspoon minced garlic

1 teaspoon Worcestershire sauce

½ teaspoon Tabasco sauce

3 tablespoons chopped fresh parsley

½ cup (55 g) chopped pecans

Press shredded carrot between paper towels to remove excess moisture; set aside. Combine cream cheese and Cheddar cheese in a medium bowl; stir well. Add carrot, garlic, Worcestershire sauce, and Tabasco sauce; stir well. Cover and chill 1 hour. These ingredients may also be combined in a food processor and mixed. Shape cheese mixture into a ball; roll in parsley and nuts. Wrap in waxed paper and chill at least 1 hour.

Yield: 24 servings

Each with: 17 g water; 97 calories (78% from Fat, 15% from protein, 6% from carb); 4 g protein; 9 g total fat; 5 g saturated fat; 3 g monounsaturated fat; 1 g polyunsaturated fat; 2 g carb; 1 g fiber; 1 g sugar; 76 mg phosphorus; 92 mg calcium; 0 mg iron; 105 mg sodium; 62 mg potassium; 1625 IU vitamin A; 62 mg vitamin E; 2 mg vitamin C; 22 mg cholesterol

Veggie Dippers

This is really not a recipe, just a reminder that you don't have to use crackers or other such things for dipping. Most of the recipes for dips and spreads in this book are great with fresh vegetables.

1 cup (116 g) radishes

1 cup (71 g) broccoli florets

1 cup (150 g) red bell pepper, cut in strips

1 cup (150 g) green bell pepper, cut in strips

1 cup (100 g) green beans, steamed until crisp-tender

1 cup (70 g) mushrooms

Arrange the assorted raw vegetables on a platter and serve with dipping sauce.

Yield: 6 servings

Each with: 103 g water; 26 calories (7% from fat, 21% from protein, 72% from carb); 2 g protein; 0 g total fat; 0 g saturated fat; 0 g monounsaturated fat; 0 g polyunsaturated fat; 6 g carb; 2 g fiber; 2 g sugar; 40 mg phosphorus; 22 mg calcium; 1 mg iron; 14 mg sodium; 255 mg potassium; 1352 IU vitamin A; 0 mg vitamin E; 69 mg vitamin C; 0 mg cholesterol

Avocado Salsa

Because it's sort of a combination of salsa and guacamole, this dip is sure to please lovers of both. If you like your salsa hotter, add another jalapeño or a few drops of Tabasco sauce.

1 avocado, peeled and diced

½ cup (90 g) chopped tomato

½ cup (80 g) chopped red onion

¼ cup (38 g) chopped green bell pepper

1 jalapeño pepper, finely chopped

½ teaspoon minced garlic

2 tablespoons (28 ml) red wine vinegar

1 tablespoon (15 ml) olive oil

Combine the vegetables in a medium bowl. Mash the garlic in a cup or small bowl. Add the vinegar and oil to the garlic. Pour the dressing over the vegetables and toss to combine the ingredients. Serve chilled or at room temperature.

Yield: 4 servings

Each with: 79 g water; 103 calories (72% from fat, 4% from protein, 23% from carb); 1 g protein; 9 g total fat; 1 g saturated fat; 6 g monounsaturated fat; 1 g polyunsaturated fat; 6 g carb; 3 g fiber; 2 g sugar; 33 mg phosphorus; 13 mg calcium; 0 mg iron; 5 mg sodium; 273 mg potassium; 268 IU vitamin A; 0 mg vitamin E; 16 mg vitamin C; 0 mg cholesterol

Pesto

This makes a fairly typical pesto.

2 cups (80 g) packed fresh basil

3 tablespoons (27 g) pine nuts

1 teaspoon finely minced garlic

¼ cup (25 g) grated Parmesan cheese

½ cup (120 ml) olive oil

Place basil leaves in small batches in food processor and whip until well chopped (process about ¾ cup at a time). Add about one-third of the nuts and garlic and blend again. Add about one-third of the Parmesan cheese; blend while slowly adding about one-third of the olive oil, stopping to scrape down sides of container. Process basil pesto until it forms a thick, smooth paste. Repeat until all ingredients are used; mix all batches together well. Serve over pasta. Basil pesto keeps in the refrigerator for 1 week or for a few months in the freezer.

Yield: 12 servings

Each with: 1 g water; 115 calories (82% from fat, 6% from protein, 13% from carb); 2 g protein; 11 g total fat; 2 g saturated fat; 7 g monounsaturated fat; 2 g polyunsaturated fat; 4 g carb; 2 g fiber; 0 g sugar; 52 mg phosphorus; 140 mg calcium; 3 mg iron; 30 mg sodium; 208 mg potassium; 536 IU vitamin A; 2 mg vitamin E; 4 mg vitamin C; 1 mg cholesterol

Broccoli Bites

This can be served as a tasty little snack or as a nice side dish.

10 ounces (280 g) frozen broccoli

1 cup (72 g) stuffing mix

½ cup (50 g) grated Parmesan cheese

3 eggs, beaten

4 tablespoons (55 g) unsalted butter, softened

¼ teaspoon black pepper

Cook broccoli according to package directions; drain well. In a medium bowl, combine cooked broccoli, stuffing mix, cheese, eggs, butter, and pepper. Shape mixture into small balls, about 1 inch (2.5 cm). Freeze, well covered, for at least 3 hours. Preheat oven to 350°F (180°C, gas mark 4). Place frozen balls on baking sheet coated with nonstick vegetable oil spray. Bake until brown, about 15 minutes.

Yield: 15 servings

Each with: 27 g water; 63 calories (72% from fat, 20% from protein, 8% from carb); 3 g protein; 5 g total fat; 3 g saturated fat; 2 g monounsaturated fat; 0 g polyunsaturated fat; 1 g carb; 1 g fiber; 0 g sugar; 56 mg phosphorus; 50 mg calcium; 0 mg iron; 116 mg sodium; 47 mg potassium; 377 IU vitamin A; 45 mg vitamin E; 8 mg vitamin C; 58 mg cholesterol

Eggplant Fingers

Fried eggplant snacks provide a big fiber boost.

1 eggplant

½ cup (120 ml) canola oil

1 cup (235 ml) skim milk

1 cup (120 g) whole wheat flour

1 cup (115 g) whole wheat bread crumbs

Peel eggplant and cut into ½-inch (1-cm) strips. Heat oil to 375°F (190°C, gas mark 5). Dip eggplant into milk, then flour, then milk again, and then bread crumbs. Deep-fry and drain completely until no trace of oil appears on paper towel.

Yield: 8 servings

Each with: 83 g water; 254 calories (52% from fat, 9% from protein, 39% from carb); 6 g protein; 15 g total fat; 1 g saturated fat; 8 g monounsaturated fat; 5 g polyunsaturated fat; 26 g carb; 4 g fiber; 2 g sugar; 123 mg phosphorus; 79 mg calcium; 1 mg iron; 39 mg sodium; 275 mg potassium; 79 IU vitamin A; 19 mg vitamin E; 2 mg vitamin C; 1 mg cholesterol

Spinach Balls

You could also serve these as a side dish, but they make a great snack or buffet item, or a spinach dip that you can carry to serve.

10 ounces (280 g) frozen spinach, thawed and drained

1 cup (72 g) stuffing mix, crushed

½ cup (50 g) grated Parmesan cheese

3 eggs, beaten

¼ cup (55 g) unsalted butter, softened

⅛ teaspoon nutmeg

Place spinach on paper towels and squeeze until barely moist. Combine spinach and next 5 ingredients in a bowl. Mix well. Shape into 2½-inch (6 cm) balls with an ice cream scoop. Place on waxed paper-lined baking sheet. Cover and refrigerate 8 hours. To bake, place spinach balls on a baking sheet coated with nonstick vegetable oil spray and bake at 350°F (180°C, gas mark 4) for 15 minutes until hot. Drain on paper towels.

Yield: 20 servings

Each with: 20 g water; 70 calories (52% from fat, 18% from protein, 29% from carb); 3 g protein; 4 g total fat; 2 g saturated fat; 1 g monounsaturated fat; 0 g polyunsaturated fat; 5 g carb; 1 g fiber; 1 g sugar; 50 mg phosphorus; 60 mg calcium; 1 mg iron; 154 mg sodium; 72 mg potassium; 1833 IU vitamin A; 34 mg vitamin E; 0 mg vitamin C; 44 mg cholesterol

Zucchini Sticks

So healthy and crunchy, these baked treats offer taste and nutrition without the fat of deep-frying.

3 medium zucchini

½ cup (56 g) wheat germ

½ cup (55 g) finely chopped almonds

¼ cup (25 g) grated Parmesan cheese

2 tablespoons (28 g) unsalted butter, melted

Cut each zucchini lengthwise into fourths, then lengthwise into halves to form sticks. Cut each stick lengthwise into halves (each zucchini makes 16 sticks). Mix wheat germ, almonds, and cheese in plastic bag. Roll about 8 zucchini sticks at a time in butter until evenly coated. Lift with fork. Shake sticks in wheat germ. Lay on an ungreased baking sheet. Cook in 350°F (180°C, gas mark 4) oven until crisp and tender, about 15 minutes.

Yield: 6 servings

Each with: 61 g water; 168 calories (62% from fat, 17% from protein, 21% from carb); 8 g protein; 12 g total fat; 4 g saturated fat; 5 g monounsaturated fat; 2 g polyunsaturated fat; 9 g carb; 3 g fiber; 2 g sugar; 221 mg phosphorus; 87 mg calcium; 2 mg iron; 74 mg sodium; 341 mg potassium; 271 IU vitamin A; 37 mg vitamin E; 11 mg vitamin C; 14 mg cholesterol

More Marinated Veggies

This version of marinated vegetables is good on a salad, but if you cut them a bit smaller, it makes a great relish for sandwiches, similar to New Orleans's muffaletta.

½ teaspoon minced garlic

½ cup (120 ml) vinegar

½ cup (120 ml) olive oil

1 teaspoon oregano

½ cup (35 g) chopped mushrooms

¼ cup (25 g) chopped black olives

¼ cup (25 g) chopped green olives

½ cup (82 g) cooked chickpeas

½ cup (80 g) chopped onion

½ cup (150 g) chopped artichoke hearts

Combine first 4 ingredients. Add any or all of the remaining ingredients, cutting raw vegetables into bite-size chunks and draining liquids from those in cans. Marinate up to 24 hours.

Yield: 24 servings

Each with: 18 g water; 53 calories (81% from fat, 3% from protein, 15% from carb); 0 g protein; 5 g total fat; 1 g saturated fat; 4 g monounsaturated fat; 1 g polyunsaturated fat; 2 g carb; 1 g fiber; 0 g sugar; 10 mg phosphorus; 7 mg calcium; 0 mg iron; 42 mg sodium; 32 mg potassium; 21 IU vitamin A; 0 mg vitamin E; 1 mg vitamin C; 0 mg cholesterol

Veggie Antipasto

This is an easy antipasto platter full of fresh veggies.

Herb Marinade

²⁄₃ cup (157 ml) red wine vinegar

¹⁄₃ cup (78 ml) olive oil

3 diced scallions

1 teaspoon basil

1 teaspoon oregano

½ teaspoon black pepper, fresh ground

½ teaspoon minced garlic

2 tablespoons fresh cilantro

Vegetables

8 ounces (225 g) mushrooms, sliced

6 ounces (170 g) artichoke hearts, halved

1 cup (130 g) sliced carrot

1 cup (150 g) sliced red bell pepper

1 cup (100 g) sliced celery

8 ounces (225 g) cherry tomatoes

4 ounces (115 g) olives

16 ounces (455 g) chickpeas

TIP *Vary the dish by using your favorite vegetables in place of or in addition to those listed.*

Mix all marinade ingredients in saucepan and boil for 2 or 3 minutes. Cool for 10 minutes and pour over vegetables in a large bowl that has a tight-fitting cover. Refrigerate covered for at least 24 hours. Invert bowl several times during the 24-hour period to make sure that all vegetables absorb flavor from the marinade.

Yield: 8 servings

Each with: 158 g water; 203 calories (50% from fat, 10% from protein, 40% from carb); 5 g protein; 12 g total fat; 2 g saturated fat; 8 g monounsaturated fat; 2 g polyunsaturated fat; 21 g carb; 6 g fiber; 2 g sugar; 105 mg phosphorus; 55 mg calcium; 2 mg iron; 330 mg sodium; 445 mg potassium; 3658 IU vitamin A; 0 mg vitamin E; 35 mg vitamin C; 0 mg cholesterol

Antipasto on a Skewer

This is handy finger food for your next outdoor meal, much easier to carry around than a plate from a typical antipasto tray.

½ teaspoon minced garlic

1 teaspoon black pepper

1 teaspoon Italian seasoning

1 teaspoon dry mustard

½ teaspoon crushed oregano

⅓ cup (78 ml) red wine vinegar

1 cup (235 ml) olive oil

8 ounces (225 g) mozzarella cheese, cut in ½ × ¼ × 2-inch (1 × 0.5 × 5 cm) sticks

12 slices salami

24 cherry tomatoes

24 black olives

12 mushrooms

10 ounces (283 g) artichoke hearts, cooked

In a tight-sealing container, combine seasonings and vinegar; shake well. Add oil and shake again for about 30 seconds. Pour marinade in a 13 × 9 × 2-inch (33 × 23 × 5 cm) baking dish. Wrap each cheese stick in one slice of salami. On each of 12 skewers, thread tomato, olive, mushroom, salami and cheese, artichoke heart, olive, and tomato. Place skewers in marinade. Marinate in refrigerator at least 24 hours, turning several times to coat all sides.

Yield: 12 servings

Each with: 72 g water; 341 calories (78% from fat, 15% from protein, 7% from carb); 13 g protein; 30 g total fat; 8 g saturated fat; 19 g monounsaturated fat; 3 g polyunsaturated fat; 6 g carb; 2 g fiber; 1 g sugar; 168 mg phosphorus; 169 mg calcium; 1 mg iron; 742 mg sodium; 317 mg potassium; 403 IU vitamin A; 24 mg vitamin E; 9 mg vitamin C; 38 mg cholesterol

Vegetable Wrap

This makes a great lunch. It's easy and quick to put together, tastes great, and packs a lot of nutrition into not many calories.

1 cup (119 g) sliced cucumber

1 cup (113 g) sliced zucchini

½ cup (65 g) sliced carrot

4 ounces (115 g) mushrooms, chopped

¼ cup (25 g) chopped scallions

½ teaspoon minced garlic

3 ounces (85 g) cream cheese

4 whole wheat tortillas

¼ cup (65 g) salsa

Combine all veggies. Spread cream cheese on tortilla. Spread veggies and salsa over cream cheese. Roll up.

Yield: 4 servings

Each with: 135 g water; 197 calories (44% from fat, 12% from protein, 44% from carb); 6 g protein; 10 g total fat; 5 g saturated fat; 3 g monounsaturated fat; 1 g polyunsaturated fat; 22 g carb; 3 g fiber; 3 g sugar; 115 mg phosphorus; 80 mg calcium; 2 mg iron; 309 mg sodium; 399 mg potassium; 3175 IU vitamin A; 76 mg vitamin E; 9 mg vitamin C; 23 mg cholesterol

Sweet Potato Chips

This is a high-fiber, fat-free snack that tastes great.

3 sweet potatoes

½ teaspoon cumin

½ teaspoon chili powder

Scrub sweet potatoes. Slice into very thin rounds. Spray baking sheet with nonstick vegetable oil spray. Lay rounds on sheet and spray the tops. Place in preheated 350°F (180°C, gas mark 4) oven and bake until crisp, about 10 minutes. Sprinkle with spices.

Yield: 6 servings

Each with: 61 g water; 59 calories (3% from fat, 7% from protein, 90% from carb); 1 g protein; 0 g total fat; 0 g saturated fat; 0 g monounsaturated fat; 0 g polyunsaturated fat; 14 g carb; 2 g fiber; 4 g sugar; 26 mg phosphorus; 23 mg calcium; 1 mg iron; 23 mg sodium; 181 mg potassium; 11948 IU vitamin A; 0 mg vitamin E; 10 mg vitamin C; 0 mg cholesterol

TIP

Vary the spices to suit your mood.

Pineapple Kabobs

Try these sweet grilled pineapple wedges with grilled ham or pork chops.

¼ cup (85 g) honey

2 tablespoons (28 g) unsalted butter

1 teaspoon cinnamon

1 pineapple

Combine honey, butter, and cinnamon. Pare and cut fresh pineapple into long wedges. Grill over medium heat 15 minutes, basting with sauce. Turn frequently.

Yield: 4 servings

Each with: 15 g water; 123 calories (40% from fat, 1% from protein, 60% from carb); 0 g protein; 6 g total fat; 4 g saturated fat; 1 g monounsaturated fat; 0 g polyunsaturated fat; 20 g carb; 1 g fiber; 19 g sugar; 4 mg phosphorus; 12 mg calcium; 0 mg iron; 2 mg sodium; 28 mg potassium; 183 IU vitamin A; 48 mg vitamin E; 1 mg vitamin C; 15 mg cholesterol

Fruit with Amaretto Cream

Use this recipe for those times when you are looking for something a little fancier for dessert.

1½ tablespoons Amaretto liqueur

2 tablespoons (30 g) packed brown sugar

½ cup (115 g) sour cream

1 cup (145 g) strawberries, halved

1 cup (145 g) blueberries

1 cup (150 g) seedless green grapes

In small mixing bowl, combine Amaretto and brown sugar. Add sour cream and mix well. Prepare at least 2 hours before serving. Stir occasionally to dissolve brown sugar. Put fruit into sherbet glasses or small soufflé dishes. Drizzle with sauce.

Yield: 4 servings

(continued on page 58)

Each with: 111 g water; 134 calories (32% from fat, 5% from protein, 63% from carb); 2 g protein; 5 g total fat; 3 g saturated fat; 1 g monounsaturated fat; 0 g polyunsaturated fat; 21 g carb; 2 g fiber; 17 g sugar; 49 mg phosphorus; 50 mg calcium; 0 mg iron; 22 mg sodium; 195 mg potassium; 196 IU vitamin A; 40 mg vitamin E; 27 mg vitamin C; 15 mg cholesterol

Banana Bites

This is a quick way to add crunch and flavor to bananas.

3 cups (450 g) sliced banana

6 ounces (213 g) orange juice concentrate

2 cups (164 g) granola

Cut bananas into bite-size pieces. Pour orange juice concentrate into mixing bowl. Spread granola on baking sheet. Dip banana bits into the orange juice. Roll in granola.

Yield: 6 servings

Each with: 103 g water; 251 calories (6% from fat, 6% from protein, 88% from carb); 4 g protein; 2 g total fat; 0 g saturated fat; 1 g monounsaturated fat; 0 g polyunsaturated fat; 59 g carb; 5 g fiber; 34 g sugar; 116 mg phosphorus; 25 mg calcium; 1 mg iron; 105 mg sodium; 671 mg potassium; 179 IU vitamin A; 0 mg vitamin E; 49 mg vitamin C; 0 mg cholesterol

5

Appetizers, Snacks, and Party Foods:
Nuts

Our appetizer, snack, and party food section is actually the only one with a whole chapter on nuts. And why not? There are lots of great ways to include nuts in your snacking, from dips and spreads to snack mixes to cookies.

Chicken Pecan Pâté

This is the kind of party food that will have everyone guessing about the ingredients. What they will be sure of is that they like it.

2 cups (280 g) chicken, cooked

8 ounces (225 g) cream cheese, cut into chunks and softened

½ teaspoon minced garlic

1 cup (110 g) finely chopped pecans

6 tablespoons (84 g) mayonnaise

4 teaspoons fresh dill

Combine chicken, cream cheese, and garlic with chopped pecans in food processor or blender and blend just until smooth. Add mayonnaise and dill and blend again. Form into a ball and arrange on a bed of lettuce. Sprinkle with additional dill.

Yield: 24 servings

Each with: 13 g water; 112 calories (80% from fat, 16% from protein, 4% from carb); 5 g protein; 10 g total fat; 3 g saturated fat; 4 g monounsaturated fat; 3 g polyunsaturated fat; 1 g carb; 1 g fiber; 0 g sugar; 47 mg phosphorus; 16 mg calcium; 0 mg iron; 58 mg sodium; 65 mg potassium; 156 IU vitamin A; 39 mg vitamin E; 0 mg vitamin C; 22 mg cholesterol

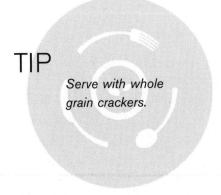

TIP

Serve with whole grain crackers.

Olive Nut Spread

This easy-to-make spread is great on either crackers or vegetables.

6 ounces (170 g) cream cheese, softened

½ cup (115 g) mayonnaise

½ cup (55 g) chopped pecans

1 cup (100 g) sliced green olives

⅛ teaspoon black pepper

Combine all ingredients. Refrigerate for a few hours until spreading consistency. This will keep for several weeks in the refrigerator.

Yield: 16 servings

Each with: 14 g water; 120 calories (91% from fat, 4% from protein, 5% from carb); 1 g protein; 12 g total fat; 3 g saturated fat; 4 g monounsaturated fat; 4 g polyunsaturated fat; 2 g carb; 1 g fiber; 0 g sugar; 23 mg phosphorus; 20 mg calcium; 1 mg iron; 144 mg sodium; 30 mg potassium; 199 IU vitamin A; 44 mg vitamin E; 0 mg vitamin C; 14 mg cholesterol

Ranch Cheese Ball

Powdered dressing mix makes ordinary cream cheese special.

8 ounces (225 g) cream cheese

1 packet ranch dressing mix (such as Hidden Valley)

2 cups (220 g) broken pecans

Soften cream cheese and then mix in dressing. Shape into ball and then roll in pecan pieces. Chill overnight.

Yield: 16 servings

Each with: 8 g water; 144 calories (88% from fat, 6% from protein, 6% from carb); 2 g protein; 15 g total fat; 4 g saturated fat; 7 g monounsaturated fat; 3 g polyunsaturated fat; 2 g carb; 1 g fiber; 1 g sugar; 53 mg phosphorus; 21 mg calcium; 1 mg iron; 42 mg sodium; 73 mg potassium; 198 IU vitamin A; 51 mg vitamin E; 0 mg vitamin C; 16 mg cholesterol

Hot Pecan Dip

Dried beef and toasted pecans provide the flavor here.

⅔ cup (74 g) pecans, toasted

2 tablespoons (28 g) unsalted butter

8 ounces (225 g) cream cheese

½ cup (115 g) sour cream

¼ teaspoon garlic powder

¼ teaspoon black pepper

½ cup (80 g) grated onion

¼ cup (38 g) chopped green bell pepper

3 ounces (85 g) chopped dried beef

Toast pecans in butter. Cream together remaining ingredients. Spread creamed mixture in buttered 9-inch (23 cm) pie plate. Top with toasted pecans and bake 20 minutes in 350°F (180°C, gas mark 4) oven.

Yield: 12 servings

Each with: 32 g water; 153 calories (81% from fat, 12% from protein, 7% from carb); 5 g protein; 14 g total fat; 7 g saturated fat; 5 g monounsaturated fat; 2 g polyunsaturated fat; 3 g carb; 1 g fiber; 1 g sugar; 63 mg phosphorus; 33 mg calcium; 1 mg iron; 258 mg sodium; 98 mg potassium; 366 IU vitamin A; 94 mg vitamin E; 3 mg vitamin C; 35 mg cholesterol

Pecan Cheese Wafers

These savory little pecan and cheese crackers are great to snack on or as dippers.

½ cup (112 g) unsalted butter, softened

2 cups (225 g) shredded Cheddar cheese

1 cup (110 g) finely chopped pecans

1 cup (120 g) whole wheat pastry flour

¼ teaspoon cayenne pepper

Cream butter and cheese. Add pecans, flour, and cayenne. Mix well. Form into 2 rolls, 1-inch (2.5 cm) diameter. Wrap in plastic and refrigerate several hours or overnight. (This can also be frozen.) Slice rolls into thin rounds and place on baking sheet coated with nonstick vegetable oil spray. Bake at 350°F (180°C, gas mark 4) for 15 minutes or until edges brown lightly. Remove to a rack to cool.

Yield: 40 servings

Each with: 3 g water; 76 calories (75% from fat, 12% from protein, 13% from carb); 2 g protein; 7 g total fat; 3 g saturated fat; 2 g monounsaturated fat; 1 g polyunsaturated fat; 3 g carb; 1 g fiber; 0 g sugar; 52 mg phosphorus; 51 mg calcium; 0 mg iron; 41 mg sodium; 31 mg potassium; 143 IU vitamin A; 36 mg vitamin E; 0 mg vitamin C; 13 mg cholesterol

Macadamia Cheese Crisps

These savory little crackers have the added bonus of macadamia nuts. You'll find it hard to limit yourself to the recommended serving size.

½ cup (112 g) unsalted butter

¼ pound (115 g) grated Swiss cheese

1 egg

1½ cups (180 g) whole wheat pastry flour

⅓ cup (45 g) chopped macadamia nuts

Preheat oven to 400°F (200°C, gas mark 6). Blend butter, cheese, and egg. Gradually work in flour and nuts. Mold into a roll 1½ inches (4 cm) in diameter. Wrap in waxed paper and chill until firm. Slice dough into ¼-inch (0.5 cm) slices. Place on lightly buttered baking sheet and bake for 10 to 15 minutes or until lightly browned.

Yield: 18 servings

Each with: 6 g water; 126 calories (64% from fat, 12% from protein, 24% from carb); 4 g protein; 9 g total fat; 5 g saturated fat; 3 g monounsaturated fat; 0 g polyunsaturated fat; 8 g carb; 1 g fiber; 0 g sugar; 84 mg phosphorus; 69 mg calcium; 1 mg iron; 7 mg sodium; 62 mg potassium; 229 IU vitamin A; 61 mg vitamin E; 0 mg vitamin C; 31 mg cholesterol

Barbecued Nuts

These are not your usual nuts. The flavor and spiciness can be varied depending on what kind of barbecue sauce you use.

4 cups (580 g) mixed nuts

1 cup (250 g) barbecue sauce

2 tablespoons grated Parmesan cheese

Heat oven to 300°F (150°C, gas mark 2). In medium bowl, combine mixed nuts and barbecue sauce; stir until evenly coated. Spread on ungreased baking sheet; sprinkle with Parmesan cheese. Bake at 350°F (180°C, gas mark 4) for 20 to 25 minutes or until nuts are dry. Transfer to waxed paper. Cool completely. Store in tightly covered container.

Yield: 16 servings

Each with: 10 g water; 254 calories (68% from fat, 10% from protein, 23% from carb); 6 g protein; 20 g total fat; 3 g saturated fat; 11 g monounsaturated fat; 5 g polyunsaturated fat; 15 g carb; 3 g fiber; 7 g sugar; 170 mg phosphorus; 47 mg calcium; 1 mg iron; 312 mg sodium; 207 mg potassium; 6 IU vitamin A; 1 mg vitamin E; 0 mg vitamin C; 1 mg cholesterol

Spicy Pecans

Tabasco adds a little heat to these pecans.

2 tablespoons (28 g) unsalted butter

½ teaspoon salt-free seasoning blend (such as Mrs. Dash)

⅛ teaspoon Tabasco sauce

1 pound (455 g) pecan halves

3 tablespoons (45 ml) Worcestershire sauce

Put butter, seasoning, and Tabasco sauce in 12 × 8 × 2-inch (30 × 20 × 5-cm) baking dish. Place in 300°F (150°C, gas mark 2) oven until butter melts. Add pecans, stirring until all are coated with butter. Bake for about 15 minutes, stirring occasionally. Sprinkle with Worcestershire sauce and stir again. Continue baking another 10 minutes until crisp.

Yield: 12 servings

Each with: 3 g water; 281 calories (87% from fat, 5% from protein, 8% from carb); 4 g protein; 29 g total fat; 4 g saturated fat; 16 g monounsaturated fat; 8 g polyunsaturated fat; 6 g carb; 4 g fiber; 2 g sugar; 109 mg phosphorus; 27 mg calcium; 1 mg iron; 37 mg sodium; 186 mg potassium; 85 IU vitamin A; 16 mg vitamin E; 7 mg vitamin C; 5 mg cholesterol

Spicy Nut Mix

Unlike the cinnamon-sugar nuts in this chapter, these are chili spiced, providing a savory snack.

1¼ cups (175 g) cashews

¾ cup (109 g) soy nuts

1 cup (145 g) sunflower seeds

2 tablespoons (28 ml) canola oil

1½ teaspoons chili powder

⅛ teaspoon garlic powder

1 teaspoon Worcestershire sauce

Combine nuts and seeds in large bowl. Place oil, spices, and Worcestershire sauce in covered container. Cover and shake. Sprinkle over nuts and seeds. Toss to coat. Spread in baking pan. Bake 20 minutes at 300°F (150°C, gas mark 2). Cool and store in covered containers in refrigerator.

Yield: 16 servings

Each with: 0 g water; 161 calories (66% from fat, 15% from protein, 19% from carb); 6 g protein; 12 g total fat; 2 g saturated fat; 5 g monounsaturated fat; 5 g polyunsaturated fat; 8 g carb; 2 g fiber; 1 g sugar; 198 mg phosphorus; 22 mg calcium; 1 mg iron; 8 mg sodium; 246 mg potassium; 71 IU vitamin A; 0 mg vitamin E; 1 mg vitamin C; 0 mg cholesterol

Party Nut Mix

Basically a sweet and spicy variation on the traditional cereal mix, this one is mostly nuts.

8 ounces (225 g) dry-roasted peanuts

8 ounces (225 g) dry-roasted cashews

6 ounces (170 g) almonds

2 cups (60 g) square wheat cereal, such as Wheat Chex

¼ cup (55 g) unsalted butter, melted

1½ tablespoons (22 ml) soy sauce

1½ tablespoons (22 ml) Worcestershire sauce

¼ teaspoon Tabasco sauce

1 cup (145 g) raisins

Combine first 4 ingredients in a large bowl; stir well. Combine butter, soy sauce, Worcestershire sauce, and Tabasco; mix well and pour over nut mixture, tossing to coat. Spread half of mixture in a 15 × 10 × 1-inch (37 × 25 × 2.5 cm) jelly-roll pan. Bake at 325°F (170°C, gas mark 3) for 15 minutes; cool and place in a large bowl. Repeat with remaining mixture. Add raisins and stir well. Store in an airtight container.

Yield: 28 servings

Each with: 3 g water; 174 calories (61% from fat, 11% from protein, 28% from carb); 5 g protein; 13 g total fat; 3 g saturated fat; 7 g monounsaturated fat; 3 g polyunsaturated fat; 13 g carb; 2 g fiber; 5 g sugar; 118 mg phosphorus; 27 mg calcium; 2 mg iron; 66 mg sodium; 209 mg potassium; 60 IU vitamin A; 14 mg vitamin E; 3 mg vitamin C; 4 mg cholesterol

Sugared Pecans

These are sweet and just slightly spicy nuts. I came up with the recipe while on a search to duplicate the spiced nuts sold at places like the Maryland Renaissance Festival. They aren't quite the same, but they're closer than the baked ones.

¾ cup (150 g) sugar

2 teaspoons cinnamon

¼ cup (60 ml) water

2 cups (220 g) pecans

Mix sugar and cinnamon in pan. Pour in water. Put in nuts. Bring to boil over medium heat; turn heat down and simmer, barely bubbling, 20 minutes or until syrup dries. Place nuts on waxed paper. Cool.

Yield: 12 servings

Each with: 6 g water; 176 calories (63% from fat, 4% from protein, 33% from carb); 2 g protein; 13 g total fat; 1 g saturated fat; 7 g monounsaturated fat; 4 g polyunsaturated fat; 15 g carb; 2 g fiber; 13 g sugar; 51 mg phosphorus; 18 mg calcium; 1 mg iron; 0 mg sodium; 77 mg potassium; 11 IU vitamin A; 0 mg vitamin E; 0 mg vitamin C; 0 mg cholesterol

Honey Nutty Snack

Kind of a healthier version of peanut brittle, this starts with honey-nut cereal for taste as well as nutrition.

1 cup (225 g) packed brown sugar

½ cup (112 g) unsalted butter, softened

¼ cup (60 ml) light corn syrup

½ teaspoon baking soda

6 cups (180 g) honey-nut-flavored round toasted oat cereal, such as Honey Nut Cheerios

1 cup (145 g) peanuts

1 cup (145 g) raisins

Heat oven to 250°F (120°C, gas mark ½). Coat 2 rectangular pans, 13 × 9 × 2 inches, (33 × 23 × 5 cm) or 1 jelly-roll pan, 15½ × 10½ × 1 inch (37 × 25 × 2.5 cm), with nonstick vegetable oil spray. Heat brown sugar, butter, and corn syrup in 2-quart (2-L) saucepan over medium heat, stirring constantly, until bubbly around edges. Cook uncovered, stirring occasionally, 2 minutes longer. Remove from heat; stir in baking soda until foamy and light colored. Pour over cereal, peanuts, and raisins in 4-quart (4 L) bowl coated with nonstick vegetable oil spray; stir until mixture is coated. Spread evenly in pans. Bake 15 minutes; stir. Let stand just until cool, about 10 minutes. Loosen mixture with metal spatula. Let stand until firm, about 30 minutes. Break into bite-size pieces.

Yield: 24 servings

Each with: 4 g water; 144 calories (30% from fat, 4% from protein, 66% from carb); 2 g protein; 5 g total fat; 3 g saturated fat; 1 g monounsaturated fat; 0 g polyunsaturated fat; 25 g carb; 1 g fiber; 17 g sugar; 49 mg phosphorus; 48 mg calcium; 2 mg iron; 90 mg sodium; 127 mg potassium; 285 IU vitamin A; 82 mg vitamin E; 2 mg vitamin C; 10 mg cholesterol

Date Chews

These are sweet little treats to nibble on.

1 cup (145 g) cut-up dates

3 teaspoons flour

1 cup (110 g) finely chopped pecans

½ cup (100 g) sugar

2 eggs

1 teaspoon vanilla extract

Combine dates with flour and stir to coat. Stir all ingredients enough to blend. Place 1 teaspoon each in mini muffin pans that have been sprayed with nonstick vegetable oil spray. Bake at 375°F (190°C, gas mark 5) for 12 to 15 minutes.

Yield: 32 servings

Each with: 4 g water; 58 calories (42% from fat, 6% from protein, 52% from carb); 1 g protein; 3 g total fat; 0 g saturated fat; 2 g monounsaturated fat; 1 g polyunsaturated fat; 8 g carb; 1 g fiber; 7 g sugar; 20 mg phosphorus; 7 mg calcium; 0 mg iron; 5 mg sodium; 56 mg potassium; 20 IU vitamin A; 5 mg vitamin E; 0 mg vitamin C; 15 mg cholesterol

Mudball Cookies

They may not sound too appetizing, but wait until you taste them.

1 cup (80 g) quick-cooking oats

½ cup (55 g) broken pecans

½ cup (45 g) instant cocoa mix

½ cup (130 g) peanut butter

½ cup (170 g) honey

1 cup (72 g) graham cracker crumbs

Mix oats, nut pieces, and instant cocoa mix in a large bowl. Add peanut butter and honey. Mix everything in the bowl until it looks like mud. Place graham cracker crumbs on a sheet of waxed paper. Take 1 teaspoon of cookie mixture at a time and roll in your hands to make a ball. Roll the cookie balls in the cracker crumbs and place on a paper plate or baking sheet. Store in the refrigerator.

Yield: 24 servings

Each with: 2 g water; 111 calories (41% from fat, 8% from protein, 51% from carb); 2 g protein; 5 g total fat; 1 g saturated fat; 2 g monounsaturated fat; 1 g polyunsaturated fat; 15 g carb; 1 g fiber; 9 g sugar; 49 mg phosphorus; 12 mg calcium; 1 mg iron; 78 mg sodium; 73 mg potassium; 2 IU vitamin A; 0 mg vitamin E; 0 mg vitamin C; 0 mg cholesterol

Peanut Butter Dip

This dip is just perfect for apple slices or celery, but don't stop there. You'll be surprised how many things it goes well with.

½ cup (130 g) crunchy peanut butter
¼ cup (85 g) honey
¼ cup (60 g) sour cream

In small bowl, combine peanut butter, honey, and sour cream; blend well. Serve with fresh vegetables or fruit dippers. Store in refrigerator.

Yield: 8 servings

Each with: 8 g water; 137 calories (55% from fat, 11% from protein, 34% from carb); 4 g protein; 9 g total fat; 2 g saturated fat; 4 g monounsaturated fat; 2 g polyunsaturated fat; 13 g carb; 1 g fiber; 10 g sugar; 59 mg phosphorus; 16 mg calcium; 0 mg iron; 82 mg sodium; 135 mg potassium; 28 IU vitamin A; 8 mg vitamin E; 0 mg vitamin C; 3 mg cholesterol

6

Appetizers, Snacks, and Party Foods:
Combinations

Finally we wrap up the appetizer and snack section with recipes that contain a combination of ingredients. They include things like more dips and roll-ups, as well as such popular items as pizzas and popcorn mixes.

Bean Hominy Dip

This seemingly unusual combination works very well.

16 ounces hominy

16 ounces (455 g) navy beans

4 ounces (115 g) cucumber

1½ cups (390 g) salsa

4 ounces (115 g) diced green chiles

1 tablespoon (15 ml) lime juice

½ teaspoon cumin

Puree hominy, beans, and cucumber in food processor until smooth. Put mixture into bowl and add remaining ingredients. Heat and serve with tortilla chips.

Yield: 36 servings

Each with: 26 g water; 65 calories (4% from fat, 14% from protein, 83% from carb); 2 g protein; 0 g total fat; 0 g saturated fat; 0 g monounsaturated fat; 0 g polyunsaturated fat; 14 g carb; 2 g fiber; 1 g sugar; 43 mg phosphorus; 13 mg calcium; 1 mg iron; 25 mg sodium; 105 mg potassium; 35 IU vitamin A; 0 mg vitamin E; 0 mg vitamin C; 0 mg cholesterol

Layered Middle Eastern Dip

Serve this Middle Eastern dip with pita bread chips.

½ cup (75 g) tabbouleh

¾ cup hummus

1 cup (180 g) chopped tomato

½ cup (80 g) chopped onion

¾ cup (113 g) feta cheese

(continued on page 76)

Layer ingredients in glass bowl so each is ½ to ¾ inch (1 to 2 cm) thick: first tabbouleh, then hummus, and then tomato-onion mix. Squeeze out extra juice before layering in the feta cheese.

Yield: 12 servings

Each with: 38 g water; 64 calories (47% from fat, 15% from protein, 38% from carb); 2 g protein; 3 g total fat; 2 g saturated fat; 1 g monounsaturated fat; 0 g polyunsaturated fat; 6 g carb; 2 g fiber; 1 g sugar; 57 mg phosphorus; 65 mg calcium; 0 mg iron; 143 mg sodium; 98 mg potassium; 172 IU vitamin A; 12 mg vitamin E; 5 mg vitamin C; 8 mg cholesterol

Texas Cheese Dip

This dip is a little on the spicy side. You can add or decrease the jalapeños to make it suit your own desired heat level.

3 ounces (85 g) cream cheese, room temperature

3 ounces (85 g) blue cheese, room temperature

8 ounces (225 g) sour cream

2½ teaspoons unflavored gelatin

¼ cup (60 ml) water

2 tablespoons (28 ml) vinegar

2 jalapeño peppers, minced

1¼ cups (138 g) chopped toasted pecans

2 ounces (55 g) pimento, drained and minced

Mix cheeses until smooth with sour cream. Add gelatin that has been softened in water and heated to dissolve. Add vinegar and let stand until slightly thickened. Add jalapeños, pecans, and pimento. Pour into mold that has been sprayed with nonstick vegetable oil spray and chill. Serve with crackers. Ritz crackers are a good choice. Garnish with fresh jalapeños, pimentos, or pecans.

Yield: 12 servings

Each with: 36 g water; 156 calories (83% from fat, 9% from protein, 8% from carb); 4 g protein; 15 g total fat; 5 g saturated fat; 7 g monounsaturated fat; 3 g polyunsaturated fat; 3 g carb; 1 g fiber; 1 g sugar; 86 mg phosphorus; 72 mg calcium; 1 mg iron; 129 mg sodium; 112 mg potassium; 370 IU vitamin A; 58 mg vitamin E; 5 mg vitamin C; 20 mg cholesterol

Deviled Nut Ball

This tasty spread is kick-started with canned deviled ham.

9 ounces (252 g) deviled ham

12 ounces (340 g) cream cheese, softened

½ cup (80 g) crushed pineapple, drained

3 tablespoons (27 g) minced green bell pepper

1 teaspoon minced onion

¼ teaspoon Tabasco sauce

½ cup (55 g) chopped pecans

½ cup (30 g) chopped fresh parsley

In a medium bowl, mix together ham and cream cheese. Stir in pineapple, bell pepper, onion, and Tabasco sauce. Chill 2 to 3 hours. On waxed paper, form mixture into a ball or log and roll in pecans and parsley to coat completely. Serve with crackers.

Yield: 16 servings

Each with: 32 g water; 137 calories (79% from fat, 10% from protein, 11% from carb); 3 g protein; 12 g total fat; 6 g saturated fat; 5 g monounsaturated fat; 1 g polyunsaturated fat; 4 g carb; 1 g fiber; 1 g sugar; 53 mg phosphorus; 25 mg calcium; 1 mg iron; 210 mg sodium; 85 mg potassium; 457 IU vitamin A; 76 mg vitamin E; 5 mg vitamin C; 29 mg cholesterol

Tuna-Pecan Ball

Tuna and veggies make this dip just a little different from the ordinary cheese ball.

8 ounces (225 g) cream cheese, softened

6½ ounces (184 g) white albacore tuna, drained and flaked

3 tablespoons (27 g) diced green bell pepper

3 tablespoons (30 g) diced onion

3 tablespoons (24 g) diced celery

5 pimento-stuffed diced olives

2 teaspoons horseradish

½ teaspoon Tabasco sauce

½ teaspoon Worcestershire sauce

½ cup (55 g) chopped pecans

Combine all ingredients except pecans; stir well. Shape into a ball; cover and chill at least 1 hour. Roll in pecans; cover and chill. Serve with assorted crackers.

Yield: 16 servings

Each with: 21 g water; 90 calories (76% from fat, 18% from protein, 5% from carb); 4 g protein; 8 g total fat; 3 g saturated fat; 3 g monounsaturated fat; 1 g polyunsaturated fat; 1 g carb; 1 g fiber; 0 g sugar; 51 mg phosphorus; 17 mg calcium; 0 mg iron; 53 mg sodium; 70 mg potassium; 209 IU vitamin A; 52 mg vitamin E; 2 mg vitamin C; 20 mg cholesterol

Black Bean Tortilla Pinwheels

While intended as an appetizer, you could make a meal of this by not cutting it into slices.

8 ounces (225 g) cream cheese, softened

1 cup (230 g) sour cream

1 cup (115 g) shredded Monterey Jack cheese

¼ cup (25 g) pimento-stuffed olives

¼ cup (40 g) chopped red onion

⅛ teaspoon garlic powder

2 cups (344 g) cooked black beans, drained

6 whole wheat tortillas

Combine cream cheese and sour cream; mix until well blended. Stir in Monterey Jack cheese, olives, onion, and garlic powder. Chill 2 hours. Spread thin layer of cream cheese mixture on each tortilla. Puree beans in food processor or blender. Starting in middle of tortilla, spread a layer covering half of tortilla with beans. Roll up tortilla tightly, starting with end that has the beans. Chill. Cut into ¾-inch (2 cm) slices. Serve with salsa.

Yield: 20 servings

Each with: 36 g water; 134 calories (56% from fat, 15% from protein, 29% from carb); 5 g protein; 8 g total fat; 5 g saturated fat; 3 g monounsaturated fat; 0 g polyunsaturated fat; 10 g carb; 2 g fiber; 0 g sugar; 89 mg phosphorus; 89 mg calcium; 1 mg iron; 146 mg sodium; 113 mg potassium; 256 IU vitamin A; 65 mg vitamin E; 0 mg vitamin C; 23 mg cholesterol

New York Goodwich Roll-Ups

I'm not sure where the name comes from, but someone told me that's what this veggie roll-up is called. Whatever you call it, it's tasty and filling.

½ cup (80 g) sliced onion

2 teaspoons (10 ml) olive oil

1 teaspoon (5 ml) barbecue sauce

2 whole wheat tortillas

1 tablespoon mayonnaise

1 cup (71 g) broccoli, cut in florets and steamed

½ cup (50 g) cauliflower, cut in florets and steamed

2 slices dill pickle

2 tablespoons grated carrot

2 tablespoons grated red cabbage

2 tablespoons grated yellow squash

½ cup (28 g) shredded lettuce

(continued on page 80)

½ cup (17 g) alfalfa sprouts

2 slices avocado

Sauté onion in oil until it begins to soften. Add barbecue sauce and sauté until tender. In hot dry skillet, heat tortillas, turning from one side to the other until soft but not crisp. Place on large sheet of plastic wrap. Spread tortillas with mayonnaise. Add broccoli in a line down center. Add cauliflower, pickle, grated vegetables, and a line of barbecued onions. Top with lettuce, sprouts, and avocado. Roll, crepe style, around vegetables. Wrap tightly until ready to serve.

Yield: 2 servings

Each with: 258 g water; 462 calories (62% from fat, 7% from protein, 31% from carb); 8 g protein; 34 g total fat; 5 g saturated fat; 19 g monounsaturated fat; 7 g polyunsaturated fat; 38 g carb; 14 g fiber; 6 g sugar; 181 mg phosphorus; 106 mg calcium; 3 mg iron; 294 mg sodium; 1076 mg potassium; 2036 IU vitamin A; 6 mg vitamin E; 75 mg vitamin C; 3 mg cholesterol

Spinach Roll-Ups

Like a spinach salad to take with you, these colorful roll-ups have spinach and bacon flavor.

10 ounces (280 g) frozen spinach

½ cup (115 g) sour cream

½ cup (115 g) mayonnaise

2 tablespoons bacon bits

3 whole wheat tortillas

Cook spinach and drain well. Mix sour cream, mayonnaise, and bacon bits. Mix in cooked spinach. Equally divide on top of tortillas. Spread mixture evenly over each tortilla. Roll up each tortilla. Store overnight in refrigerator. Slice into 1-inch (2.5-cm) slices.

Yield: 15 servings

Each with: 26 g water; 92 calories (71% from fat, 8% from protein, 21% from carb); 2 g protein; 7 g total fat; 2 g saturated fat; 2 g monounsaturated fat; 3 g polyunsaturated fat; 5 g carb; 1 g fiber; 0 g sugar; 27 mg phosphorus; 48 mg calcium; 1 mg iron; 124 mg sodium; 80 mg potassium; 2330 IU vitamin A; 14 mg vitamin E; 1 mg vitamin C; 6 mg cholesterol

Vegetable Quesadillas

If you have an indoor grill like the George Foreman models, it is perfect for making these quesa-dillas. If not, place them on a baking sheet in a 350°F (180°C, gas mark 4) oven until crisp. Serve them with salsa and sour cream.

¼ cup (55 g) unsalted butter

2½ teaspoons chili powder

1 teaspoon minced garlic

1 teaspoon oregano

8 ounces (225 g) mushrooms, sliced

1 cup (150 g) sliced green bell pepper

⅔ cup (110 g) finely chopped onion

½ cup chopped fresh cilantro

1½ cups (175 g) shredded Monterey Jack cheese

2 tablespoons (28 ml) olive oil

16 corn tortillas, 5½ inch (14 cm)

Melt the butter in a large skillet over medium-high heat. Add chili powder, garlic, and oregano and sauté about 1 minute. Add mushrooms and sauté until tender, about 10 minutes. Remove from heat and mix in the bell pepper, onion, and cilantro. Cool for 10 minutes and then mix in the cheese. Lightly brush oil on one side of 8 of the tortillas. Divide vegetable mixture among tortillas, spreading to even thickness. Top with the remaining 8 tortillas and brush tops with oil. Grill quesadillas until heated through and golden brown, about 3 minutes per side. Cut into wedges (4 to 6) to serve.

Yield: 12 servings

Each with: 62 g water; 205 calories (52% from fat, 13% from protein, 35% from carb); 7 g protein; 12 g total fat; 6 g saturated fat; 4 g monounsaturated fat; 1 g polyunsaturated fat; 19 g carb; 3 g fiber; 1 g sugar; 207 mg phosphorus; 193 mg calcium; 1 mg iron; 101 mg sodium; 184 mg potassium; 569 IU vitamin A; 63 mg vitamin E; 12 mg vitamin C; 25 mg cholesterol

Vegetable Pita Pockets

I just love it when things that are good for you also taste great. This is one of those things.

1 cup (71 g) sliced broccoli

1 cup (100 g) sliced cauliflower

1 cup (130 g) sliced carrot

½ cup (80 g) sliced onion

1 tablespoon unsalted butter

1 cup (180 g) chopped tomato

¼ teaspoon oregano leaves

¼ teaspoon basil leaves

1 cup (110 g) shredded Swiss cheese

4 whole wheat pitas

Sauté broccoli, cauliflower, carrot, and onion in butter for 3 to 4 minutes until crisp and tender. Toss sautéed vegetables with tomato, oregano, basil, and cheese. Cut pita bread in half to form two half-circle pockets. Divide vegetable mixture evenly in all the pita halves.

Yield: 4 servings

Each with: 163 g water; 364 calories (33% from fat, 19% from protein, 48% from carb); 18 g protein; 14 g total fat; 8 g saturated fat; 3 g monounsaturated fat; 1 g polyunsaturated fat; 46 g carb; 8 g fiber; 4 g sugar; 367 mg phosphorus; 361 mg calcium; 3 mg iron; 384 mg sodium; 478 mg potassium; 6123 IU vitamin A; 93 mg vitamin E; 47 mg vitamin C; 38 mg cholesterol

Stuffed Artichokes

Walnuts give this appetizer both crunch and extra fiber.

10 ounces (280 g) frozen spinach

¼ cup (30 g) chopped walnuts

1 cup (235 ml) fat-free evaporated milk

½ teaspoon crushed garlic

1 can artichoke bottoms, drained and rinsed

2 tablespoons (30 ml) lemon juice

¼ cup (25 g) grated Parmesan cheese

Cook and drain spinach. Process spinach in blender with chopped walnuts, evaporated milk, and crushed garlic until coarsely chopped. Arrange artichoke bottoms in baking dish coated with nonstick vegetable oil spray. Drizzle with lemon juice. Stuff with spinach mixture and top with Parmesan cheese. Bake in oven at 350°F (180°C, gas mark 4) for 20 to 25 minutes.

Yield: 4 servings

Each with: 181 g water; 301 calories (44% from fat, 32% from protein, 25% from carb); 25 g protein; 15 g total fat; 7 g saturated fat; 4 g monounsaturated fat; 3 g polyunsaturated fat; 19 g carb; 6 g fiber; 9 g sugar; 493 mg phosphorus; 701 mg calcium; 2 mg iron; 710 mg sodium; 680 mg potassium; 9058 IU vitamin A; 116 mg vitamin E; 9 mg vitamin C; 33 mg cholesterol

Veggie Pizza Bites

Like miniature pieces of pizza, these small wedges are sure to be a hit with nibblers of all ages.

2 teaspoons chopped garlic

1 cup (180 g) sliced tomato

2 tablespoons (28 ml) olive oil

⅛ teaspoon black pepper

6 ounces (170 g) mozzarella cheese, sliced

2 whole wheat tortillas

2 tablespoons minced fresh basil

½ cup (50 g) grated Parmesan cheese

In a small bowl, place the garlic, tomato, olive oil, and pepper. Thoroughly coat the tomatoes. Place the cheese slices over the tortillas. Place the soaked tomatoes on top. Sprinkle on the basil and Parmesan cheese. Preheat the oven to 350°F (180°C, gas mark 4). Place the tortillas on a baking sheet and bake them for 8 minutes or until the cheese is melted. Cut each pizza into 3 wedges.

Yield: 6 servings

Each with: 43 g water; 201 calories (63% from fat, 21% from protein, 16% from carb); 11 g protein; 14 g total fat; 6 g saturated fat; 6 g monounsaturated fat; 1 g polyunsaturated fat; 8 g carb; 1 g fiber; 1 g sugar; 184 mg phosphorus; 267 mg calcium; 1 mg iron; 372 mg sodium; 131 mg potassium; 449 IU vitamin A; 59 mg vitamin E; 7 mg vitamin C; 30 mg cholesterol

Pizza Pitas

Pizza snacks are always a hit. And you don't have to tell anyone that these are actually good for them.

1 whole wheat pita

2 tablespoons pizza sauce

⅛ teaspoon crushed dried oregano

½ cup (75 g) sliced red bell pepper

½ cup (80 g) sliced onion

2 ounces (56 g) shredded mozzarella cheese

Split pita bread round in half, forming 2 thin circles. Spread each circle with half of the sauce. Sprinkle half of the oregano over each. Top each circle with half of the veggies and half of the cheese. Place pita bread halves on a baking sheet. Bake in a 375°F (190°C, gas mark 5) oven for 8 to 10 minutes or until cheese is bubbly and edges of pita bread are crisp. Remove from baking sheet; cool slightly.

Yield: 2 servings

Each with: 109 g water; 189 calories (26% from fat, 22% from protein, 52% from carb); 11 g protein; 6 g total fat; 3 g saturated fat; 1 g monounsaturated fat; 1 g polyunsaturated fat; 26 g carb; 4 g fiber; 5 g sugar; 216 mg phosphorus; 241 mg calcium; 1 mg iron; 434 mg sodium; 278 mg potassium; 1434 IU vitamin A; 35 mg vitamin E; 53 mg vitamin C; 18 mg cholesterol

Veggie Bars

This makes both a pretty and a tasty appetizer. It's light enough that people won't get filled up on it, so it's also a good choice before a meal. We've used it to satisfy the family munchies while roast beef is cooking for New Year's dinner.

1 package crescent rolls

¼ cup (60 g) sour cream

1 tablespoon (15 ml) ranch dressing

8 ounces (225 g) cream cheese

½ cup (75 g) finely chopped green bell pepper

½ cup (80 g) finely chopped onion

½ cup (36 g) finely chopped broccoli

½ cup (65 g) finely chopped carrot

½ cup (50 g) finely chopped cauliflower

¼ cup (25 g) finely chopped black olives

½ cup (35 g) finely chopped mushrooms

½ cup (58 g) shredded Cheddar cheese

Carefully unroll crescent rolls and place dough in 8 × 13-inch (20 × 33 cm) pan. Gently press and shape to cover bottom. Bake at 350°F (180°C, gas mark 4) for 8 minutes. Let cool. Mix sour cream, dressing, and cream cheese. Spread on cooled crust. Sprinkle remaining ingredients on top, cover with plastic wrap, and press vegetables down into cream. Chill for 3 to 4 hours. Cut into bars and serve.

Yield: 16 servings

Each with: 35 g water; 90 calories (73% from fat, 12% from protein, 15% from carb); 3 g protein; 7 g total fat; 4 g saturated fat; 2 g monounsaturated fat; 0 g polyunsaturated fat; 3 g carb; 1 g fiber; 1 g sugar; 51 mg phosphorus; 55 mg calcium; 0 mg iron; 108 mg sodium; 78 mg potassium; 965 IU vitamin A; 65 mg vitamin E; 9 mg vitamin C; 22 mg cholesterol

Pecan-Stuffed Mushrooms

This appetizer always disappears fast. Something about the crunch of pecans just makes these different from other mushrooms.

12 large mushrooms

2 tablespoons (20 g) chopped onion

2 tablespoons (28 g) unsalted butter

½ cup (55 g) chopped pecans

½ cup (60 g) whole wheat bread crumbs

1 teaspoon lemon juice

Wash mushrooms gently in cool water or wipe with damp cloth. Remove stems and chop. Sauté onion in butter; add chopped stems, pecans, bread crumbs, and lemon juice. Mix well. Mound mushroom caps with stuffing. Broil 4 minutes about 4 inches (10 cm) from heat or cook in microwave oven on 100 percent power 2 to 3 minutes until heated through.

Yield: 12 servings

Each with: 14 g water; 70 calories (68% from fat, 8% from protein, 24% from carb); 1 g protein; 5 g total fat; 2 g saturated fat; 2 g monounsaturated fat; 1 g polyunsaturated fat; 4 g carb; 1 g fiber; 1 g sugar; 31 mg phosphorus; 13 mg calcium; 0 mg iron; 7 mg sodium; 68 mg potassium; 62 IU vitamin A; 16 mg vitamin E; 1 mg vitamin C; 5 mg cholesterol

Pecan Crunch Snack

This easy-to-make snack mix is full of nuts and crunchy cereal.

1 cup (225 g) unsalted butter

1 cup (225 g) brown sugar

8 cups mini shredded wheat cereal

1 pound (455 g) pecans

Melt butter and brown sugar; boil 2 minutes. Place cereal and nuts in two 9 × 13-inch
(23 × 33 cm) cake pans. Pour butter-sugar mixture over cereal-nuts mixture. Bake at 375°F
(190°C, gas mark 5) for 8 minutes. Stir occasionally. Store in covered container.

Yield: 20 servings

Each with: 3 g water; 280 calories (78% from fat, 3% from protein, 19% from carb); 2 g protein; 26 g total
fat; 7 g saturated fat; 12 g monounsaturated fat; 5 g polyunsaturated fat; 14 g carb; 2 g fiber; 11 g sugar;
68 mg phosphorus; 28 mg calcium; 1 mg iron; 6 mg sodium; 134 mg potassium; 296 IU vitamin A; 76 mg
vitamin E; 0 mg vitamin C; 24 mg cholesterol

Fruit and Nut Popcorn

This sweetly spiced popcorn-and-fruit mixture is perfect with a glass of apple cider.

2 quarts (64 g) popped popcorn

1 cup (86 g) chopped dried apples

1 cup (130 g) chopped dried apricots

1 cup (145 g) raisins

1 cup (120 g) coarsely chopped walnuts

¼ teaspoon confectioners' sugar

1½ teaspoons cinnamon

½ teaspoon nutmeg

In a large bowl, combine hot popcorn, fruits, and nuts. Combine sugar, cinnamon, and nutmeg. Sprinkle over popcorn mixture to coat. Store in an airtight container. This will keep for up to 3 days.

Yield: 12 servings

Each with: 28 g water; 164 calories (48% from fat, 8% from protein, 44% from carb); 4 g protein; 9 g total fat; 1 g saturated fat; 2 g monounsaturated fat; 5 g polyunsaturated fat; 19 g carb; 2 g fiber; 11 g sugar; 87 mg phosphorus; 20 mg calcium; 1 mg iron; 80 mg sodium; 214 mg potassium; 364 IU vitamin A; 0 mg vitamin E; 2 mg vitamin C; 0 mg cholesterol

Cinnamon Apple Popcorn

This is a nice sweet treat to nibble while you are watching television.

1 cup (86 g) chopped dried apples

5 cups (40 g) popped popcorn

1 cup (55 g) halved pecans

4 tablespoons (55 g) unsalted butter, melted

1 teaspoon cinnamon

¼ teaspoon nutmeg

2 tablespoons (30 g) brown sugar

¼ teaspoon vanilla extract

Preheat oven to 250°F (120°C, gas mark ½). Place apples in a large shallow baking pan. Bake 20 minutes. Remove pan from oven and stir in popcorn and pecans. In a small bowl, combine remaining ingredients. Drizzle butter mixture over popcorn mixture, stirring well. Bake for 30 minutes, stirring every 10 minutes. Pour onto waxed paper to cool. Store in an airtight container.

Yield: 14 servings

Each with: 8 g water; 118 calories (77% from fat, 3% from protein, 19% from carb); 1 g protein; 11 g total fat; 3 g saturated fat; 4 g monounsaturated fat; 3 g polyunsaturated fat; 6 g carb; 1 g fiber; 3 g sugar; 32 mg phosphorus; 11 mg calcium; 0 mg iron; 43 mg sodium; 55 mg potassium; 115 IU vitamin A; 27 mg vitamin E; 0 mg vitamin C; 9 mg cholesterol

Apricot Chews

These sweet little treats are perfect when you just want a little something sweet.

2 ounces (57 g) cream cheese, softened

1 tablespoon confectioners' sugar

¼ teaspoon vanilla extract

8 ounces (225 g) dried apricots

1 tablespoon wheat germ

3 tablespoons (27 g) slivered almonds

Blend cream cheese, confectioners' sugar, and vanilla until softened. Place small amount of mixture between two halves of apricots. Combine wheat germ and almonds. Roll apricots in mixture. Chill for 15 minutes.

Yield: 15 servings

Each with: 15 g water; 35 calories (57% from fat, 10% from protein, 33% from carb); 1 g protein; 2 g total fat; 1 g saturated fat; 1 g monounsaturated fat; 0 g polyunsaturated fat; 3 g carb; 1 g fiber; 2 g sugar; 21 mg phosphorus; 10 mg calcium; 0 mg iron; 12 mg sodium; 47 mg potassium; 307 IU vitamin A; 14 mg vitamin E; 1 mg vitamin C; 4 mg cholesterol

Apple Nut Dip

This is a great dip for apples, pears, grapes, and other fruit. It is also good as a spread for raisin bread or other sweet breakfast breads.

1 cup (230 g) sour cream

8 ounces (225 g) cream cheese, softened

¼ teaspoon cinnamon

1 cup (150 g) shredded apple

½ cup (55 g) chopped pecans

2 tablespoons (30 g) brown sugar

Beat sour cream, cream cheese, and cinnamon in medium bowl. Stir in remaining ingredients. Chill. Serve with fruit dippers.

Yield: 16 servings

Each with: 26 g water; 103 calories (78% from fat, 7% from protein, 15% from carb); 2 g protein; 9 g total fat; 4 g saturated fat; 3 g monounsaturated fat; 1 g polyunsaturated fat; 4 g carb; 1 g fiber; 3 g sugar; 40 mg phosphorus; 32 mg calcium; 0 mg iron; 49 mg sodium; 63 mg potassium; 252 IU vitamin A; 66 mg vitamin E; 0 mg vitamin C; 21 mg cholesterol

Orange and Nut Spread

This is a nice sweet fruity dip or spread.

1 orange

1 cup (110 g) broken pecans

2½ cups (365 g) raisins

¾ cup (175 g) mayonnaise

Do not peel orange. Quarter and seed orange. In a food processor bowl, process orange and pecans, covered, until finely chopped. Add half of the raisins and all of the mayonnaise. Cover; process until raisins are chopped. Add remaining raisins; cover and process until finely chopped. Transfer to a covered container; chill.

Yield: 28 servings

Each with: 9 g water; 117 calories (54% from fat, 3% from protein, 43% from carb); 1 g protein; 8 g total fat; 1 g saturated fat; 3 g monounsaturated fat; 3 g polyunsaturated fat; 13 g carb; 1 g fiber; 10 g sugar; 28 mg phosphorus; 14 mg calcium; 0 mg iron; 35 mg sodium; 140 mg potassium; 34 IU vitamin A; 5 mg vitamin E; 4 mg vitamin C; 2 mg cholesterol

TIP

To serve, spread on orange slices, celery, or crackers.

7

Breakfast:
Grains

Breakfast is a key meal to get your day started right, and grains are a natural way to do that. Of course, you could choose the quick and easy solution of a high-fiber cereal. But sometimes you want something a little different. At least I know I do. In this chapter we have some ways to spice up your plain old oatmeal, as well as a variety of recipes for pancakes, waffles, scones, and homemade granola.

Baked Oatmeal

Okay, it seems like a strange idea, but this really works. What you end up with is not at all the same as just microwaving your oatmeal. Try it and see if it's not worth the effort.

½ cup (125 g) applesauce

¾ cup (170 g) brown sugar

2 eggs

1 cup (235 ml) skim milk

3 cups (240 g) quick-cooking oats

2 teaspoons baking powder

½ teaspoon cinnamon

²/₃ cup (80 g) chopped walnuts

Combine applesauce, sugar, eggs, and milk; mix well. Mix remaining ingredients together and then combine with first mixture. Bake in a 9 × 13-inch (23 × 33 cm) pan coated with nonstick vegetable oil spray for 30 minutes at 350°F (180°C, gas mark 4). Serve with hot milk.

Yield: 6 servings

Each with: 72 g water; 406 calories (27% from fat, 13% from protein, 60% from carb); 14 g protein; 13 g total fat; 2 g saturated fat; 4 g monounsaturated fat; 6 g polyunsaturated fat; 63 g carb; 5 g fiber; 31 g sugar; 386 mg phosphorus; 215 mg calcium; 3 mg iron; 226 mg sodium; 423 mg potassium; 183 IU vitamin A; 51 mg vitamin E; 1 mg vitamin C; 80 mg cholesterol

Homestyle Pancake Mix

Make up a batch of this mix and you'll always be ready to make pancakes in a flash.

6 cups (720 g) whole wheat pastry flour

1½ cups (210 g) cornmeal

½ cup (100 g) sugar

1½ cups (102 g) nonfat dry milk

2 tablespoons (28 g) baking powder

Combine all ingredients and store in tightly covered jar. To cook, add 1 cup water to 1 cup mix; use less water if you want a thicker pancake. Stir only until lumps disappear. Lightly coat a nonstick skillet or griddle with nonstick vegetable oil spray and preheat until drops of cold water bounce and sputter. Drop batter to desired size and cook until bubbles form and edges begin to dry. Turn only once.

Yield: 16 servings

Each with: 7 g water; 256 calories (4% from fat, 14% from protein, 82% from carb); 9 g protein; 1 g total fat; 0 g saturated fat; 0 g monounsaturated fat; 0 g polyunsaturated fat; 55 g carb; 6 g fiber; 10 g sugar; 272 mg phosphorus; 196 mg calcium; 3 mg iron; 221 mg sodium; 314 mg potassium; 187 IU vitamin A; 45 mg vitamin E; 0 mg vitamin C; 1 mg cholesterol

Multigrain Pancakes

These are great pancakes, thicker and full of much more flavor than regular ones. Try them with the apple topping in chapter 8.

1½ cups (180 g) whole wheat pastry flour

¼ cup (35 g) cornmeal

¼ cup (20 g) rolled oats

2 tablespoons oat bran

2 tablespoons wheat germ

2 tablespoons (18 g) toasted wheat cereal, such as Wheatena

1 teaspoon baking soda

½ teaspoon baking powder

1 teaspoon vanilla extract

1½ cups (355 ml) skim milk

2 egg whites

Mix all dry ingredients. Add milk to make batter. Thicker batter makes thicker pancakes. Set aside to rest for a half an hour. Beat egg whites until stiff peaks form. Gently fold into batter after it has

(continued on page 96)

rested. Spoon onto moderate griddle and cook until bubbles break. Turn and cook until done. Bake more slowly than with regular pancakes because of the heavy batter.

Yield: 6 servings

Each with: 70 g water; 195 calories (6% from fat, 20% from protein, 74% from carb); 10 g protein; 1 g total fat; 0 g saturated fat; 0 g monounsaturated fat; 1 g polyunsaturated fat; 37 g carb; 5 g fiber; 1 g sugar; 249 mg phosphorus; 127 mg calcium; 2 mg iron; 101 mg sodium; 316 mg potassium; 154 IU vitamin A; 40 mg vitamin E; 1 mg vitamin C; 1 mg cholesterol

Cinnamon–Oat Bran Pancakes

These are the kind of pancakes you want on a snowy day, warm and flavorful. The good news is they are also a lot better for you than the regular boring pancakes.

¾ cup (75 g) oat bran

¾ cup (90 g) whole wheat pastry flour

1 tablespoon sugar

½ teaspoon baking powder

½ teaspoon cinnamon

¼ teaspoon baking soda

1¼ cups (295 ml) buttermilk

1 tablespoon (15 ml) canola oil

½ cup (55 g) finely chopped pecans

In medium mixing bowl, combine dry ingredients. Set bowl aside. In a small mixing bowl, combine buttermilk and oil. Add to dry ingredients, stirring until just combined. Stir in pecans. Cook on hot griddle. Use ¼ cup batter for each pancake.

Yield: 4 servings

Each with: 72 g water; 277 calories (46% from fat, 11% from protein, 43% from carb); 8 g protein; 15 g total fat; 2 g saturated fat; 8 g monounsaturated fat; 4 g polyunsaturated fat; 32 g carb; 5 g fiber; 9 g sugar; 241 mg phosphorus; 160 mg calcium; 4 mg iron; 174 mg sodium; 302 mg potassium; 113 IU vitamin A; 30 mg vitamin E; 2 mg vitamin C; 3 mg cholesterol

Whole Wheat Buttermilk Pancakes

This is a great tasty, old-fashioned pancake. It reminds me of the kind of things my grandmother used to make.

1 cup (120 g) whole wheat pastry flour

½ teaspoon baking soda

¼ teaspoon cinnamon

1¼ cups (295 ml) buttermilk

2 eggs

3 tablespoons (45 ml) canola oil

Blend dry ingredients. Blend wet ingredients except oil. Mix the two mixtures together. It will be slightly lumpy. Heat oil in cast-iron skillet. Pour one-quarter of the batter into pan. When pancake bubbles, turn and cook 1 to 2 minutes more.

Yield: 4 servings

Each with: 93 g water; 266 calories (48% from fat, 15% from protein, 38% from carb); 10 g protein; 15 g total fat; 2 g saturated fat; 8 g monounsaturated fat; 4 g polyunsaturated fat; 26 g carb; 4 g fiber; 4 g sugar; 226 mg phosphorus; 116 mg calcium; 2 mg iron; 121 mg sodium; 275 mg potassium; 159 IU vitamin A; 44 mg vitamin E; 1 mg vitamin C; 122 mg cholesterol

Cornmeal Pancakes

Another of those old-fashioned breakfast meals. Do you suppose that I keep saying that because people ate more healthy food in the good old days?

1 cup (235 ml) boiling water

¾ cup (105 g) cornmeal

1¼ cups (295 ml) buttermilk

2 eggs

1 cup (120 g) whole wheat pastry flour

1 tablespoon baking powder

(continued on page 98)

¼ teaspoon baking soda

¼ cup (60 ml) canola oil

Pour water over cornmeal, stir until thick. Add buttermilk; beat in eggs. Mix flour, baking powder, and baking soda. Add to cornmeal mixture. Stir in canola oil. Bake on hot griddle.

Yield: 7 servings

Each with: 89 g water; 233 calories (40% from fat, 12% from protein, 48% from carb); 7 g protein; 11 g total fat; 1 g saturated fat; 6 g monounsaturated fat; 3 g polyunsaturated fat; 29 g carb; 3 g fiber; 3 g sugar; 190 mg phosphorus; 182 mg calcium; 2 mg iron; 280 mg sodium; 184 mg potassium; 127 IU vitamin A; 25 mg vitamin E; 0 mg vitamin C; 69 mg cholesterol

Oven-Baked Pancake

Mix it up, stick it in the oven, and enjoy it. This makes a great weekend breakfast choice.

3 eggs

½ cup (60 g) whole wheat pastry flour

½ cup (120 ml) skim milk

¼ cup (55 g) unsalted butter, divided

2 tablespoons (26 g) sugar

2 tablespoons (18 g) slivered almonds, toasted

2 tablespoons (30 ml) lemon juice

Beat eggs with an electric mixer at medium speed until well blended. Gradually add flour, beating until smooth. Add milk and 2 tablespoons (28 g) melted butter; beat until batter is smooth. Pour batter into a 10-inch (25 cm) skillet coated with nonstick vegetable oil spray. Bake at 400°F (200°C, gas mark 6) for 15 minutes or until pancake is puffed and golden brown. Sprinkle with sugar and toasted almonds. Combine remaining butter and lemon juice; heat until butter melts. Serve over hot pancake.

Yield: 3 servings

Each with: 94 g water; 370 calories (58% from fat, 13% from protein, 29% from carb); 13 g protein; 24 g total fat; 12 g saturated fat; 8 g monounsaturated fat; 2 g polyunsaturated fat; 28 g carb; 3 g fiber; 9 g sugar; 255 mg phosphorus; 116 mg calcium; 2 mg iron; 106 mg sodium; 291 mg potassium; 832 IU vitamin A; 230 mg vitamin E; 5 mg vitamin C; 278 mg cholesterol

Baked Pancake

This is a German-style pancake, baked in one large pan in the oven, then cut into serving-size pieces.

1½ cups (180 g) whole wheat pastry flour

1½ cups (355 ml) skim milk

4 eggs, slightly beaten

¼ cup (55 g) unsalted butter

1 cup (170 g) sliced strawberries

Gradually add flour and milk to eggs. Melt butter in 9 × 13-inch (23 × 33 cm) pan. Pour batter over melted butter. Bake at 400°F (200°C, gas mark 6) for about 30 minutes. Serve with fresh sliced strawberries.

Yield: 4 servings

Each with: 167 g water; 378 calories (42% from fat, 17% from protein, 41% from carb); 17 g protein; 18 g total fat; 9 g saturated fat; 5 g monounsaturated fat; 2 g polyunsaturated fat; 41 g carb; 6 g fiber; 7 g sugar; 368 mg phosphorus; 169 mg calcium; 3 mg iron; 201 mg sodium; 462 mg potassium; 823 IU vitamin A; 229 mg vitamin E; 22 mg vitamin C; 269 mg cholesterol

Wheat Waffles

You can certainly have these for breakfast, but we also like them for dinner, topped with something like chicken à la king.

2 cups (240 g) whole wheat pastry flour

4 teaspoons (18 g) baking powder

2 tablespoons (40 g) honey

1¾ cups (410 ml) skim milk

4 tablespoons (60 ml) canola oil

2 eggs

Mix dry ingredients together. Stir in remaining ingredients. For lighter waffles, separate eggs. Beat egg whites and carefully fold in. Pour into a waffle iron coated with nonstick vegetable oil spray.

Yield: 8 servings

Each with: 63 g water; 223 calories (35% from fat, 14% from protein, 51% from carb); 8 g protein; 9 g total fat; 1 g saturated fat; 5 g monounsaturated fat; 3 g polyunsaturated fat; 30 g carb; 4 g fiber; 5 g sugar; 241 mg phosphorus; 230 mg calcium; 2 mg iron; 297 mg sodium; 241 mg potassium; 180 IU vitamin A; 52 mg vitamin E; 1 mg vitamin C; 60 mg cholesterol

Oatmeal Waffles

These great waffles are easy to make. They don't require the separated eggs and beaten whites that most waffle recipes call for. This and the whole grains make them a little crisper than some waffles, but the taste is wonderful.

1½ cups (180 g) whole wheat pastry flour

1 cup (80 g) quick-cooking oats

1 tablespoon baking powder

1 teaspoon cinnamon

2 tablespoons (30 g) brown sugar

3 tablespoons (42 g) unsalted butter

1½ cups (355 ml) skim milk

2 eggs, slightly beaten

In large bowl, mix all dry ingredients together and set aside. Melt butter and add milk and eggs. Mix well and then add to flour mixture. Stir until well blended. Pour into a waffle iron coated with nonstick vegetable oil spray.

Yield: 5 servings

Each with: 91 g water; 326 calories (29% from fat, 15% from protein, 56% from carb); 13 g protein; 11 g total fat; 5 g saturated fat; 3 g monounsaturated fat; 1 g polyunsaturated fat; 47 g carb; 6 g fiber; 10 g sugar; 382 mg phosphorus; 299 mg calcium; 3 mg iron; 360 mg sodium; 371 mg potassium; 476 IU vitamin A; 133 mg vitamin E; 0 mg vitamin C; 115 mg cholesterol

Bran Applesauce Muffins

Most people tend to think of bran muffins as something you need to force yourself to eat. These are not like that. They are moist and flavorful.

1¼ cups (150 g) whole wheat pastry flour

¾ cup (30 g) bran flakes cereal, crushed

½ cup (100 g) sugar

1 teaspoon baking soda

1 teaspoon cinnamon

½ teaspoon nutmeg

1 cup (245 g) applesauce

½ cup (120 ml) canola oil

1 teaspoon vanilla extract

2 eggs

½ cup (75 g) raisins

1 tablespoon sugar

½ teaspoon cinnamon

(continued on page 102)

Heat oven to 400°F (200°C, gas mark 6). Line 12 muffin cups with paper baking cups or spray with nonstick vegetable oil spray. Lightly spoon flour into measuring cup; level off. In large bowl, combine all ingredients except the sugar and cinnamon; mix well. Spoon batter into prepared muffin cups, filling two-thirds full. In small bowl, combine the sugar and cinnamon; sprinkle over top of each muffin. Bake at 400°F (200°C, gas mark 6) for 15 to 20 minutes or until toothpick inserted in center comes out clean. Immediately remove from pan. Serve warm.

Yield: 12 servings

Each with: 27 g water; 224 calories (41% from fat, 6% from protein, 53% from carb); 4 g protein; 11 g total fat; 1 g saturated fat; 6 g monounsaturated fat; 3 g polyunsaturated fat; 31 g carb; 3 g fiber; 17 g sugar; 87 mg phosphorus; 19 mg calcium; 1 mg iron; 44 mg sodium; 148 mg potassium; 185 IU vitamin A; 13 mg vitamin E; 2 mg vitamin C; 39 mg cholesterol

Oat Bran Muffins

These are so good you won't guess that they are good for you.

2¼ cups (225 g) oat bran

1 tablespoon baking powder

¼ cup (35 g) raisins

¼ cup (28 g) chopped pecans

2 eggs

2 tablespoons (28 ml) olive oil

¼ cup (85 g) honey

1¼ cups (295 ml) water

TIP

Cover when cooled, as they dry quickly.

Preheat oven to 425°F (220°C, gas mark 7). Put dry ingredients, raisins, and pecans in mixing bowl. Beat eggs, olive oil, honey, and water lightly. Add this mixture to dry ingredients and stir until moistened. Line muffin pans with paper liners or spray with nonstick vegetable oil spray and fill about half full. Bake for 15 to 17 minutes.

Yield: 12 servings

Each with: 34 g water; 113 calories (39% from fat, 9% from protein, 52% from carb); 3 g protein; 5 g total fat; 1 g saturated fat; 3 g monounsaturated fat; 1 g polyunsaturated fat; 16 g carb; 1 g fiber; 9 g sugar; 97 mg phosphorus; 93 mg calcium; 3 mg iron; 168 mg sodium; 89 mg potassium; 129 IU vitamin A; 38 mg vitamin E; 1 mg vitamin C; 39 mg cholesterol

Orange Bran Muffins

These are good, moist bran muffins with just a hint of orange flavor.

2½ cups (300 g) whole wheat pastry flour

1 tablespoon baking soda

3 cups (177 g) raisin bran cereal

½ cup (100 g) sugar

1 teaspoon cinnamon

1½ tablespoons orange peel

2 cups (460 g) plain fat-free yogurt

2 eggs, beaten

½ cup (120 ml) canola oil

In large bowl, mix flour and baking soda. Add the cereal, sugar, cinnamon, and orange peel, mixing well. Briefly but thoroughly mix in yogurt, beaten eggs, and cooking oil. Spoon into muffin tins lined with paper liners or sprayed with nonstick vegetable oil spray. Bake for 20 minutes in a 375°F (190°C, gas mark 5) oven.

Yield: 12 servings

Each with: 46 g water; 283 calories (33% from fat, 11% from protein, 56% from carb); 8 g protein; 11 g total fat; 2 g saturated fat; 3 g monounsaturated fat; 6 g polyunsaturated fat; 42 g carb; 5 g fiber; 17 g sugar; 233 mg phosphorus; 106 mg calcium; 2 mg iron; 136 mg sodium; 314 mg potassium; 183 IU vitamin A; 53 mg vitamin E; 2 mg vitamin C; 40 mg cholesterol

Pasta Fritters

This is a different sort of use for leftover pasta. We called them breakfast, but they could just as easily be a side dish at dinner.

2 cups (280 g) leftover spaghetti

¼ cup (25 g) chopped scallions

½ cup (56 g) shredded zucchini

⅓ cup (78 ml) canola oil

1 egg

1 cup (120 g) whole wheat pastry flour

⅛ teaspoon black pepper

1 cup (235 ml) water

About 35 minutes before serving, coarsely chop cooked spaghetti, chop onions, and shred zucchini; set aside. In 12-inch (30-cm) skillet, over high heat, heat canola oil until very hot. Meanwhile prepare batter. In medium bowl, with wire whisk or fork, mix egg, flour, pepper, and water. Stir in spaghetti mixture. Drop mixture into hot oil in skillet by ¼ cups into 4 mounds about 2 inches (5 cm) apart. With spatula, flatten each to make 3-inch (7.5 cm) pancake. Cook fritters until golden brown on both sides; drain fritters on paper towels. Keep warm. Repeat with remaining mixture, adding more oil to skillet if needed.

Yield: 6 servings

Each with: 92 g water; 254 calories (48% from fat, 10% from protein, 42% from carb); 6 g protein; 14 g total fat; 1 g saturated fat; 8 g monounsaturated fat; 4 g polyunsaturated fat; 28 g carb; 5 g fiber; 1 g sugar; 132 mg phosphorus; 24 mg calcium; 2 mg iron; 21 mg sodium; 152 mg potassium; 123 IU vitamin A; 15 mg vitamin E; 3 mg vitamin C; 35 mg cholesterol

Cinnamon Honey Scones

These are sort of a free-form scone, rather than the more traditional wedges. Serve warm with honey and butter to bring out the flavor of the scones even more.

1¾ cups (220 g) whole wheat pastry flour

1½ teaspoons baking powder

¼ teaspoon cinnamon

6 tablespoons (85 g) unsalted butter, softened

1 tablespoon (20 g) honey

½ cup (120 ml) skim milk

1 egg

Preheat oven to 450°F (230°C, gas mark 8). Line baking sheet with aluminum foil. In a bowl, mix the flour, baking powder, and cinnamon with a wooden spoon. Work butter into mixture by hand until mixture is yellow. Add honey and milk, then egg. Stir with wooden spoon until thoroughly mixed. Scoop spoonful of dough and drop onto baking sheet. Leave 1 inch (2.5 cm) between each. Bake 15 minutes or until golden brown. Cool 5 minutes.

Yield: 8 servings

Each with: 23 g water; 192 calories (45% from fat, 10% from protein, 45% from carb); 5 g protein; 10 g total fat; 6 g saturated fat; 3 g monounsaturated fat; 1 g polyunsaturated fat; 22 g carb; 3 g fiber; 2 g sugar; 142 mg phosphorus; 89 mg calcium; 1 mg iron; 115 mg sodium; 147 mg potassium; 342 IU vitamin A; 92 mg vitamin E; 0 mg vitamin C; 49 mg cholesterol

Oatmeal Raisin Scones

I've learned to like scones in recent years. This version not only tastes great, but it is healthy too.

2 cups (240 g) whole wheat pastry flour

3 tablespoons (45 g) brown sugar

1 teaspoon baking powder

½ teaspoon baking soda

½ cup (112 g) unsalted butter, chilled

1½ cups (120 g) rolled oats

½ cup (75 g) raisins

1 cup (235 ml) buttermilk

2 tablespoons cinnamon

2 tablespoons (26 g) sugar

Preheat the oven to 375°F (190°C, gas mark 5). Combine flour, brown sugar, baking powder, and baking soda. Cut in butter until the mixture resembles coarse crumbs. Stir in oats and raisins. Add the buttermilk and mix with a fork until dough forms a ball. Turn out on lightly floured board and knead 6 to 8 minutes. Pat dough into ½-inch (1 cm) thickness. Cut 8 to 10 rounds or wedges and place them on ungreased baking sheet. Sprinkle with sugar and cinnamon. Bake 20 to 25 minutes.

Yield: 10 servings

Each with: 29 g water; 273 calories (34% from fat, 9% from protein, 57% from carb); 6 g protein; 11 g total fat; 6 g saturated fat; 3 g monounsaturated fat; 1 g polyunsaturated fat; 41 g carb; 5 g fiber; 13 g sugar; 185 mg phosphorus; 97 mg calcium; 2 mg iron; 80 mg sodium; 262 mg potassium; 296 IU vitamin A; 78 mg vitamin E; 1 mg vitamin C; 25 mg cholesterol

Whole Grain Scones

The mornings we have these for breakfast, I forgo my usual coffee for a cup of tea.

1 egg

½ cup (100 g) sugar

5 tablespoons (75 ml) canola oil

⅛ teaspoon lemon peel

½ cup (40 g) rolled oats

¼ cup (25 g) wheat bran

1½ cups (180 g) whole wheat pastry flour

2 tablespoons poppyseeds

1 tablespoon baking powder

½ teaspoon cinnamon

½ cup (120 ml) skim milk

Lemon Topping

3 tablespoons (45 ml) lemon juice

¼ cup (25 g) confectioners' sugar

Preheat oven to 375°F (190°C, gas mark 5). Whisk the egg, sugar, and oil together in a bowl. Mix the lemon peel and all of the dry ingredients together in a separate bowl and stir with a wooden spoon until all of them are evenly dispersed throughout. Slowly add the dry ingredients into the egg, sugar, and oil, and mix to create a thick dough. Add the milk and mix well. Coat a baking sheet with nonstick vegetable oil spray. Scoop up tablespoons of the dough and drop them one by one in mounds onto the baking sheet, leaving 2 inches (5 cm) of space between. Bake for 15 to 20 minutes, just until the crust is barely golden brown and the dough is dry. Remove from the oven and let cool for 10 minutes. With a fork, mix the lemon topping ingredients until the sugar is completely melded in. Drizzle 1 tablespoon ever each scone.

Yield: 10 servings

Each with: 21 g water; 218 calories (36% from fat, 8% from protein, 56% from carb); 5 g protein; 9 g total fat; 1 g saturated fat; 5 g monounsaturated fat; 3 g polyunsaturated fat; 32 g carb; 3 g fiber; 14 g sugar; 165 mg phosphorus; 138 mg calcium; 1 mg iron; 164 mg sodium; 152 mg potassium; 61 IU vitamin A; 16 mg vitamin E; 2 mg vitamin C; 21 mg cholesterol

Granola

Some healthy cereals are available if you are careful about reading the ingredient labels. But it would be hard to find one healthier or tastier than this homemade granola.

6 cups (480 g) rolled oats

6 cups rolled wheat

2 cups (290 g) sunflower seeds

4 ounces (113 g) sesame seeds

2 cups (190 g) peanuts

3 cups (255 g) coconut

1 cup (112 g) wheat germ

1½ cups (355 ml) canola oil

1 cup (340 g) honey

½ cup (170 g) molasses

1 tablespoon (15 ml) vanilla extract

1 cup (145 g) raisins

Mix all dry ingredients together in large bowl. Put aside. Heat the oil, honey, molasses, and vanilla together and mix with dry ingredients. Spread mixture on baking sheets. Bake at 350°F (180°C, gas mark 4) for 30 to 40 minutes or until light brown. Stir frequently to brown evenly. Remove from oven and add raisins or any other dried fruit.

Yield: 30 servings

Each with: 10 g water; 391 calories (49% from fat, 8% from protein, 43% from carb); 8 g protein; 22 g total fat; 4 g saturated fat; 9 g monounsaturated fat; 8 g polyunsaturated fat; 44 g carb; 5 g fiber; 18 g sugar; 290 mg phosphorus; 75 mg calcium; 5 mg iron; 75 mg sodium; 372 mg potassium; 205 IU vitamin A; 60 mg vitamin E; 1 mg vitamin C; 0 mg cholesterol

Toasty Nut Granola

This is great both as a snack or breakfast cereal.

6 cups (480 g) rolled oats

1 cup (110 g) chopped pecans

¾ cup (84 g) wheat germ

½ cup (115 g) firmly packed brown sugar

½ cup (40 g) shredded coconut

½ cup (72 g) sesame seeds

½ cup (120 ml) canola oil

½ cup (170 g) honey

1½ teaspoons vanilla extract

Toast oats in a 9 × 13-inch (23 × 33 cm) pan at 350°F (180°C, gas mark 4) for 10 minutes. Combine remaining ingredients in a large bowl and add toasted oats. Bake on 2 baking sheets at 350°F (180°C, gas mark 4) for 20 to 25 minutes. Stir when cool and store in refrigerator.

Yield: 28 servings

Each with: 4 g water; 194 calories (44% from fat, 9% from protein, 47% from carb); 5 g protein; 10 g total fat; 2 g saturated fat; 4 g monounsaturated fat; 4 g polyunsaturated fat; 24 g carb; 3 g fiber; 9 g sugar; 146 mg phosphorus; 42 mg calcium; 2 mg iron; 3 mg sodium; 139 mg potassium; 6 IU vitamin A; 0 mg vitamin E; 0 mg vitamin C; 0 mg cholesterol

Breakfast Bars

These contain a little more nutrition than commercial granola bars and are equally good for a breakfast on the run.

1 cup (80 g) quick-cooking oats

½ cup (60 g) whole wheat flour

½ cup (58 g) crunchy wheat-barley cereal, such as Grape-Nuts

½ teaspoon cinnamon

1 egg

¼ cup (60 g) applesauce

¼ cup (85 g) honey

3 tablespoons (45 g) brown sugar

2 tablespoons (28 ml) canola oil

¼ cup (36 g) sunflower seeds, unsalted

¼ cup (30 g) chopped walnuts

7 ounces (198 g) dried fruit

Preheat oven to 325°F (170°C, gas mark 3). Line a 9-inch (23 cm) square baking pan with aluminum foil. Spray the foil with nonstick vegetable oil spray. In a large bowl, stir together the oats, flour, cereal, and cinnamon. Add the egg, applesauce, honey, brown sugar, and oil. Mix well. Stir in the sunflower seeds, walnuts, and dried fruit. Spread mixture evenly in the prepared pan. Bake 30 minutes or until firm and lightly browned around the edges. Let cool. Use the foil to lift from the pan. Cut into bars and store in the refrigerator.

Yield: 12 servings

Each with: 16 g water; 222 calories (26% from fat, 9% from protein, 65% from carb); 6 g protein; 7 g total fat; 1 g saturated fat; 2 g monounsaturated fat; 3 g polyunsaturated fat; 38 g carb; 4 g fiber; 10 g sugar; 164 mg phosphorus; 27 mg calcium; 3 mg iron; 43 mg sodium; 284 mg potassium; 492 IU vitamin A; 6 mg vitamin E; 1 mg vitamin C; 20 mg cholesterol

Whole Wheat Coffee Cake

This is a nice whole wheat coffee cake with a crunchy filling.

1¾ cups (210 g) whole wheat pastry flour

1 teaspoon baking powder

1 teaspoon baking soda

½ cup (112 g) unsalted butter, softened

⅔ cup (133 g) sugar

2 eggs

1 teaspoon vanilla extract

1 cup (230 g) sour cream

Bran Nut Filling

⅓ cup (75 g) packed brown sugar

½ cup bran flakes (20 g) cereal

½ cup (60 g) chopped walnuts

1 teaspoon cinnamon

Mix flour, baking powder, and baking soda; set aside. In large bowl beat butter, sugar, eggs, and vanilla until light and fluffy. At low speed stir in sour cream alternately with flour mixture until blended. To make the bran nut filling, combine all filling ingredients in a small bowl. To assemble the cake, spread one-third of the sour cream mixture in a 9-inch (23 cm) square pan coated with nonstick vegetable oil spray. Sprinkle on about ½ cup filling. Repeat layering twice. Bake in preheated 350°F (180°C, gas mark 4) oven for 30 to 45 minutes. Cool slightly.

Yield: 12 servings

Each with: 27 g water; 275 calories (45% from fat, 8% from protein, 46% from carb); 6 g protein; 14 g total fat; 7 g saturated fat; 4 g monounsaturated fat; 2 g polyunsaturated fat; 33 g carb; 3 g fiber; 17 g sugar; 148 mg phosphorus; 68 mg calcium; 2 mg iron; 85 mg sodium; 174 mg potassium; 451 IU vitamin A; 97 mg vitamin E; 1 mg vitamin C; 68 mg cholesterol

Crunchy Breakfast Topping

You can sprinkle this over oatmeal, toast, fresh fruit, yogurt, pancakes, waffles, or French toast.

¼ cup (55 g) unsalted butter

1¼ cups (140 g) wheat germ

½ cup (115 g) packed brown sugar

½ cup (47 g) ground almonds

1 tablespoon grated orange peel

½ teaspoon cinnamon

Melt butter in a 9 × 13-inch (23 × 33 cm) baking pan in oven about 4 minutes. Add remaining ingredients and mix well. Bake 10 to 12 minutes or until deep golden brown. Stir. Cool and store in the refrigerator for up to 3 months.

Yield: 12 servings

Each with: 2 g water; 149 calories (47% from fat, 12% from protein, 41% from carb); 5 g protein; 8 g total fat; 3 g saturated fat; 3 g monounsaturated fat; 2 g polyunsaturated fat; 16 g carb; 3 g fiber; 10 g sugar; 167 mg phosphorus; 29 mg calcium; 2 mg iron; 6 mg sodium; 187 mg potassium; 133 IU vitamin A; 32 mg vitamin E; 1 mg vitamin C; 10 mg cholesterol

8

Breakfast:
Vegetables and Fruits

Vegetables and fruits are another natural choice for breakfast. You can add them to omelets, pancakes, and quiches. You can have fruit in a variety of ways. And you can make smoothies and shakes, giving breakfast options that are packed with fiber and other good things.

Frittata

This frittata cooks completely in the oven. It's great for breakfast or dinner.

¼ cup (60 ml) olive oil

2 baking potatoes, peeled and thinly sliced

1 cup (160 g) thinly sliced onion

2 cups (226 g) thinly sliced zucchini

1 cup (150 g) red bell pepper, cut in ½-inch (1-cm) cubes

1 cup (150 g) green bell pepper, cut in ½-inch (1-cm) cubes

12 eggs

2 tablespoons chopped fresh parsley

Preheat oven to 450°F (230°C, gas mark 8). Pour oil into 12-inch (30 cm) square or round baking dish. Heat oil in oven for 5 minutes and then remove. Place potatoes and onion over bottom of dish and bake until potatoes are just tender, 20 minutes. Arrange zucchini slices over potatoes and onion and then sprinkle peppers over all. Beat eggs and season with salt and pepper. Add chopped parsley to eggs. Pour eggs over vegetables. Bake until eggs are set and sides are "puffy," about 25 minutes. Top should be golden brown. Serve hot or at room temperature.

Yield: 6 servings

Each with: 293 g water; 364 calories (50% from fat, 19% from protein, 31% from carb); 18 g protein; 20 g total fat; 5 g saturated fat; 11 g monounsaturated fat; 3 g polyunsaturated fat; 29 g carb; 5 g fiber; 5 g sugar; 320 mg phosphorus; 92 mg calcium; 4 mg iron; 172 mg sodium; 918 mg potassium; 1606 IU vitamin A; 156 mg vitamin E; 87 mg vitamin C; 474 mg cholesterol

Cinnamon Apple Omelet

This is a different version of an omelet. I remember years ago there were often recipes for omelets with jelly or other sweet fillings, but you don't see them much any more. This one makes me think they are still a good idea.

1 tablespoon unsalted butter, divided

1 apple, peeled and sliced thin

½ teaspoon cinnamon

1 tablespoon (15 g) brown sugar

3 eggs

1 tablespoon cream

1 tablespoon sour cream

Melt 2 teaspoons butter in a skillet. Add apple, cinnamon, and brown sugar. Sauté until tender. Pour into a bowl and set aside. Clean skillet. Whip eggs and cream until fluffy; set aside. Melt remaining butter and pour in egg mixture. Cook as you would for an omelet. When eggs are ready to flip, turn them. Add the sour cream to the center of the eggs and top that with the apple mixture. Fold it onto a plate.

Yield: 2 servings

Each with: 129 g water; 252 calories (57% from fat, 17% from protein, 25% from carb); 11 g protein; 16 g total fat; 8 g saturated fat; 5 g monounsaturated fat; 1 g polyunsaturated fat; 16 g carb; 1 g fiber; 14 g sugar; 181 mg phosphorus; 73 mg calcium; 2 mg iron; 126 mg sodium; 211 mg potassium; 695 IU vitamin A; 187 mg vitamin E; 3 mg vitamin C; 379 mg cholesterol

Zucchini Pancakes

These make a great side dish with almost any kind of meat, but I have to admit to having them for breakfast a time or two also. Maybe that's just because I get desperate when the garden is really producing zucchini.

4 cups (452 g) shredded zucchini

4 eggs

½ cup (62 g) flour

⅛ teaspoon black pepper

¼ teaspoon garlic powder

¼ cup chopped fresh parsley

3 tablespoons (45 ml) canola oil

Wash zucchini and trim the ends. Grate or grind into a bowl. Squeeze dry. In a bowl, combine the zucchini and all the other ingredients except the oil. (If mixture is thin, add more flour.) Heat the oil in a heavy skillet over medium heat. Drop zucchini mixture by heaping tablespoons into hot oil. Flatten them a little and fry until golden brown on bottom. Turn and brown second side. Drain on paper towels.

Yield: 6 servings

Each with: 110 g water; 168 calories (58% from fat, 16% from protein, 26% from carb); 7 g protein; 11 g total fat; 2 g saturated fat; 6 g monounsaturated fat; 3 g polyunsaturated fat; 11 g carb; 1 g fiber; 2 g sugar; 116 mg phosphorus; 37 mg calcium; 2 mg iron; 62 mg sodium; 293 mg potassium; 560 IU vitamin A; 52 mg vitamin E; 17 mg vitamin C; 158 mg cholesterol

Spinach Quiche

This versatile dish can work for breakfast, lunch, or dinner.

8 slices low-sodium bacon

1 cup (160 g) chopped onion

4 eggs, beaten

1 cup (235 ml) light cream

1 cup (235 ml) skim milk

1 tablespoon flour

⅛ teaspoon nutmeg

12 ounces (340 g) frozen spinach, thawed and chopped

4 ounces (115 g) mushrooms, sliced

1 cup (115 g) shredded Monterey Jack cheese

1 cup (115 g) shredded Cheddar cheese

1 prepared piecrust

Cook together bacon and onion. Crumble bacon. Mix all ingredients together. Place piecrust into pie pan. Pour ingredients into piecrust. Bake at 325°F (170°C, gas mark 3) for 50 minutes. Let stand 10 minutes before serving.

Yield: 8 servings

Each with: 141 g water; 296 calories (65% from fat, 25% from protein, 11% from carb); 19 g protein; 22 g total fat; 12 g saturated fat; 7 g monounsaturated fat; 1 g polyunsaturated fat; 8 g carb; 2 g fiber; 2 g sugar; 338 mg phosphorus; 382 mg calcium; 2 mg iron; 379 mg sodium; 387 mg potassium; 5775 IU vitamin A; 174 mg vitamin E; 3 mg vitamin C; 177 mg cholesterol

Spinach Pie

This side dish goes great with chicken, turkey, or beef.

10 ounces (280 g) frozen spinach

6 eggs, stirred

2 cups (450 g) cottage cheese

¼ cup (55 g) unsalted butter, melted

6 tablespoons (48 g) flour

10 ounces (283 g) Cheddar cheese, cut into cubes

Preheat oven to 350°F (180°C, gas mark 4). Cook spinach according to package directions; drain thoroughly and squeeze dry. Mix all ingredients together in a 9 × 13-inch (23 × 33 cm) pan. Bake for 1 hour.

Yield: 6 servings

Each with: 143 g water; 423 calories (62% from fat, 28% from protein, 10% from carb); 30 g protein; 29 g total fat; 17 g saturated fat; 9 g monounsaturated fat; 2 g polyunsaturated fat; 10 g carb; 2 g fiber; 2 g sugar; 433 mg phosphorus; 462 mg calcium; 3 mg iron; 425 mg sodium; 290 mg potassium; 6696 IU vitamin A; 268 mg vitamin E; 1 mg vitamin C; 310 mg cholesterol

Baked Stuffed Peaches

The coconut-almond flavor of macaroons just seems to go with peaches. So here we combine the two in a treat that can be a dessert as well as breakfast.

6 peaches, peeled and halved

½ cup (100 g) sugar

½ pound (225 g) macaroons, crushed (about 2 cups crumbs)

4 egg yolks

Scoop out about 1 teaspoon of the center pulp of each peach half. Mash pulp; mix with sugar, macaroon crumbs, and egg yolks. Place halves close together, cut side up, in a baking dish about 8 × 12 inches (20 × 30 cm) coated with nonstick vegetable oil spray. Spoon macaroon mixture into center of each. Bake in a slow 300°F (150°C, gas mark 2) oven for 30 minutes or until peaches are tender.

Yield: 6 servings

Each with: 141 g water; 329 calories (26% from fat, 8% from protein, 66% from carb); 7 g protein; 10 g total fat; 6 g saturated fat; 2 g monounsaturated fat; 1 g polyunsaturated fat; 57 g carb; 3 g fiber; 55 g sugar; 106 mg phosphorus; 29 mg calcium; 1 mg iron; 156 mg sodium; 351 mg potassium; 647 IU vitamin A; 59 mg vitamin E; 9 mg vitamin C; 140 mg cholesterol

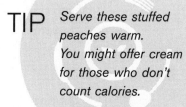

TIP *Serve these stuffed peaches warm. You might offer cream for those who don't count calories.*

Latkes

You don't need to be Jewish to enjoy these.

4 potatoes

1 tablespoon finely chopped onion

1 egg

½ cup (60 g) bread crumbs

2 tablespoons (28 ml) canola oil

Peel and grate potatoes. Squeeze in a kitchen towel to remove excess moisture. Mix all ingredients together. Heat oil in heavy skillet. Drop batter onto hot skillet in ¼-cup measures and flatten with fork into pancakes. Cook until browned. Turn over and finish cooking.

Yield: 4 servings

Each with: 11 g water; 139 calories (61% from fat, 10% from protein, 29% from carb); 3 g protein; 9 g total fat; 1 g saturated fat; 5 g monounsaturated fat; 3 g polyunsaturated fat; 10 g carb; 1 g fiber; 1 g sugar; 47 mg phosphorus; 32 mg calcium; 1 mg iron; 42 mg sodium; 47 mg potassium; 84 IU vitamin A; 22 mg vitamin E; 0 mg vitamin C; 53 mg cholesterol

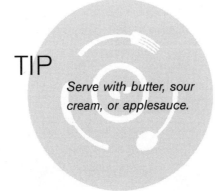

TIP

Serve with butter, sour cream, or applesauce.

Oat Baked Apple

Stick these in the oven before dinner and by the time you are finished you'll have a great dessert waiting for you. Or have them for breakfast, as we like to do on a weekend.

4 ounces (113 g) Cheddar cheese, divided

3 tablespoons quick-cooking oats

2 tablespoons (30 g) brown sugar

1 tablespoon oat bran

1 tablespoon coarsely chopped pecans

1 tablespoon raisins

¼ teaspoon cinnamon

4 apples, cored

½ cup (120 ml) cold water

Preheat oven to 375°F (190°C, gas mark 5). Cut half of cheese into small cubes; shred remainder. Mix cheese cubes, oats, brown sugar, oat bran, pecans, raisins, and cinnamon until well blended. Place baking apples in 8-inch (20 cm) square pan; fill with oat mixture. Pour water in bottom of pan. Cover with foil; bake 30 minutes. Uncover and continue baking 15 minutes or until tender. Sprinkle with shredded cheese. Continue baking until cheese is melted.

Yield: 4 servings

Each with: 152 g water; 239 calories (40% from fat, 13% from protein, 46% from carb); 8 g protein; 11 g total fat; 6 g saturated fat; 3 g monounsaturated fat; 1 g polyunsaturated fat; 29 g carb; 2 g fiber; 21 g sugar; 190 mg phosphorus; 225 mg calcium; 1 mg iron; 183 mg sodium; 211 mg potassium; 341 IU vitamin A; 75 mg vitamin E; 5 mg vitamin C; 30 mg cholesterol

Pineapple Boats

We like these for breakfast, but they would make a great luncheon dish, or even a full dinner, perfect for those hot summer evenings when you don't feel like cooking.

2 pineapples

4 kiwifruits

1 cup (150 g) seedless green grapes

2 cups (300 g) sliced banana

¼ cup (60 g) packed brown sugar

1 teaspoon poppyseeds

½ pound (225 g) ham, thinly sliced

¼ pound (115 g) Swiss cheese

Slice pineapple lengthwise in half, crown to stem. Leave leafy crown on. Remove tough core. Loosen fruit by cutting to rind; cut in bite-size pieces. Place in large bowl. Peel kiwifruit and bananas and slice into wedges. Cut grapes in half and add all other fruit to pineapple. Toss with brown sugar and poppyseeds. Line pineapple shells with ham. Spoon in fruit mixture. Dice Swiss cheese and tuck among fruit.

Yield: 4 servings

Each with: 248 g water; 441 calories (27% from fat, 20% from protein, 53% from carb); 23 g protein; 14 g total fat; 7 g saturated fat; 4 g monounsaturated fat; 1 g polyunsaturated fat; 61 g carb; 6 g fiber; 42 g sugar; 366 mg phosphorus; 342 mg calcium; 2 mg iron; 620 mg sodium; 1039 mg potassium; 415 IU vitamin A; 60 mg vitamin E; 97 mg vitamin C; 49 mg cholesterol

Breakfast Citrus Cups

It may be quick and easy, but the citrus and grape combination and the addition of the almonds make it a little more than just grapefruit and oranges.

4 grapefruits

2 cups (300 g) seedless green grapes

2 oranges, sectioned

¼ cup (27 g) slivered almonds, toasted

Cut grapefruits in half. Remove sections and membrane, leaving shells intact. Combine grapefruit sections, grapes, and oranges; mix lightly. Chill. Add nuts to fruit mixture just before serving. Spoon fruit mixture onto grapefruit shells.

Yield: 8 servings

Each with: 210 g water; 116 calories (18% from fat, 8% from protein, 74% from carb); 3 g protein; 3 g total fat; 0 g saturated fat; 1 g monounsaturated fat; 1 g polyunsaturated fat; 24 g carb; 4 g fiber; 20 g sugar; 44 mg phosphorus; 51 mg calcium; 0 mg iron; 2 mg sodium; 389 mg potassium; 1666 IU vitamin A; 0 mg vitamin E; 82 mg vitamin C; 0 mg cholesterol

Apple and Banana Fritters

A search for something for breakfast that would use up some overripe bananas was rewarded with the this recipe. They are incredibly light and very tasty. Sprinkle with confectioners' sugar or dip in honey if you don't mind adding a few more calories to the ones they already have.

1 cup (120 g) whole wheat pastry flour

1 tablespoon sugar

1 tablespoon baking powder

½ cup (120 ml) skim milk

1 egg

1 tablespoon (15 ml) canola oil

½ cup (75 g) chopped banana

½ cup (62 g) chopped apple

½ teaspoon nutmeg

Stir together flour, sugar, and baking powder. Combine the milk, egg, and oil. Add banana, apple, and nutmeg. Stir into dry ingredients, stirring until just moistened. Drop by tablespoons into hot oil. Fry for 2 to 3 minutes on a side until golden brown. Drain.

Yield: 4 servings

Each with: 74 g water; 212 calories (23% from fat, 13% from protein, 64% from carb); 7 g protein; 6 g total fat; 1 g saturated fat; 3 g monounsaturated fat; 1 g polyunsaturated fat; 36 g carb; 5 g fiber; 8 g sugar; 249 mg phosphorus; 267 mg calcium; 2 mg iron; 405 mg sodium; 311 mg potassium; 157 IU vitamin A; 38 mg vitamin E; 3 mg vitamin C; 60 mg cholesterol

Fruit with Orange Cream Dip

This is a nice dip with fruit for a party or company, but it wouldn't be a bad idea to have it for breakfast also since it's got so many good things for you.

1 cup (230 g) sour cream

2 tablespoons (30 g) firmly packed brown sugar

1 tablespoon (15 ml) orange juice

1 teaspoon orange peel

1 cup (165 g) pineapple chunks

1 cup (195 g) orange sections

1 cup (177 g) sliced kiwifruit

1 cup (145 g) strawberries

In medium-size serving bowl, stir together all ingredients except fruit. Cover; refrigerate at least 2 hours. Serve with skewered fresh fruit for dipping.

Yield: 6 servings

Each with: 120 g water; 112 calories (39% from fat, 6% from protein, 55% from carb); 2 g protein; 5 g total fat; 3 g saturated fat; 1 g monounsaturated fat; 0 g polyunsaturated fat; 16 g carb; 2 g fiber; 11 g sugar; 57 mg phosphorus; 67 mg calcium; 0 mg iron; 20 mg sodium; 256 mg potassium; 198 IU vitamin A; 40 mg vitamin E; 47 mg vitamin C; 16 mg cholesterol

Fruit Sauce

This is a simple, uncooked fruit sauce. For a real treat, try this over the multigrain pancakes in the Breakfast: Grains chapter.

1 cup (235 ml) apple juice

4 apples, peeled and cored

2 cups (300 g) sliced banana

1 pear, peeled and cored

1 teaspoon cinnamon

1 teaspoon nutmeg

(continued on page 126)

Put apple juice and fruits in blender. Blend until smooth. Then add spices and mix.

Yield: 6 servings

Each with: 183 g water; 138 calories (4% from fat, 3% from protein, 93% from carb); 1 g protein; 1 g total fat; 0 g saturated fat; 0 g monounsaturated fat; 0 g polyunsaturated fat; 35 g carb; 4 g fiber; 24 g sugar; 32 mg phosphorus; 17 mg calcium; 1 mg iron; 4 mg sodium; 423 mg potassium; 82 IU vitamin A; 0 mg vitamin E; 11 mg vitamin C; 0 mg cholesterol

Banana-Peach-Blueberry Smoothie

Smoothies make a quick and easy breakfast, and they are packed with nutrition. The fiber and protein will help to keep you from being hungry as the morning goes on.

2 cups (490 g) peach low-fat yogurt

1 cup (145 g) blueberries

2 cups (300 g) sliced banana

Mix all ingredients in a blender and serve.

Yield: 2 servings

Each with: 415 g water; 485 calories (7% from fat, 10% from protein, 83% from carb); 13 g protein; 4 g total fat; 2 g saturated fat; 1 g monounsaturated fat; 0 g polyunsaturated fat; 108 g carb; 8 g fiber; 81 g sugar; 325 mg phosphorus; 354 mg calcium; 1 mg iron; 133 mg sodium; 1296 mg potassium; 282 IU vitamin A; 27 mg vitamin E; 28 mg vitamin C; 12 mg cholesterol

Chocolate-Raspberry Smoothie

How could anyone not like the taste of chocolate and raspberries for breakfast?

1 cup (235 ml) skim milk

½ cup (141 g) chocolate syrup

3 cups (750 g) frozen raspberries

Pour the milk and chocolate syrup into a blender. Slowly add the raspberries, 1 cup at a time, and blend for 15 to 30 seconds after adding each cup. Do not overmix, as this will thin the drink down. Serve immediately.

Yield: 2 servings

TIP *Substitute other frozen fruit for the raspberries (strawberry, banana, etc.).*

Each with: 268 g water; 146 calories (9% from fat, 18% from protein, 73% from carb); 7 g protein; 2 g total fat; 0 g saturated fat; 0 g monounsaturated fat; 1 g polyunsaturated fat; 29 g carb; 12 g fiber; 8 g sugar; 191 mg phosphorus; 222 mg calcium; 1 mg iron; 74 mg sodium; 502 mg potassium; 311 IU vitamin A; 75 mg vitamin E; 50 mg vitamin C; 2 mg cholesterol

Raspberry-Banana Smoothie

This is another great-tasting smoothie. The raspberries give this one a special boost in fiber.

2 cups (500 g) fresh raspberries

2 cups (300 g) sliced banana

2 cups (475 ml) skim milk

¼ cup (60 g) low-fat vanilla yogurt

1 tablespoon (20 g) honey

Combine all ingredients in a blender or food processor and process until smooth.

Yield: 2 servings

(continued on page 128)

Each with: 496 g water; 397 calories (5% from fat, 13% from protein, 83% from carb); 14 g protein; 2 g total fat; 1 g saturated fat; 0 g monounsaturated fat; 1 g polyunsaturated fat; 88 g carb; 14 g fiber; 42 g sugar; 361 mg phosphorus; 394 mg calcium; 2 mg iron; 149 mg sodium; 1444 mg potassium; 684 IU vitamin A; 150 mg vitamin E; 55 mg vitamin C; 5 mg cholesterol

Bananaberry Breakfast Shake

So why not a shake for breakfast? Besides, it's really just a smoothie.

1 cup (145 g) strawberries

1 cup (150 g) sliced banana

1½ cups (355 ml) skim milk

1 cup (230 g) vanilla yogurt

1 tablespoon (20 g) honey

TIP

This is great with toast or muffins.

Place all ingredients in a blender. Process until well blended.

Yield: 2 servings

Each with: 417 g water; 336 calories (7% from fat, 17% from protein, 76% from carb); 15 g protein; 3 g total fat; 1 g saturated fat; 1 g monounsaturated fat; 0 g polyunsaturated fat; 67 g carb; 4 g fiber; 43 g sugar; 415 mg phosphorus; 492 mg calcium; 1 mg iron; 192 mg sodium; 1129 mg potassium; 508 IU vitamin A; 127 mg vitamin E; 58 mg vitamin C; 10 mg cholesterol

9

Breakfast:
Combinations

Breakfast combination recipes offer a wide variety of choices. We have breakfast burritos, fruit- and vegetable-filled muffins and pancakes, breakfast cookies and bars, and even more great granola recipes.

Black Bean and Spinach Breakfast Burrito

This recipe is almost as quick as fast food and will get your day off to a good start with something a little different providing 12 grams of fiber while doing it.

1 egg

1 egg white

1 cup (30 g) fresh spinach

¼ cup (45 g) diced tomato

¼ cup (43 g) cooked black beans, drained

1 tablespoon grated Cheddar cheese

1 tablespoon (16 g) salsa

1 whole wheat tortilla

Preheat the oven to 350°F (180°C, gas mark 4). Mix the egg and egg white and scramble them quickly in a small frying pan. Fold in all the other ingredients. Place this mixture in the middle of the tortilla. Wrap the two sides over tightly and place the roll, seam side down, on a baking sheet coated with nonstick vegetable oil spray. Bake at 350°F (180°C, gas mark 4) for about 6 minutes until the tortilla is crisp and the filling is heated through.

Yield: 1 serving

Each with: 320 g water; 363 calories (32% from fat, 28% from protein, 41% from carb); 26 g protein; 13 g total fat; 5 g saturated fat; 5 g monounsaturated fat; 2 g polyunsaturated fat; 39 g carb; 12 g fiber; 4 g sugar; 349 mg phosphorus; 438 mg calcium; 7 mg iron; 616 mg sodium; 1040 mg potassium; 23694 IU vitamin A; 110 mg vitamin E; 9 mg vitamin C; 219 mg cholesterol

Breakfast Burrito

This breakfast burrito is filled with good things. It also is perfect for grabbing on your way out the door.

2 ounces (55 g) chorizo, finely chopped

¼ cup (40 g) chopped onion

¼ cup (38 g) chopped red bell pepper

1 whole wheat tortilla

1 egg, beaten

2 tablespoons (30 g) sour cream

2 ounces (55 g) Monterey Jack cheese, shredded or crumbled

Preheat oven to 400°F (200°C, gas mark 6). In a small pan, cook the chorizo, onion, and bell pepper over medium heat until cooked through. Drain excess fat. Place the tortilla on a baking sheet covered with a very damp, clean dish towel. Let the tortilla cook for about 3 minutes. Whisk together the egg and sour cream. Pour the egg mixture into the pan over the chorizo and cook over medium heat; stir while cooking to scramble the eggs. Take the tortilla out of the oven and place eggs down the center; then top with shredded cheese. Fold up the burrito and let it sit for about 1 minute to let the burrito mold itself closed.

Yield: 1 serving

Each with: 187 g water; 710 calories (64% from fat, 22% from protein, 14% from carb); 39 g protein; 51 g total fat; 24 g saturated fat; 20 g monounsaturated fat; 4 g polyunsaturated fat; 25 g carb; 2 g fiber; 5 g sugar; 531 mg phosphorus; 539 mg calcium; 4 mg iron; 1289 mg sodium; 569 mg potassium; 1988 IU vitamin A; 217 mg vitamin E; 51 mg vitamin C; 349 mg cholesterol

Breakfast Enchiladas

As a make-ahead breakfast, you can assemble this the night before and then just bake it in the morning. This and the large number of servings make it a great choice when you have company staying overnight.

12 ounces (340 g) ham, finely chopped

½ cup (50 g) chopped scallions

2 cups (300 g) chopped green bell pepper

1 cup (160 g) chopped onion

2½ cups (300 g) grated Cheddar cheese

8 whole wheat tortillas

4 eggs

2 cups (475 ml) skim milk

1 tablespoon flour

¼ teaspoon garlic powder

1 teaspoon Tabasco sauce

TIP

Serve with dollop of sour cream, salsa, and avocado slices.

Preheat oven to 350°F (180°C, gas mark 4). Mix together ham, scallions, bell pepper, onion, and cheese. Put 5 tablespoons of mixture on each tortilla and roll up. Place seam side down in a 12 × 7 × 2-inch (30 × 18 × 5 cm) pan coated with nonstick vegetable oil spray. In separate bowl, beat together eggs and milk, flour, garlic, and Tabasco. Pour over enchiladas. Place in refrigerator overnight. Cover with foil and bake for 30 minutes, uncovering for the last 10 minutes.

Yield: 8 servings

Each with: 188 g water; 418 calories (49% from fat, 27% from protein, 24% from carb); 28 g protein; 23 g total fat; 11 g saturated fat; 8 g monounsaturated fat; 2 g polyunsaturated fat; 25 g carb; 2 g fiber; 3 g sugar; 482 mg phosphorus; 455 mg calcium; 3 mg iron; 984 mg sodium; 500 mg potassium; 885 IU vitamin A; 183 mg vitamin E; 33 mg vitamin C; 180 mg cholesterol

California Breakfast Sandwich

A Mexican version of eggs Benedict—this is a great weekend breakfast.

6 eggs

¾ cup (120 g) chopped onion

1 tablespoon unsalted butter

2 ounces (55 g) mushrooms, sliced

1 avocado, sliced

½ cup (90 g) chopped tomato

½ cup (60 g) grated Cheddar cheese

6 whole wheat English muffins

Mix eggs with wire whisk. In large skillet, brown onion with butter until clear and limp. Add mushrooms, avocado, and tomato. Stir. Add beaten eggs. Cook until almost set; add grated cheese. Spoon onto toasted English muffins.

Yield: 6 servings

Each with: 126 g water; 319 calories (43% from fat, 19% from protein, 37% from carb); 16 g protein; 16 g total fat; 6 g saturated fat; 6 g monounsaturated fat; 2 g polyunsaturated fat; 31 g carb; 5 g fiber; 3 g sugar; 254 mg phosphorus; 220 mg calcium; 3 mg iron; 368 mg sodium; 396 mg potassium; 581 IU vitamin A; 122 mg vitamin E; 5 mg vitamin C; 254 mg cholesterol

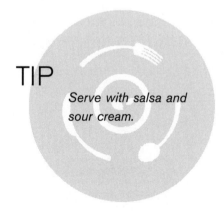

TIP

Serve with salsa and sour cream.

Easy Breakfast Strata

This is another great fix-ahead breakfast. We usually have some variation of this on special holidays when there is a lot to do in the morning, but we want a special family breakfast.

1 pound (455 g) sausage

8 eggs

10 slices whole wheat bread, cubed

3 cups (710 g) skim milk

2 cups (225 g) shredded Cheddar cheese

10 ounces (280 g) frozen chopped broccoli, thawed

2 tablespoons (28 g) unsalted butter, melted

2 tablespoons (16 g) flour

1 tablespoon dry mustard

2 teaspoons basil

In large skillet, brown sausage and drain. In large bowl, beat eggs. Add remaining ingredients and mix well. Spoon into 13 × 9-inch (33 × 23 cm) baking pan coated with nonstick vegetable oil spray. Cover and refrigerate 8 hours or overnight. Preheat oven to 350°F (180°C, gas mark 4). Bake 60 to 70 minutes or until knife inserted near center comes out clean.

Yield: 8 servings

Each with: 181 g water; 379 calories (49% from fat, 25% from protein, 26% from carb); 24 g protein; 21 g total fat; 11 g saturated fat; 6 g monounsaturated fat; 2 g polyunsaturated fat; 24 g carb; 2 g fiber; 3 g sugar; 449 mg phosphorus; 462 mg calcium; 3 mg iron; 593 mg sodium; 396 mg potassium; 1293 IU vitamin A; 243 mg vitamin E; 15 mg vitamin C; 281 mg cholesterol

Apple Pancakes

This makes a great breakfast for a weekend (or maybe when you are snowed in). They're kind of like apple fritters, only the syrup flavor gets baked right into the pancakes.

4 cups (440 g) sliced apple

½ cup (120 ml) maple syrup

2 tablespoons (28 g) unsalted butter

1½ cups (192 g) biscuit baking mix

1 cup (235 ml) skim milk

2 eggs

½ teaspoon cinnamon

¼ teaspoon nutmeg

Combine apples in skillet with syrup and butter. Cook until tender but firm, about 25 minutes. Meanwhile combine rest of ingredients and mix until smooth. Remove apples from skillet with slotted spoon and add to batter. Fold gently until apples are covered. Lift batter-covered apples onto hot griddle coated with nonstick vegetable oil spray. Grill until edges are cooked. Turn pancakes once. Serve with remaining syrup in which apples were cooked.

Yield: 6 servings

Each with: 126 g water; 306 calories (30% from fat, 8% from protein, 62% from carb); 7 g protein; 10 g total fat; 4 g saturated fat; 4 g monounsaturated fat; 1 g polyunsaturated fat; 48 g carb; 2 g fiber; 27 g sugar; 258 mg phosphorus; 145 mg calcium; 2 mg iron; 417 mg sodium; 269 mg potassium; 323 IU vitamin A; 83 mg vitamin E; 4 mg vitamin C; 91 mg cholesterol

High-Protein Blueberry Pancakes

When you are looking for a great-tasting breakfast but want something that also is good for you, you should give these pancakes a try.

4 eggs

1 cup (225 g) cottage cheese

¼ cup (28 g) wheat germ

¼ cup (20 g) quick-cooking oats

2 tablespoons (28 ml) canola oil

1 cup (145 g) blueberries

Place all the ingredients except blueberries in a blender and mix thoroughly. Stir in blueberries. Drop by tablespoons onto a hot frying pan or griddle coated with nonstick vegetable oil spray.

Yield: 4 servings

Each with: 103 g water; 240 calories (51% from fat, 27% from protein, 22% from carb); 16 g protein; 14 g total fat; 3 g saturated fat; 7 g monounsaturated fat; 3 g polyunsaturated fat; 13 g carb; 2 g fiber; 5 g sugar; 254 mg phosphorus; 49 mg calcium; 2 mg iron; 84 mg sodium; 200 mg potassium; 311 IU vitamin A; 81 mg vitamin E; 4 mg vitamin C; 239 mg cholesterol

Praline French Toast

This breakfast treat is like a taste of old New Orleans and will definitely be on your list to make again.

8 eggs

1½ cups (355 ml) skim milk

½ cup (115 g) brown sugar, divided

2 teaspoons vanilla extract

8 slices whole wheat bread

¼ cup (55 g) unsalted butter

¼ cup (60 ml) maple syrup

½ cup (55 g) chopped pecans

Thoroughly blend eggs, milk, 1 tablespoon brown sugar, and vanilla. Pour half of egg mixture into 9 × 13-inch (23 × 33 cm) baking dish. Place bread slices in mixture. Pour remaining egg mixture over bread. Cover and refrigerate several hours or overnight. Preheat oven to 350°F (180°C, gas mark 4). Remove bread from baking dish and set aside. Place butter in 9 × 13-inch (23 × 33-cm) baking dish and put in oven until butter melts. Stir in remaining brown sugar and syrup. Sprinkle with pecans. Carefully place reserved bread slices on pecans. Pour any remaining egg mixture over bread. Bake uncovered until puffed and lightly brown, 30 to 35 minutes. Invert slices to serve.

Yield: 8 servings

Each with: 98 g water; 345 calories (45% from fat, 14% from protein, 41% from carb); 12 g protein; 17 g total fat; 6 g saturated fat; 7 g monounsaturated fat; 3 g polyunsaturated fat; 36 g carb; 2 g fiber; 22 g sugar; 221 mg phosphorus; 156 mg calcium; 2 mg iron; 243 mg sodium; 304 mg potassium; 547 IU vitamin A; 154 mg vitamin E; 1 mg vitamin C; 253 mg cholesterol

Banana Pumpkin Muffins

These moist pumpkin muffins have a spiced brown sugar topping.

½ cup (112 g) pureed banana

½ cup (123 g) canned pumpkin

½ cup (100 g) sugar

¼ cup (60 ml) skim milk

¼ cup (60 ml) canola oil

1 egg

1¾ cups (210 g) whole wheat pastry flour

2 teaspoons baking powder

1 teaspoon pumpkin pie spice

Topping

½ cup (115 g) packed brown sugar

½ cup (40 g) rolled oats

½ teaspoon pumpkin pie spice

Mix pureed banana, pumpkin, sugar, milk, oil, and egg until well blended. Combine flour, baking powder, and pumpkin pie spice. Spoon into muffin pans coated with nonstick vegetable oil spray. Top each with 1 tablespoon of the sugar-spice mixture. Bake in preheated 375°F (190°C, gas mark 5) oven for 20 minutes or until toothpick inserted into muffin comes out clean.

Yield: 12 servings

Each with: 19 g water; 195 calories (26% from fat, 7% from protein, 67% from carb); 4 g protein; 6 g total fat; 1 g saturated fat; 3 g monounsaturated fat; 2 g polyunsaturated fat; 34 g carb; 3 g fiber; 18 g sugar; 112 mg phosphorus; 74 mg calcium; 1 mg iron; 96 mg sodium; 151 mg potassium; 1629 IU vitamin A; 11 mg vitamin E; 0 mg vitamin C; 18 mg cholesterol

Blueberry Oatmeal Muffins

Here are some quick muffins with a great blueberry taste.

3 cups (384 g) biscuit baking mix

½ cup (115 g) packed brown sugar

¾ cup (60 g) quick-cooking oats

1 teaspoon cinnamon

2 eggs, well beaten

1½ cups (355 ml) skim milk

¼ cup (55 g) unsalted butter, melted

2 cups (290 g) blueberries

TIP *To up the fiber even more, use the whole wheat baking mix in chapter 18.*

Combine biscuit mix, brown sugar, oats, and cinnamon. Mix eggs, milk, and butter. Add dry ingredients all at once and stir until just blended; fold in blueberries. Spoon into muffin pans coated with nonstick vegetable oil spray, filling each cup two-thirds full. Bake in preheated 400°F (200°C, gas mark 6) oven for 15 to 20 minutes. Remove from pans and place on rack to cool.

Yield: 18 servings

Each with: 40 g water; 167 calories (34% from fat, 9% from protein, 57% from carb); 4 g protein; 6 g total fat; 3 g saturated fat; 3 g monounsaturated fat; 1 g polyunsaturated fat; 24 g carb; 2 g fiber; 10 g sugar; 166 mg phosphorus; 77 mg calcium; 1 mg iron; 266 mg sodium; 124 mg potassium; 161 IU vitamin A; 43 mg vitamin E; 2 mg vitamin C; 34 mg cholesterol

Carrot Apple Muffins

These are one of my all-time favorite muffins—very moist and tasty. I like to make a batch on the weekend so I have them available for quick breakfasts during the week.

½ cup (75 g) raisins

2 cups (240 g) whole wheat pastry flour

1 cup (200 g) sugar

2 teaspoons baking soda

2 teaspoons cinnamon

¾ cup (83 g) grated carrot

1 green apple, grated

½ cup (55 g) sliced almonds

½ cup (40 g) sweet shredded coconut

3 eggs

⅔ cup (160 ml) vegetable oil

2 teaspoons vanilla extract

Soak raisins in hot water to cover for 30 minutes; drain thoroughly. Preheat oven to 350°F (180°C, gas mark 4). Mix flour, sugar, baking soda, and cinnamon in bowl. Stir in raisins, carrot, apple, almonds, and coconut. Beat eggs with oil and vanilla to blend. Stir into flour mixture until just combined. Divide into muffin cups. Bake until golden brown 20 to 22 minutes. Cool 5 minutes before removing from pan.

Yield: 12 servings

Each with: 31 g water; 343 calories (45% from fat, 7% from protein, 48% from carb); 6 g protein; 18 g total fat; 3 g saturated fat; 6 g monounsaturated fat; 8 g polyunsaturated fat; 42 g carb; 4 g fiber; 24 g sugar; 140 mg phosphorus; 39 mg calcium; 2 mg iron; 39 mg sodium; 244 mg potassium; 1420 IU vitamin A; 19 mg vitamin E; 1 mg vitamin C; 59 mg cholesterol

Peanut Butter Banana Muffins

This is a tasty way to use up leftover bananas.

2 cups (240 g) whole wheat pastry flour

½ cup (100 g) sugar

1 tablespoon baking powder

½ cup (130 g) crunchy peanut butter

2 tablespoons (28 g) unsalted butter

½ cup (120 ml) skim milk

2 eggs

1 cup (225 g) mashed banana

½ cup (73 g) chopped unsalted dry-roasted peanuts

Combine first 3 ingredients in a mixing bowl. Cut in peanut butter and butter until mixture resembles coarse crumbs. Add milk, eggs, banana, and peanuts and stir until just mixed. Fill muffin pans coated with nonstick vegetable oil spray two-thirds full. Bake at 400°F (200°C, gas mark 6) for 15 to 17 minutes.

Yield: 12 servings

Each with: 33 g water; 251 calories (39% from fat, 13% from protein, 48% from carb); 9 g protein; 12 g total fat; 3 g saturated fat; 5 g monounsaturated fat; 3 g polyunsaturated fat; 32 g carb; 4 g fiber; 12 g sugar; 184 mg phosphorus; 104 mg calcium; 1 mg iron; 195 mg sodium; 300 mg potassium; 139 IU vitamin A; 35 mg vitamin E; 2 mg vitamin C; 45 mg cholesterol

Raspberry Almond Muffins

These are a real taste treat, with their hidden raspberry and almond surprise.

5 ounces (140 g) almond paste

½ cup (112 g) unsalted butter, room temperature

¾ cup (150 g) sugar

2 eggs

1 teaspoon baking powder

½ teaspoon baking soda

1 teaspoon almond extract

2 cups (240 g) whole wheat pastry flour

1 cup (235 ml) buttermilk

¼ cup (80 g) raspberry preserves

Heat oven to 350°F (180°C, gas mark 4). Line muffin pans with paper baking cups or spray with nonstick vegetable oil spray. Cut almond paste into 12 pieces and pat each piece into a round disk about 1½ inches (4 cm) across. In a large bowl, beat butter until creamy. Beat in sugar until pale and fluffy. Beat in eggs, one at a time. Then mix in baking powder, baking soda, and almond extract. With a rubber spatula, fold in 1 cup (120 g) of flour, then the buttermilk, and lastly the remaining flour until well blended. Spoon about 2 tablespoons of batter into each cup and smooth the surface with spatula or spoon. Top with a level teaspoon of raspberry preserves and then with a piece of almond paste. Top each muffin with another 2 tablespoons of batter. Bake 25 to 30 minutes or until lightly browned. Turn out onto a rack and let stand at least 10 minutes.

Yield: 12 servings

Each with: 33 g water; 280 calories (39% from fat, 8% from protein, 53% from carb); 6 g protein; 12 g total fat; 6 g saturated fat; 5 g monounsaturated fat; 1 g polyunsaturated fat; 39 g carb; 3 g fiber; 21 g sugar; 148 mg phosphorus; 82 mg calcium; 1 mg iron; 80 mg sodium; 170 mg potassium; 289 IU vitamin A; 78 mg vitamin E; 1 mg vitamin C; 61 mg cholesterol

Cranberry–Oat Bran Muffins

This recipe combines cranberry-orange flavor with a good-for-you muffin.

2 cups (200 g) cranberries

1½ cups (150 g) oat bran

1 teaspoon orange peel

1 cup (200 g) sugar

⅓ cup (75 g) brown sugar

2½ cups (300 g) whole wheat pastry flour

1 tablespoon baking powder

½ teaspoon allspice

¼ cup (60 ml) canola oil

½ cup (120 ml) skim milk

2 eggs

½ cup (55 g) chopped pecans

Preheat oven to 350°F (180°C, gas mark 4). Chop cranberries and add to oat bran along with orange peel and both sugars. Combine flour, baking powder, and allspice. Combine oil, milk, and eggs. Add to flour mixture. Blend in nuts and cranberry mixture. Fill mini muffin pans and bake 10 to 12 minutes.

Yield: 12 servings

Each with: 23 g water; 348 calories (24% from fat, 7% from protein, 69% from carb); 6 g protein; 10 g total fat; 1 g saturated fat; 5 g monounsaturated fat; 3 g polyunsaturated fat; 63 g carb; 5 g fiber; 37 g sugar; 186 mg phosphorus; 118 mg calcium; 3 mg iron; 166 mg sodium; 207 mg potassium; 127 IU vitamin A; 36 mg vitamin E; 1 mg vitamin C; 40 mg cholesterol

Strawberry-Rhubarb Muffins

These muffins taste like spring—that's really the only way to say it.

1¾ cups (210 g) whole wheat pastry flour

¾ cup (150 g) sugar, divided

2½ teaspoons baking powder

1 egg, lightly beaten

¾ cup (175 ml) skim milk

⅓ cup (80 ml) canola oil

¾ cup (80 g) minced rhubarb

½ cup (85 g) sliced strawberries

Heat oven to 400°F (200°C, gas mark 6). Mix flour, ½ cup (100 g) sugar, and the baking powder in large bowl. Combine egg, milk, and oil in small bowl; stir into flour mixture with fork just until moistened. Fold rhubarb and sliced strawberries into batter. Fill muffin pans coated with nonstick vegetable oil spray two-thirds full with batter. Sprinkle tops with remaining sugar. Bake until golden, 20 to 25 minutes. Remove from pans; cool on wire racks.

Yield: 12 servings

Each with: 31 g water; 181 calories (34% from fat, 8% from protein, 58% from carb); 4 g protein; 7 g total fat; 1 g saturated fat; 4 g monounsaturated fat; 2 g polyunsaturated fat; 27 g carb; 2 g fiber; 13 g sugar; 109 mg phosphorus; 94 mg calcium; 1 mg iron; 120 mg sodium; 137 mg potassium; 69 IU vitamin A; 17 mg vitamin E; 5 mg vitamin C; 18 mg cholesterol

Whole Wheat Strawberry-Banana Muffins

These are a seasonal sort of thing, good with fresh strawberries.

1½ cups (180 g) whole wheat pastry flour

¼ cup (50 g) sugar

¼ cup (28 g) wheat germ

2½ teaspoons baking powder

½ teaspoon baking soda

1 egg

¾ cup (175 ml) skim milk

⅓ cup (80 ml) canola oil

½ cup (112 g) mashed banana

½ cup (85 g) chopped strawberries

Stir together the dry ingredients. Mix together the rest of the ingredients and stir into dry mixture, stirring until just moistened. Spoon into sprayed or paper-lined muffin pans. Bake at 350°F (180°C, gas mark 4) for 20 to 25 minutes, until done.

Yield: 12 servings

Each with: 34 g water; 157 calories (41% from fat, 9% from protein, 50% from carb); 4 g protein; 7 g total fat; 1 g saturated fat; 4 g monounsaturated fat; 2 g polyunsaturated fat; 20 g carb; 3 g fiber; 6 g sugar; 122 mg phosphorus; 89 mg calcium; 1 mg iron; 120 mg sodium; 163 mg potassium; 71 IU vitamin A; 17 mg vitamin E; 5 mg vitamin C; 18 mg cholesterol

Apple Coffee Cake

This is the kind of coffee cake you can find in old-fashioned bakeries, if you can find an old-fashioned bakery.

2½ cups (300 g) whole wheat pastry flour

2 teaspoons sugar

2 teaspoons baking powder

1 cup (225 g) unsalted butter

1 egg

¼ cup (60 ml) skim milk

6 apples, sliced

Topping

1½ cups (300 g) sugar

1 tablespoon flour

½ teaspoon cinnamon

Combine dry ingredients. Cut in butter with a pastry blender until crumbly and then add egg and milk; beat and blend. Spread evenly on foil-lined 10 × 15-inch (25 × 37 cm) jelly-roll pan and up the sides. Put sliced apples in rows, overlapping them slightly with pointed edges down. Combine the topping ingredients and sprinkle over apples. Bake at 375°F (190°C, gas mark 5) about 25 minutes, until crust is golden brown.

Yield: 15 servings

Each with: 55 g water; 291 calories (39% from fat, 5% from protein, 56% from carb); 4 g protein; 13 g total fat; 8 g saturated fat; 3 g monounsaturated fat; 1 g polyunsaturated fat; 43 g carb; 3 g fiber; 26 g sugar; 103 mg phosphorus; 58 mg calcium; 1 mg iron; 76 mg sodium; 144 mg potassium; 430 IU vitamin A; 110 mg vitamin E; 2 mg vitamin C; 47 mg cholesterol

Oatmeal Breakfast Cake

Serve this cake with warm milk and cinnamon.

1 cup (235 ml) canola oil

1½ cups (300 g) sugar

4 eggs, beaten

2 cups (475 ml) skim milk

4 teaspoons (18 g) baking powder

6 cups (480 g) rolled oats

1 teaspoon cinnamon

1 cup (86 g) dried apples

1 cup (110 g) slivered almonds

TIP

This recipe freezes well and is excellent to make ahead of time.

Thoroughly mix all ingredients together. Pour into 10 × 13-inch (25 × 33 cm) pan. Bake 30 minutes at 350°F (180°C, gas mark 4).

Yield: 12 servings

Each with: 60 g water; 377 calories (61% from fat, 6% from protein, 32% from carb); 6 g protein; 27 g total fat; 2 g saturated fat; 16 g monounsaturated fat; 7 g polyunsaturated fat; 31 g carb; 2 g fiber; 29 g sugar; 168 mg phosphorus; 185 mg calcium; 1 mg iron; 206 mg sodium; 185 mg potassium; 178 IU vitamin A; 51 mg vitamin E; 0 mg vitamin C; 80 mg cholesterol

Baked Breakfast Cereal

Baking softens the apple and raisins and allows the flavors to blend more with the oatmeal.

2 cups (467 g) cooked rolled oats

1½ cups (225 g) diced apple

1 cup (110 g) chopped pecans

½ cup (75 g) raisins

¼ cup (85 g) molasses

2 tablespoons (40 g) honey

1 teaspoon cinnamon

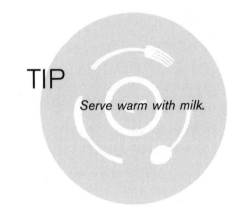

TIP

Serve warm with milk.

Combine all ingredients in an 8-inch × 8-inch (20.3 × 20.3 cm) casserole dish coated with nonstick vegetable oil spray and bake in a 400°F (200°C, gas mark 6) oven for 20 minutes.

Yield: 6 servings

Each with: 31 g water; 244 calories (45% from fat, 3% from protein, 51% from carb); 2 g protein; 13 g total fat; 1 g saturated fat; 7 g monounsaturated fat; 4 g polyunsaturated fat; 34 g carb; 3 g fiber; 25 g sugar; 72 mg phosphorus; 55 mg calcium; 2 mg iron; 7 mg sodium; 414 mg potassium; 22 IU vitamin A; 0 mg vitamin E; 2 mg vitamin C; 0 mg cholesterol

Breakfast Couscous

We usually think of couscous as a dinner item, perhaps with curry or some other savory topping. But this sweeter version makes a great breakfast.

¼ cup (55 g) unsalted butter, divided

¼ teaspoon cinnamon

¼ teaspoon cardamom

2¼ cups (535 ml) orange juice

½ cup (75 g) currants

1½ cups (263 g) whole wheat couscous

¼ cup (35 g) chopped cashews

Melt 2 tablespoons butter, add spices, and cook 2 minutes. Add juice and currants. Bring to a boil. Mix in couscous and add remaining butter. Cover. Remove from heat and let stand 5 minutes. Fluff with fork and put in bowl. Add cashews. Serve.

Yield: 4 servings

Each with: 144 g water; 466 calories (31% from fat, 9% from protein, 59% from carb); 11 g protein; 16 g total fat; 8 g saturated fat; 5 g monounsaturated fat; 1 g polyunsaturated fat; 69 g carb; 4 g fiber; 0 g sugar; 180 mg phosphorus; 47 mg calcium; 2 mg iron; 11 mg sodium; 473 mg potassium; 496 IU vitamin A; 95 mg vitamin E; 71 mg vitamin C; 31 mg cholesterol

Banana Cereal Cookie

Bananas and oatmeal are a great combination. These cookies are great either for breakfast or as a snack.

1¼ cups (281 g) shortening

2 cups (400 g) sugar

3 eggs

3 cups (360 g) whole wheat pastry flour

½ teaspoon nutmeg

1¼ teaspoons cinnamon

3½ cups (280 g) quick-cooking oats

1 teaspoon baking soda

2 cups (450 g) mashed banana

1 cup (110 g) chopped pecans

Cream shortening and sugar. Add eggs; cream well. Sift flour, soda, nutmeg, and cinnamon together. Add oats to shortening mixture. Add flour mixture alternately with mashed banana. Add chopped pecans. Drop on baking sheet coated with nonstick vegetable oil spray. Bake at 375°F (190°C, gas mark 5) for 12 to 15 minutes.

Yield: 48 servings

Each with: 11 g water; 157 calories (43% from fat, 7% from protein, 50% from carb); 3 g protein; 8 g total fat; 2 g saturated fat; 4 g monounsaturated fat; 2 g polyunsaturated fat; 20 g carb; 2 g fiber; 10 g sugar; 69 mg phosphorus; 10 mg calcium; 1 mg iron; 6 mg sodium; 99 mg potassium; 25 IU vitamin A; 5 mg vitamin E; 1 mg vitamin C; 15 mg cholesterol

Breakfast Cookies

Personally, I like the idea of cookies for breakfast. It makes me feel like I'm getting away with something, especially when they taste as good as these do.

½ cup (112 g) unsalted butter

1 cup (225 g) firmly packed brown sugar

2 eggs

1 tablespoon (15 ml) skim milk

1 teaspoon vanilla extract

1¼ cups (150 g) whole wheat pastry flour

½ teaspoon baking soda

2 cups (164 g) granola

½ cup (43 g) dried apples

½ cup (55 g) chopped pecans

Preheat oven to 350°F (180°C, gas mark 4). Coat baking sheets with nonstick vegetable oil spray. Cream together butter and brown sugar in a large bowl. Add eggs, milk, and vanilla. Beat well. In a medium bowl, combine flour and baking soda. Mix well and add to sugar mixture. Stir in granola, apples, and pecans. Drop by teaspoons onto prepared baking sheets. Bake 10 to 12 minutes until edges are browned.

Yield: 36 servings

Each with: 6 g water; 94 calories (40% from fat, 6% from protein, 54% from carb); 2 g protein; 4 g total fat; 2 g saturated fat; 2 g monounsaturated fat; 1 g polyunsaturated fat; 13 g carb; 1 g fiber; 8 g sugar; 40 mg phosphorus; 12 mg calcium; 0 mg iron; 25 mg sodium; 64 mg potassium; 97 IU vitamin A; 26 mg vitamin E; 0 mg vitamin C; 20 mg cholesterol

Cereal Breakfast Cookies

These are tasty little things and keep well. This recipe makes a lot, but they freeze well and you can save time by making a big batch—then just take out a bagful whenever you need more.

1 cup (235 ml) canola oil

1 cup (225 g) brown sugar

1 cup (200 g) sugar

1 teaspoon vanilla extract

2 eggs

4 cups (480 g) whole wheat pastry flour

1 teaspoon baking powder

1 teaspoon baking soda

1 cup (80 g) rolled oats

1 cup (40 g) bran flakes cereal

1 cup (110 g) chopped pecans

Mix together oil, sugars, vanilla, and eggs. Add the flour, baking powder, baking soda, oats, and bran flakes. Mix well. Batter will be sticky. Flour your hands and roll into 1-inch (2.5 cm) balls (go easy on the flour on your hands or your cookies will come out dry). Bake on ungreased baking sheet at 350°F (180°C, gas mark 4) for 8 to 9 minutes. Do not overbake—cookies should be chewy in the middle.

Yield: 80 servings

Each with: 2 g water; 81 calories (44% from fat, 6% from protein, 50% from carb); 1 g protein; 4 g total fat; 0 g saturated fat; 2 g monounsaturated fat; 1 g polyunsaturated fat; 10 g carb; 1 g fiber; 5 g sugar; 34 mg phosphorus; 10 mg calcium; 0 mg iron; 9 mg sodium; 45 mg potassium; 8 IU vitamin A; 2 mg vitamin E; 0 mg vitamin C; 6 mg cholesterol

Breakfast Carrot Cookies

This is another quick grab-and-go breakfast option.

1 cup (110 g) grated carrot

½ cup (115 g) plain fat-free yogurt

¼ cup (60 g) brown sugar

2 tablespoons (28 ml) canola oil

1 teaspoon vanilla extract

1½ cups (220 g) chopped dates

1½ cups (180 g) whole wheat pastry flour

¼ cup (29 g) crunchy wheat-barley cereal, such as Grape-Nuts

½ teaspoon baking soda

TIP
You can substitute raisins or other dried fruit for the dates.

Preheat oven to 350°F (180°C, gas mark 4). Spray baking sheets with nonstick vegetable oil spray or line with parchment paper or silicone sheet. In medium mixing bowl, stir carrot, yogurt, sugar, oil, vanilla, and dates. Let stand 15 minutes. Stir in remaining dry ingredients until well blended. Drop tablespoons of mixture onto baking sheets, spacing 1½ inches (4 cm) apart. Bake 15 minutes or until cookie top springs back when lightly touched. Cool.

Yield: 30 servings

Each with: 10 g water; 69 calories (14% from fat, 8% from protein, 78% from carb); 1 g protein; 1 g total fat; 0 g saturated fat; 1 g monounsaturated fat; 0 g polyunsaturated fat; 14 g carb; 2 g fiber; 8 g sugar; 36 mg phosphorus; 16 mg calcium; 1 mg iron; 13 mg sodium; 115 mg potassium; 733 IU vitamin A; 1 mg vitamin E; 0 mg vitamin C; 0 mg cholesterol

Peanut Granola Bars

These easy–to-make no-bake bars are better than the ones you get in the store.

¾ cup (255 g) honey

½ cup (130 g) crunchy peanut butter

2 eggs

¼ cup (55 g) unsalted butter

1 cup (145 g) chopped peanuts

3 cups (245 g) granola

Mix honey and peanut butter in a saucepan. Beat in eggs, one at a time. Stir over medium heat until mixture boils and leaves sides of pan. Remove from heat and stir in butter. Add peanuts and granola. Mix well. Press into oiled 9-inch (23 cm) square pan and refrigerate. Cut into bars.

Yield: 18 servings

Each with: 10 g water; 181 calories (39% from fat, 9% from protein, 53% from carb); 4 g protein; 8 g total fat; 3 g saturated fat; 3 g monounsaturated fat; 2 g polyunsaturated fat; 25 g carb; 2 g fiber; 17 g sugar; 81 mg phosphorus; 15 mg calcium; 1 mg iron; 122 mg sodium; 114 mg potassium; 109 IU vitamin A; 30 mg vitamin E; 0 mg vitamin C; 33 mg cholesterol

No-Bake Breakfast Bars

These bars are good tasting and good for you—plus quick and easy to make.

1½ cups (390 g) crunchy peanut butter

1 cup (340 g) honey

¾ cup (170 g) brown sugar

5 cups (200 g) bran flakes cereal

6 ounces (170 g) dried apples, chopped

Combine peanut butter, honey, and brown sugar in large saucepan. Bring to a boil, stirring constantly. Remove from heat and quickly stir in cereal and fruit bits. Mix well. Using buttered spatula or waxed paper, press mixture evenly into a 13 × 9 × 2-inch (33 × 23 × 5 cm) pan sprayed with nonstick vegetable oil spray. Cool 15 minutes before cutting.

Yield: 18 servings

Each with: 12 g water; 267 calories (34% from fat, 9% from protein, 57% from carb); 7 g protein; 11 g total fat; 2 g saturated fat; 5 g monounsaturated fat; 3 g polyunsaturated fat; 41 g carb; 4 g fiber; 27 g sugar; 148 mg phosphorus; 25 mg calcium; 3 mg iron; 236 mg sodium; 290 mg potassium; 604 IU vitamin A; 0 mg vitamin E; 8 mg vitamin C; 0 mg cholesterol

Raisin Nut Breakfast Bars

These not only make a good breakfast on the run, but I've also been known to sneak one in the evening too.

¾ cup (90 g) whole wheat pastry flour

¾ cup (84 g) wheat germ

¼ cup (50 g) sugar

½ teaspoon baking powder

½ teaspoon cinnamon

¼ cup (55 g) unsalted butter, melted

¼ cup (85 g) honey

1 egg

½ teaspoon vanilla extract

1 cup (145 g) raisins

½ cup (60 g) chopped walnuts

Heat oven to 350°F (180°C, gas mark 4). Coat an 8-inch (20 cm) square pan with nonstick vegetable oil spray. Combine flour, wheat germ, sugar, baking powder, and cinnamon. Stir in butter, honey, egg, and vanilla; mix well. Stir in raisins and walnuts. Press mixture firmly into greased pan. Bake at 350°F (180°C, gas mark 4) for 20 to 25 minutes or until lightly browned.

Yield: 12 servings

Each with: 8 g water; 206 calories (35% from fat, 10% from protein, 56% from carb); 5 g protein; 8 g total fat; 3 g saturated fat; 2 g monounsaturated fat; 3 g polyunsaturated fat; 31 g carb; 3 g fiber; 19 g sugar; 161 mg phosphorus; 32 mg calcium; 2 mg iron; 31 mg sodium; 239 mg potassium; 156 IU vitamin A; 39 mg vitamin E; 1 mg vitamin C; 28 mg cholesterol

Apple-Coconut Granola

Apple juice adds a whole different flavor to this granola mix.

8 cups (640 g) rolled oats

1 pound (455 g) coconut

1½ cups (150 g) wheat bran

1 tablespoon cinnamon

⅔ cup (230 g) honey

⅔ cup (160 ml) canola oil

6 ounces (170 g) apple juice concentrate

Mix all the ingredients together well. Place in shallow baking pan. Bake at 225°F for 2½ hours; stir every 30 minutes.

Yield: 24 servings

Each with: 13 g water; 291 calories (42% from fat, 7% from protein, 51% from carb); 6 g protein; 14 g total fat; 6 g saturated fat; 4 g monounsaturated fat; 3 g polyunsaturated fat; 39 g carb; 5 g fiber; 11 g sugar; 186 mg phosphorus; 25 mg calcium; 2 mg iron; 7 mg sodium; 237 mg potassium; 1 IU vitamin A; 0 mg vitamin E; 6 mg vitamin C; 0 mg cholesterol

Cashew Granola

Cashews are my favorite nuts, and this granola is a real treat, just full of good things.

8 cups (640 g) rolled oats

1 cup (80 g) shredded coconut

1½ cups (168 g) wheat germ

⅔ cup (93 g) chopped cashews

1 cup (144 g) sesame seeds

1 cup (145 g) sunflower seeds

½ teaspoon vanilla extract

1¼ cups (295 ml) canola oil

1 cup (340 g) honey

Combine first 6 ingredients in large bowl; mix well. Blend vanilla, oil, and honey in small bowl. Add to oats mixture; mix quickly until evenly coated. Spread on 3 ungreased baking sheets. Bake at 350°F (180°C, gas mark 4) for 10 minutes. Turn mixture over with spatula. Bake for 10 minutes longer. Reduce heat to 250°F (120°C, gas mark ½). Bake until brown. Cool. Store in airtight container.

Yield: 32 servings

Each with: 6 g water; 358 calories (45% from fat, 11% from protein, 44% from carb); 10 g protein; 18 g total fat; 3 g saturated fat; 8 g monounsaturated fat; 6 g polyunsaturated fat; 41 g carb; 6 g fiber; 9 g sugar; 356 mg phosphorus; 72 mg calcium; 3 mg iron; 3 mg sodium; 302 mg potassium; 6 IU vitamin A; 0 mg vitamin E; 0 mg vitamin C; 0 mg cholesterol

Date Granola

This recipe is great as a cereal, a snack, or a topping for oatmeal, ice cream, or whatever pleases you.

6 cups (480 g) rolled oats

1 cup (80 g) shredded coconut, unsweetened

1 cup (112 g) wheat germ

1 cup (145 g) sunflower seeds

½ cup (72 g) sesame seeds

⅔ cup (45 g) powdered milk

1 cup (340 g) honey

1 cup (110 g) slivered almonds

1 cup (145 g) chopped dates, lightly floured

In a large bowl, combine oats, coconut, wheat germ, sunflower seeds, sesame seeds, and powdered milk. Warm the honey until it pours easily. Add honey to dry ingredients, stirring until well mixed. Pour mixture into a large shallow baking pan that has been generously brushed with oil. Spread mixture evenly in the pan. Bake at 325°F (170°C, gas mark 3) for 1 hour, stirring every 15 minutes. When lightly browned, remove from oven and add almonds and dates. Allow to cool completely before storing in airtight container.

Yield: 24 servings

Each with: 7 g water; 265 calories (32% from fat, 12% from protein, 56% from carb); 8 g protein; 10 g total fat; 2 g saturated fat; 4 g monounsaturated fat; 4 g polyunsaturated fat; 39 g carb; 5 g fiber; 20 g sugar; 286 mg phosphorus; 88 mg calcium; 2 mg iron; 23 mg sodium; 319 mg potassium; 51 IU vitamin A; 13 mg vitamin E; 1 mg vitamin C; 0 mg cholesterol

Oat Bran–Berry Smoothie

Adding oat bran to a smoothie is probably not something you'd thought about doing. But it really works, adding flavor, texture, and lots of good nutrition.

1 cup (235 ml) cranberry juice

1 cup (255 g) strawberries, frozen

8 ounces (225 g) vanilla yogurt

⅔ cup (66 g) oat bran

1 cup ice cubes

Place all ingredients except ice in blender. Cover. Blend on high about 2 minutes or until smooth. Gradually add ice, blending on high until smooth. Serve immediately.

Yield: 2 servings

Each with: 267 g water; 246 calories (9% from fat, 13% from protein, 79% from carb); 8 g protein; 2 g total fat; 1 g saturated fat; 1 g monounsaturated fat; 0 g polyunsaturated fat; 50 g carb; 3 g fiber; 22 g sugar; 251 mg phosphorus; 241 mg calcium; 5 mg iron; 135 mg sodium; 449 mg potassium; 217 IU vitamin A; 58 mg vitamin E; 60 mg vitamin C; 6 mg cholesterol

10

Main Dishes:
Legumes

Moving into main dishes, we start with legumes. You probably think of chili immediately. And we have some chili recipes, but we also have a variety of other soups, casseroles, and main-dish salads containing a wide variety of different kinds of beans.

Beef with Chili Dumplings

This is a great southwestern meal in a pot. With the dumplings, nothing else is even needed.

2 pound (900 g) beef round steak

¼ cup (31 g) flour

1 teaspoon chili powder

½ teaspoon cumin

¼ teaspoon black pepper

2 tablespoons (28 ml) olive oil

1 cup (160 g) chopped onion

2 cups (200 g) cooked kidney beans

10 ounces (280 g) frozen corn

Dumplings

1 tablespoon unsalted butter

1 teaspoon chili powder

¾ cup (175 ml) skim milk

2 cups (128 g) biscuit baking mix

Trim fat from beef and cut into 1-inch (2.5 cm) cubes. Shake meat with flour, chili powder, cumin, and pepper in a resealable plastic bag to coat well. Heat oil in a large Dutch oven. Add beef cubes to oil, a few at a time, and brown. Remove beef from pot. Stir onion into the pot and sauté until soft. Return beef to pot. Drain liquid from beans into a large measuring container and add water to make 3 cups. Stir into beef mixture and cover. Heat to boiling. Lower heat and simmer for 2 hours or until beef is tender. Stir in corn and beans; heat to boiling again. To make chili dumplings, heat butter with chili powder in a small saucepan until bubbly. In large bowl add milk and chili-butter mix to baking mix all at once and stir with a fork until evenly moist. Drop batter by tablespoon on top of boiling stew to make 12 mounds. Cook uncovered, 10 minutes. Cover. Cook 10 minutes longer or until dumplings are done.

Yield: 8 servings

Each with: 143 g water; 624 calories (21% from fat, 37% from protein, 42% from carb); 58 g protein; 15 g total fat; 4 g saturated fat; 7 g monounsaturated fat; 2 g polyunsaturated fat; 65 g carb; 14 g fiber; 3 g sugar; 678 mg phosphorus; 201 mg calcium; 10 mg iron; 118 mg sodium; 1438 mg potassium; 486 IU vitamin A; 56 mg vitamin E; 7 mg vitamin C; 106 mg cholesterol

Brisket of Beef with Beans

This recipe is kind of like baked beans with beef. The cooking liquid gives the beef a nice flavor, and the beans go well with it.

1 pound (455 g) navy beans

2 pound (900 g) beef brisket

2 slices bacon

½ teaspoon black pepper, freshly ground

2 cups (475 ml) water

¼ cup (60 ml) maple syrup

½ cup (115 g) packed brown sugar

½ teaspoon dry mustard

TIP

The beef also makes great sandwiches.

Soak beans in water overnight. Drain the beans. Brown the fat side of the brisket in a Dutch oven or heavy skillet over medium-high heat. Add the bacon and brown the other side. Add the pepper, water, and beans. Reduce heat to medium and cook, covered, for 2 hours or until the beef and beans are tender, stirring occasionally to prevent sticking. Remove the beef and keep warm. Add the maple syrup, brown sugar, and mustard to the beans. Mix thoroughly, and simmer over medium heat for another 10 minutes. Slice the brisket thinly and serve with the beans.

Yield: 6 servings

Each with: 221 g water; 644 calories (49% from fat, 22% from protein, 29% from carb); 35 g protein; 35 g total fat; 14 g saturated fat; 15 g monounsaturated fat; 2 g polyunsaturated fat; 47 g carb; 8 g fiber; 26 g sugar; 379 mg phosphorus; 103 mg calcium; 5 mg iron; 165 mg sodium; 829 mg potassium; 2 IU vitamin A; 0 mg vitamin E; 0 mg vitamin C; 125 mg cholesterol

Cornbread-Topped Bean Casserole

This casserole is a complete meal in one pan. Preparation is made easier by using canned pork and beans, but the flavor definitely says homemade.

1 pound (455 g) ground beef

½ cup (80 g) chopped onion

2 cups (506 g) pork and beans

4 ounces (115 g) chopped green chiles, drained

2 tablespoons taco seasoning mix

¼ cup (60 ml) water

1¼ cups (175 g) cornmeal

¼ cup (31 g) flour

1 tablespoon baking powder

1 tablespoon sugar

1 cup (115 g) shredded Cheddar cheese

1 cup (235 ml) skim milk

1 egg

3 tablespoons (45 ml) canola oil

Brown ground beef and onion; drain. Stir in pork and beans, chiles, seasoning mix, and water. Spread in 8-inch (20 cm) glass baking dish. Heat oven to 350°F (180°C, gas mark 4). Combine dry ingredients. Add cheese, tossing to coat. Add remaining ingredients, stirring just until dry ingredients are moistened. Spread topping evenly over ground beef mixture. Bake 30 to 35 minutes or until wooden pick comes out clean. Let stand 5 minutes before cutting to serve.

Yield: 9 servings

Each with: 136 g water; 402 calories (37% from fat, 22% from protein, 41% from carb); 20 g protein; 15 g total fat; 5 g saturated fat; 6 g monounsaturated fat; 2 g polyunsaturated fat; 36 g carb; 4 g fiber; 5 g sugar; 317 mg phosphorus; 281 mg calcium; 4 mg iron; 669 mg sodium; 445 mg potassium; 440 IU vitamin A; 64 mg vitamin E; 7 mg vitamin C; 78 mg cholesterol

Tex-Mex Meat Loaf

We love meat loaf and we love food with a Mexican flavor, so it's no surprise that this turned out to be a big hit around our house.

1½ pounds (675 g) ground beef

2 cups (200 g) cooked kidney beans, rinsed and drained

1½ cups (390 g) salsa, divided

1 cup (160 g) chopped onion

½ teaspoon minced garlic

½ cup (60 g) bread crumbs

2 eggs

1½ teaspoons ground cumin

2 tablespoons (30 g) brown sugar

Combine beef, beans, 1 cup (260 g) salsa, onion, garlic, bread crumbs, eggs, and cumin. Mix well. Press into a loaf shape on a broiler pan or roasting pan. Bake 1 hour at 350°F (180°C, gas mark 4). Carefully pour off any drippings. Combine remaining salsa and brown sugar; mix well. Spread over top of meat loaf. Continue baking 15 minutes; remove and let stand 10 minutes.

Yield: 6 servings

Each with: 176 g water; 579 calories (20% from fat, 34% from protein, 46% from carb); 41 g protein; 10 g total fat; 4 g saturated fat; 4 g monounsaturated fat; 1 g polyunsaturated fat; 55 g carb; 17 g fiber; 10 g sugar; 492 mg phosphorus; 155 mg calcium; 9 mg iron; 223 mg sodium; 1484 mg potassium; 287 IU vitamin A; 26 mg vitamin E; 6 mg vitamin C; 157 mg cholesterol

Country Beef Stew

This hearty stew of beef and beans is perfect for a winter day.

2 tablespoons (28 ml) olive oil

2 pound (900 g) boneless beef chuck, cut into 1-inch (2.5 cm) cubes

2 cups (480 g) canned no-salt-added tomatoes

1 cup (160 g) coarsely chopped onion

1½ cups (355 ml) water

1 tablespoon (15 ml) Worcestershire sauce

¾ teaspoon tarragon

½ teaspoon black pepper

½ teaspoon garlic powder

2 cups (260 g) sliced carrot

5 cups (885 g) cooked great northern beans, drained

In large kettle or Dutch oven, heat oil until hot. Add half of the beef and brown on all sides. Remove with slotted spoon and repeat with remaining beef. Return meat to kettle. Add tomatoes, onion, water, Worcestershire sauce, tarragon, black pepper, and garlic powder. Bring to a boil. Reduce heat and simmer, covered, until meat is almost tender, about 1 hour. Add carrot. Simmer, covered, until carrot and meat are tender, about 20 minutes. Stir in beans and cook until beans are heated through, about 5 minutes.

Yield: 8 servings

Each with: 321 g water; 587 calories (40% from fat, 31% from protein, 29% from carb); 46 g protein; 26 g total fat; 9 g saturated fat; 10 g monounsaturated fat; 3 g polyunsaturated fat; 42 g carb; 10 g fiber; 4 g sugar; 452 mg phosphorus; 141 mg calcium; 6 mg iron; 110 mg sodium; 1102 mg potassium; 5455 IU vitamin A; 0 mg vitamin E; 15 mg vitamin C; 108 mg cholesterol

Southwestern Pie

This is like a Mexican quiche with lots of flavor and good nutrition. Serve topped with salsa with cornbread on the side.

1 cup (160 g) chopped onion

1 tablespoon (15 ml) olive oil

1 teaspoon chili powder

1 teaspoon cumin

½ teaspoon garlic powder

2 cups (200 g) cooked kidney beans

1½ cups (330 g) cooked brown rice

1 cup (115 g) shredded Cheddar cheese

¾ cup (175 ml) skim milk

2 eggs, beaten

In saucepan, cook onion in oil. Stir in chili powder, cumin, and garlic powder. Cook 1 minute. Cool. Stir in beans, rice, cheese, milk, and eggs. Spray a 10-inch (25 cm) oven-safe pie pan with nonstick vegetable oil spray. Add rice mixture. Bake to 350°F (180°C, gas mark 4) until heated through, about 20 minutes. Serve garnished with chopped green pepper if desired.

Yield: 6 servings

Each with: 86 g water; 537 calories (22% from fat, 20% from protein, 57% from carb); 28 g protein; 14 g total fat; 6 g saturated fat; 5 g monounsaturated fat; 2 g polyunsaturated fat; 78 g carb; 18 g fiber; 3 g sugar; 598 mg phosphorus; 321 mg calcium; 7 mg iron; 205 mg sodium; 1123 mg potassium; 502 IU vitamin A; 101 mg vitamin E; 5 mg vitamin C; 103 mg cholesterol

Mexican Layered Casserole

For a Mexican version of lasagna, tortillas are layered with meat, beans, and cheese.

1 pound (455 g) ground beef

1 cup (160 g) chopped onion

1 cup (150 g) chopped bell pepper

4 ounces (115 g) chopped green chiles

16 ounces (455 g) no-salt-added tomato sauce

2 cups (342 g) cooked pinto beans

½ teaspoon garlic powder

2 tablespoons taco seasoning

1 cup (235 ml) water

2 cups (240 g) grated Cheddar cheese

6 flour tortillas

In a large pot, brown beef, onion, and bell pepper. Add remaining ingredients except cheese and tortillas. Simmer 10 minutes. In a large casserole dish, alternately layer meat mixture, cheese, and tortillas, beginning with meat and ending with cheese. Bake at 350°F (180°C, gas mark 4) for 30 minutes.

Yield: 6 servings

Each with: 280 g water; 583 calories (40% from fat, 27% from protein, 33% from carb); 35 g protein; 22 g total fat; 12 g saturated fat; 7 g monounsaturated fat; 1 g polyunsaturated fat; 42 g carb; 9 g fiber; 6 g sugar; 494 mg phosphorus; 414 mg calcium; 5 mg iron; 688 mg sodium; 949 mg potassium; 1640 IU vitamin A; 114 mg vitamin E; 51 mg vitamin C; 98 mg cholesterol

Three Bean Casserole

If you like baked beans but are one of those people who want meat with their meal, this one-dish bean and beef dinner should be just the thing for you.

15 ounces (420 g) kidney beans, rinsed and drained

15 ounces (420 g) chickpeas, rinsed and drained

15 ounces (420 g) lima beans, rinsed and drained

1 pound (455 g) ground beef, extra lean

1 cup (160 g) chopped onion

½ teaspoon minced garlic

¼ cup (60 g) brown sugar

½ teaspoon black pepper

2 tablespoons (28 ml) mustard

½ cup (120 ml) low-sodium ketchup

1 teaspoon cumin

¼ cup (60 ml) water

1 tablespoon (15 ml) cider vinegar

In 2½-quart (2.5 L) casserole dish, combine beans; set aside. In a skillet, cook beef, onion, and garlic. Remove from heat and drain. Add remaining ingredients. Mix well. Stir beef mix into beans. Bake at 350°F (180°C, gas mark 4) for 45 minutes.

Yield: 6 servings

Each with: 246 g water; 495 calories (26% from fat, 24% from protein, 50% from carb); 30 g protein; 14 g total fat; 5 g saturated fat; 6 g monounsaturated fat; 1 g polyunsaturated fat; 63 g carb; 15 g fiber; 15 g sugar; 366 mg phosphorus; 120 mg calcium; 7 mg iron; 295 mg sodium; 1092 mg potassium; 333 IU vitamin A; 0 mg vitamin E; 13 mg vitamin C; 52 mg cholesterol

Bean Salad Burrito

Want a salad you can pick up and go with? Here beans are layered with salad ingredients in a tortilla, giving you a handy, tasty meal to go.

1 cup (100 g) cooked kidney beans

1 cup (182 g) cooked navy beans

1 cup (172 g) cooked black beans

¼ cup (38 g) chopped green bell pepper

½ cup (50 g) sliced scallions

½ cup (90 g) chopped tomato

1 cup (260 g) salsa

3 cups (115 g) shredded lettuce

1 cup (230 g) plain fat-free yogurt

1 cup (115 g) shredded Cheddar cheese

6 flour tortillas

Drain and rinse beans and place in a large mixing bowl. Add bell pepper, scallions, tomato, and salsa; chill. Layer lettuce, beans, yogurt, and cheese on a tortilla and wrap like a burrito.

Yield: 6 servings

Each with: 177 g water; 486 calories (20% from fat, 23% from protein, 58% from carb); 28 g protein; 11 g total fat; 5 g saturated fat; 3 g monounsaturated fat; 1 g polyunsaturated fat; 71 g carb; 18 g fiber; 9 g sugar; 548 mg phosphorus; 407 mg calcium; 7 mg iron; 400 mg sodium; 1359 mg potassium; 742 IU vitamin A; 58 mg vitamin E; 13 mg vitamin C; 24 mg cholesterol

Bean and Cheddar Cheese Pie

Beans and cheese combine to make a filling and tasty meatless main dish with a south western accent.

¾ cup (93 g) flour

1½ cups (175 g) shredded Cheddar cheese, divided

1½ teaspoons baking powder

⅓ cup (80 ml) skim milk

1 egg, beaten

2 cups (328 g) cooked chickpeas, drained

2 cups (200 g) cooked kidney beans, drained

8 ounces (225 g) no-salt-added tomato sauce

½ cup (75 g) chopped green bell pepper

¼ cup (40 g) chopped onion

2 teaspoons chili powder

½ teaspoon dried oregano leaves

¼ teaspoon garlic powder

Heat oven to 375°F (190°C, gas mark 5). Spray a 10-inch (25 cm) pie pan with nonstick vegetable oil spray. Mix flour, ½ cup (58 g) cheese, and baking powder in a medium bowl. Stir in milk and egg until blended. Spread over bottom and up sides of pie pan. Mix ½ cup (58 g) of the remaining cheese and the remaining ingredients; spoon into pie pan. Sprinkle with remaining cheese. Bake about 25 minutes or until edges are puffy and light brown. Let stand 10 minutes before cutting.

Yield: 8 servings

Each with: 109 g water; 400 calories (23% from fat, 23% from protein, 54% from carb); 23 g protein; 10 g total fat; 6 g saturated fat; 3 g monounsaturated fat; 1 g polyunsaturated fat; 55 g carb; 15 g fiber; 3 g sugar; 438 mg phosphorus; 343 mg calcium; 6 mg iron; 464 mg sodium; 957 mg potassium; 648 IU vitamin A; 81 mg vitamin E; 16 mg vitamin C; 52 mg cholesterol

Bean Soup with Dumplings

Whole wheat dumplings give this soup extra flavor and nutrition.

1 pound (455 g) dried navy beans

8 ounces (225 g) no-salt-added tomato sauce

2 cups (360 g) chopped tomato

1 cup (160 g) chopped onion

3 quarts (2.8 L) water

4 potatoes, diced

¾ cup (90 g) whole wheat flour

2 teaspoons baking powder

1 egg, beaten

2 tablespoons (28 ml) skim milk

Use a large soup pot. Add beans, tomato sauce, tomato, and onion. Cover with water and cook on low until beans are tender, about 2 hours. Add additional water if necessary. Add potatoes. Let cook about 1 additional hour. Sift the flour and baking powder together. Add the egg and milk and mix well. Drop in bean soup. Cover and cook at medium boil for 15 minutes. Do not take the lid off the pan until the 15 minutes are up.

Yield: 8 servings

Each with: 630 g water; 271 calories (6% from fat, 16% from protein, 78% from carb); 11 g protein; 2 g total fat; 0 g saturated fat; 0 g monounsaturated fat; 1 g polyunsaturated fat; 55 g carb; 9 g fiber; 4 g sugar; 293 mg phosphorus; 146 mg calcium; 4 mg iron; 419 mg sodium; 1285 mg potassium; 394 IU vitamin A; 13 mg vitamin E; 31 mg vitamin C; 26 mg cholesterol

Black Bean Turkey Chili

This makes a rather mild chili, but you can easily add more chili powder or some red pepper flakes to spice it up if that's the way you like your chili.

1 pound (455 g) ground turkey

1 tablespoon (15 ml) olive oil

¾ cup (120 g) chopped onion

½ cup (75 g) seeded and chopped green bell pepper

½ teaspoon minced garlic

4 cups (688 g) cooked no-salt-added black beans, rinsed and drained

2 cups (510 g) no-salt-added stewed tomatoes

8 ounces (225 g) no-salt-added tomato sauce

1 cup (235 ml) dark beer or low-sodium beef broth

1 tablespoon chili powder

1 tablespoon ground cumin

1 teaspoon ground coriander

1 teaspoon dried oregano, crushed

Heat a large, heavy saucepan or Dutch oven to medium-high, and brown the turkey until done. Drain meat and set aside. In the saucepan, add the oil and bring to medium heat. Add the onion, bell pepper, and garlic, and cook until vegetables are tender, about 5 to 6 minutes. Return meat to pan. Add remaining ingredients. Bring chili to a boil; then reduce heat and simmer for 30 to 45 minutes or until thickened, stirring occasionally. Taste to adjust seasonings.

Yield: 6 servings

Each with: 301 g water; 368 calories (18% from fat, 39% from protein, 44% from carb); 35 g protein; 7 g total fat; 2 g saturated fat; 3 g monounsaturated fat; 2 g polyunsaturated fat; 40 g carb; 14 g fiber; 5 g sugar; 374 mg phosphorus; 134 mg calcium; 6 mg iron; 92 mg sodium; 1108 mg potassium; 733 IU vitamin A; 0 mg vitamin E; 25 mg vitamin C; 57 mg cholesterol

Chili with Beans

This makes a nice thick, moderately spicy chili. Like most chili it's best if it simmers for a while.

2 pounds (900 g) ground beef

1 tablespoon (15 ml) olive oil

1 cup (160 g) chopped onion

1 cup (150 g) chopped red bell pepper

½ teaspoon minced garlic

½ teaspoon black pepper, fresh ground

1 teaspoon ground cumin

1 ounce (28 g) dried ground chipotle pepper

1 teaspoon cayenne pepper

1 tablespoon chili powder

3 cups (710 ml) water

6 ounces (170 g) no-salt-added tomato paste

4 cups (1 kg) no-salt-added canned tomatoes

4 cups (1 kg) dried kidney beans

Brown beef in 2 batches in thick-bottomed soup kettle. Drain off fat and set browned beef aside. Heat oil in kettle over medium-high heat, adding onion when hot. Sauté for 4 to 5 minutes, stirring often. Add bell pepper and garlic, continuing to cook 2 to 3 more minutes. Add black pepper, cumin, chipotle, and cayenne to taste plus chili powder. Stir continually until spices begin to stick to bottom of kettle and brown. Quickly add water. Add tomato paste and tomatoes with the juice they were packed in. Add kidney beans. Add the beef but try not to include any fat that may have accumulated. Stir. When chili begins to boil, reduce heat to low and cover. Ideally, chili should be simmered 3 hours to let all the flavors blend together. Stir about every 15 minutes. Check each time to make sure heat is not too high, causing chili to stick to the bottom of kettle. If you don't have 3 hours to cook the chili, use less chipotle and cayenne or else they will overpower the other flavors.

Yield: 8 servings

Each with: 375 g water; 486 calories (38% from fat, 34% from protein, 28% from carb); 42 g protein; 21 g total fat; 7 g saturated fat; 9 g monounsaturated fat; 1 g polyunsaturated fat; 34 g carb; 12 g fiber; 7 g sugar; 425 mg phosphorus; 130 mg calcium; 8 mg iron; 274 mg sodium; 1365 mg potassium; 2149 IU vitamin A; 0 mg vitamin E; 43 mg vitamin C; 98 mg cholesterol

Cholent

Cholent is a European delicacy that enabled Jews to prepare a warm Sabbath meal without violating the prohibition against cooking since the dish is prepared on Friday and slow cooks until Sabbath lunch. If you are not using it in the traditional manner, it will be done in 10 to 12 hours, but the longer cooking time makes the meat even more tender and the flavors more developed.

1 cup (250 g) dried kidney beans

1 cup (208 g) dried navy beans

1 cup (225 g) dried split peas

3 pound (1¼ kg) beef brisket, cut into large chunks

1½ cups (240 g) sliced onion

1 cup (200 g) pearl barley

4 potatoes, peeled and sliced

½ cup (120 ml) water

¼ teaspoon black pepper

Boil all beans in a large pot of water for 5 minutes and then drain and rinse beans. Arrange in a slow cooker layers of meat, onion, beans, barley, and potatoes. Add pepper, then water. Cover tightly. Set slow cooker on lowest setting. Replenish water during cooking time, if necessary. It will be done within 24 hours.

Yield: 10 servings

Each with: 253 g water; 710 calories (40% from fat, 22% from protein, 38% from carb); 40 g protein; 31 g total fat; 12 g saturated fat; 13 g monounsaturated fat; 2 g polyunsaturated fat; 68 g carb; 16 g fiber; 4 g sugar; 551 mg phosphorus; 107 mg calcium; 7 mg iron; 101 mg sodium; 1749 mg potassium; 16 IU vitamin A; 0 mg vitamin E; 16 mg vitamin C; 110 mg cholesterol

Dutch Pea Soup

This is a hearty pea soup with smoked sausage. We like this with a dark bread like pumpernickel.

2 cups (450 g) dried split peas

3½ quarts (3.3 L) water

4 leeks, chopped

1½ cups (150 g) chopped celery

½ pound (225 g) smoked sausage, sliced

Soak peas in 3 cups (710 ml) cold water for 12 hours; drain. Add water to make 3½ quarts (3.3 L) and bring to boil. Add leeks and celery and simmer 3 to 5 hours until tender. Thirty minutes before soup is done, add sausage.

Yield: 6 servings

Each with: 694 g water; 203 calories (31% from fat, 22% from protein, 47% from carb); 11 g protein; 7 g total fat; 2 g saturated fat; 3 g monounsaturated fat; 1 g polyunsaturated fat; 24 g carb; 7 g fiber; 5 g sugar; 92 mg phosphorus; 71 mg calcium; 3 mg iron; 504 mg sodium; 415 mg potassium; 1107 IU vitamin A; 0 mg vitamin E; 14 mg vitamin C; 26 mg cholesterol

Green Pea Soup

If you are thinking split pea soup, think again. This chilled soup is made with green peas, yogurt, and dill. It is perfect for a summer luncheon.

10 ounces (280 g) frozen peas

¼ cup (25 g) chopped scallions

2 cups (475 ml) low-sodium chicken broth, divided

½ teaspoon dill

¾ cup (180 g) plain fat-free yogurt

Place peas, scallions, 2 tablespoons (28 ml) of the chicken broth, and the dill in a heavy nonstick pan over medium-high heat. Cover and cook 5 to 6 minutes or until peas are tender. Remove from heat and cool. Stir in remaining chicken broth. Working in batches, transfer pea mixture to a blender or food processor and process until smooth. Pour blended mixture into a bowl and repeat process until whole mixture is pureed. Cover and refrigerate until chilled. Just before serving, whisk yogurt into pea soup. Pour into individual serving bowls and top with an extra spoonful of yogurt, if desired.

Yield: 3 servings

Each with: 288 g water; 137 calories (9% from fat, 33% from protein, 58% from carb); 12 g protein; 1 g total fat; 0 g saturated fat; 0 g monounsaturated fat; 0 g polyunsaturated fat; 21 g carb; 5 g fiber; 10 g sugar; 233 mg phosphorus; 160 mg calcium; 2 mg iron; 402 mg sodium; 481 mg potassium; 2082 IU vitamin A; 1 mg vitamin E; 12 mg vitamin C; 1 mg cholesterol

Pinto Bean and Squash Stew

This unexpected combination makes a great meatless meal. Serve with crusty French bread or cornbread.

1 pound (455 g) dried pinto beans

¼ cup (40 g) chopped onion

½ teaspoon minced garlic

4 slices bacon, cubed

1 jalapeño pepper, seeded and chopped

¼ cup (25 g) minced scallions

1 butternut squash, peeled and diced

1 cup (235 ml) low-sodium beef broth

½ cup finely diced red onion

¼ cup chopped fresh cilantro

¾ cup (180 g) sour cream

Cover pinto beans with 3 inches (7.5 cm) of boiling water in large pot. Add onion and garlic. Cover and bake at 250°F (120°C, gas mark ½) until beans are cooked, 2 to 2½ hours. Keep warm. Cook bacon with jalapeño and scallions over low heat in large sauté pan until bacon is crisp. Add squash and broth. Cover and cook until squash is just tender, about 30 minutes. Combine beans and squash and mix gently but well. Spoon beans and squash into 6 serving bowls. Sprinkle each with red onion, cilantro, and 2 tablespoons (30 g) sour cream.

Yield: 6 servings

Each with: 137 g water; 192 calories (16% from fat, 26% from protein, 58% from carb); 11 g protein; 3 g total fat; 1 g saturated fat; 1 g monounsaturated fat; 0 g polyunsaturated fat; 24 g carb; 7 g fiber; 1 g sugar; 183 mg phosphorus; 79 mg calcium; 2 mg iron; 163 mg sodium; 477 mg potassium; 293 IU vitamin A; 31 mg vitamin E; 5 mg vitamin C; 18 mg cholesterol

Senate Bean Soup

Bean soup is on the menu in the U.S. Senate's restaurant every day. According to the Senate website, there are several stories about the origin of that mandate. According to one story, the Senate's bean soup tradition began early in the twentieth-century at the request of Senator Fred Dubois of Idaho. Another story attributes the request to Senator Knute Nelson of Minnesota, who expressed his fondness for the soup in 1903. The recipe attributed to Dubois includes mashed potatoes (from his home state). The recipe served in the Senate today does not include mashed potatoes but does include a braised onion. The recipe below has the mashed potatoes because I like the way they thicken the soup.

1 pound (455 g) dried navy beans

½ pound (225 g) ham, diced

1½ cups (337 g) mashed potatoes

1 cup (160 g) chopped onion

¼ cup (25 g) chopped celery

½ teaspoon chopped garlic

Clean the beans and then cover them with water and cook until nearly done. Drain. Add ham and 1 quart (946 ml) water and bring to a boil. Add potatoes and mix thoroughly. Add chopped vegetables and bring to a boil. Simmer for 1 hour before serving.

Yield: 6 servings

Each with: 102 g water; 390 calories (15% from fat, 24% from protein, 61% from carb); 24 g protein; 7 g total fat; 2 g saturated fat; 2 g monounsaturated fat; 1 g polyunsaturated fat; 60 g carb; 13 g fiber; 5 g sugar; 424 mg phosphorus; 135 mg calcium; 5 mg iron; 578 mg sodium; 1230 mg potassium; 88 IU vitamin A; 18 mg vitamin E; 8 mg vitamin C; 21 mg cholesterol

Slow Cooker Split Pea Soup

I'm not sure what I like best about this soup, the great taste or the fact that it cooks while you are away. It also freezes well, adding to the convenience.

1 pound (455 g) dried green split peas, rinsed

2 cups (300 g) diced ham

1½ cups (195 g) peeled, sliced carrot

1 cup (160 g) chopped onion

½ cup (50 g) chopped celery

½ teaspoon minced garlic

1 bay leaf

¼ cup chopped fresh parsley

½ teaspoon black pepper

1½ quarts (1.4 L) water

TIP

Serve garnished with croutons.

Layer ingredients in slow cooker and pour in water. Do not stir. Cover and cook on high 4 to 5 hours or on low 8 to 10 hours until peas are very soft. Remove bay leaf before serving.

Yield: 6 servings

Each with: 338 g water; 363 calories (12% from fat, 32% from protein, 56% from carb); 29 g protein; 5 g total fat; 1 g saturated fat; 2 g monounsaturated fat; 1 g polyunsaturated fat; 52 g carb; 21 g fiber; 9 g sugar; 403 mg phosphorus; 77 mg calcium; 4 mg iron; 548 mg sodium; 1088 mg potassium; 5742 IU vitamin A; 0 mg vitamin E; 9 mg vitamin C; 19 mg cholesterol

Spicy Bean Soup

If you like your bean soup with a little kick, this could be the recipe for you. (If not, just replace the spicy vegetable juice with regular and leave out the Tabasco.)

6 cups (1.4 L) water

1 cup (210 g) dried beans, assorted (navy, red, and pinto.)

½ cup (95 g) brown rice

1 cup (160 g) diced onion

1 cup (130 g) diced carrot

½ cup (75 g) diced green bell pepper

6 ounces (175 ml) spicy vegetable juice, such as V8

¼ teaspoon Tabasco sauce

¾ cup (90 g) diced celery

1 teaspoon black pepper

1 cup (150 g) diced ham

Combine all ingredients in a large pot. Simmer for at least 3 hours.

Yield: 6 servings

Each with: 350 g water; 239 calories (11% from fat, 23% from protein, 66% from carb); 14 g protein; 3 g total fat; 1 g saturated fat; 1 g monounsaturated fat; 1 g polyunsaturated fat; 39 g carb; 7 g fiber; 4 g sugar; 256 mg phosphorus; 77 mg calcium; 3 mg iron; 426 mg sodium; 733 mg potassium; 3779 IU vitamin A; 0 mg vitamin E; 16 mg vitamin C; 10 mg cholesterol

White Bean Soup

This is a simple pureed bean soup that is both filling and tasty. Serve with multigrain bread and a salad.

½ cup (80 g) minced onion

½ cup (60 g) minced celery

¼ cup (38 g) chopped green bell pepper

2 tablespoons (28 ml) olive oil

½ pound (225 g) smoked sausage, cut in ½-inch (1 cm) slices

8 ounces (225 g) no-salt-added tomato sauce

4 cups (728 g) cooked navy beans

4 cups (950 ml) water

1 teaspoon black pepper

In large saucepan, cook onion, celery, and bell pepper in oil until soft. Add sausage and tomato sauce; simmer 15 to 20 minutes. In a separate saucepan, bring navy beans to boil. Puree beans and their liquid in a food processor or blender; add to vegetable mixture. Add the water and pepper and simmer for 1 hour.

Yield: 4 servings

Each with: 477 g water; 477 calories (34% from fat, 19% from protein, 47% from carb); 24 g protein; 18 g total fat; 5 g saturated fat; 10 g monounsaturated fat; 3 g polyunsaturated fat; 57 g carb; 21 g fiber; 4 g sugar; 292 mg phosphorus; 154 mg calcium; 6 mg iron; 705 mg sodium; 1006 mg potassium; 290 IU vitamin A; 0 mg vitamin E; 25 mg vitamin C; 40 mg cholesterol

Winter Bean Soup

This is a flavorful soup with smoked sausage and just a hint of chili flavor.

2 cups (420 g) dried mixed beans

2 quarts (1.9 L) water

½ pound (225 g) smoked sausage, sliced

1 cup (160 g) chopped onion

½ teaspoon minced garlic

1 teaspoon chili powder

4 cups (1 kg) no-salt-added canned tomatoes

2 tablespoons (30 ml) lemon juice

TIP *Use a variety of beans (great northern, navy, black, chickpeas, split peas, pinto, red beans, or lentils).*

Rinse beans and cover with water. Soak overnight. Drain and add 2 quarts (1.9 L) water and sausage and simmer until tender. Add onion, garlic, chili powder, tomatoes, and lemon juice and simmer 45 minutes more.

Yield: 6 servings

Each with: 526 g water; 350 calories (19% from fat, 25% from protein, 57% from carb); 22 g protein; 8 g total fat; 3 g saturated fat; 3 g monounsaturated fat; 1 g polyunsaturated fat; 52 g carb; 12 g fiber; 7 g sugar; 243 mg phosphorus; 229 mg calcium; 9 mg iron; 500 mg sodium; 1567 mg potassium; 312 IU vitamin A; 0 mg vitamin E; 25 mg vitamin C; 26 mg cholesterol

Sausage and Bean Soup

This is such a quick and easy soup to make for lunch or dinner. The bean, potato, and sausage mixture reminds me of the bean and ham meals we sometimes had when I was growing up.

¾ teaspoon olive oil

⅓ cup (55 g) chopped onion

⅔ cup (87 g) sliced carrot

1 potato, peeled and cubed

1 cup (235 ml) low-sodium beef broth

5 ounces (142 g) smoked sausage, cut into ½-inch (1 cm) slices

10 ounces (280 g) great northern beans, undrained

10 ounces (180 g) green beans, frozen

Heat oil in a saucepan over medium heat. Sauté onion 4 to 5 minutes, stirring frequently, until tender. Add carrot, potato, and broth. Bring to a boil. Reduce heat to low, cover, and simmer about 15 minutes or until vegetables are tender. Add sausage and beans. Cook until thoroughly heated.

Yield: 4 servings

Each with: 282 g water; 275 calories (25% from fat, 20% from protein, 56% from carb); 14 g protein; 8 g total fat; 3 g saturated fat; 4 g monounsaturated fat; 1 g polyunsaturated fat; 39 g carb; 8 g fiber; 4 g sugar; 196 mg phosphorus; 84 mg calcium; 3 mg iron; 492 mg sodium; 924 mg potassium; 4083 IU vitamin A; 0 mg vitamin E; 29 mg vitamin C; 25 mg cholesterol

Bean Chalupa

Kind of like a super pot of nachos, pork and pinto beans are slow cooked until falling apart, served over corn chips, and topped with cheese, lettuce, tomato, avocado, and hot sauce.

1 pound (455 g) dried pinto beans

3 pound (1¼ kg) pork loin roast

7 cups (1.6 L) water

½ cup (80 g) chopped onion

½ teaspoon minced garlic

2 tablespoons chili powder

1 tablespoon cumin

1 teaspoon oregano

4 ounces (115 g) chopped green chiles

Mix all together in heavy pan and cook, covered, on low heat for 5 hours. Break up roast and cook uncovered 30 minutes more.

Yield: 12 servings

Each with: 241 g water; 287 calories (18% from fat, 46% from protein, 36% from carb); 32 g protein; 6 g total fat; 2 g saturated fat; 2 g monounsaturated fat; 1 g polyunsaturated fat; 26 g carb; 7 g fiber; 1 g sugar; 412 mg phosphorus; 76 mg calcium; 4 mg iron; 118 mg sodium; 1003 mg potassium; 403 IU vitamin A; 2 mg vitamin E; 8 mg vitamin C; 71 mg cholesterol

Two-Bean Pita Pizzas

This is not an Italian pizza, but its preparation and the look of the finished product makes it a pizza in my mind.

4 whole wheat pitas

2 tablespoons (28 ml) olive oil

1 cup (160 g) thinly sliced onion

¾ teaspoon finely chopped garlic

16 ounces (455 g) kidney beans

16 ounces (455 g) chickpeas

12 ounces (340 g) salsa

1 teaspoon crumbled basil

½ teaspoon crumbled thyme

½ teaspoon crumbled oregano

1 cup (113 g) shredded mozzarella cheese, divided

¼ cup (25 g) grated Parmesan cheese

Preheat oven to 375°F (190°C, gas mark 5). Heat pitas on foil for 8 to 10 minutes. Heat oil in skillet over medium heat. Sauté onion for 3 minutes. Add garlic and sauté 2 more minutes. Drain and rinse beans. Add to skillet with salsa and herbs. Cook until heated. With serrated knife, slice pitas in half. Place pita rounds, inside facing up and overlapping slightly, around surface of 12-inch (30 cm) pizza pan. Sprinkle with ¾ cup (90 g) mozzarella. Spoon bean mixture on top and spread to cover. Sprinkle with remaining mozzarella and Parmesan cheese. Bake 10 to 15 minutes.

Yield: 8 servings

Each with: 152 g water; 323 calories (22% from fat, 20% from protein, 58% from carb); 17 g protein; 8 g total fat; 3 g saturated fat; 4 g monounsaturated fat; 1 g polyunsaturated fat; 48 g carb; 11 g fiber; 3 g sugar; 295 mg phosphorus; 226 mg calcium; 4 mg iron; 577 mg sodium; 566 mg potassium; 237 IU vitamin A; 21 mg vitamin E; 5 mg vitamin C; 12 mg cholesterol

Chicken and Bean Skillet

This is a great, quick dinner for those nights when you don't have something planned and everyone is hungry. It is simple and fast but loaded with flavor and nutrition.

1 cup (160 g) chopped onion

⅓ cup (50 g) chopped red bell pepper

¾ teaspoon crushed garlic

2 teaspoons (10 ml) olive oil

½ pound (225 g) boneless chicken breast, cut in 1-inch (2.5 cm) cubes

¾ teaspoon cumin

½ teaspoon cinnamon

10 ounces (280 g) navy beans, drained

10 ounces (280 g) kidney beans, drained

2 cups (510 g) no-salt-added stewed tomatoes, undrained

TIP *This dish is delicious served over cooked rice, couscous, or pasta.*

Sauté onion, pepper, and garlic in oil in medium saucepan 2 to 3 minutes. Add chicken, cumin, and cinnamon; cook over medium-high heat until chicken is lightly browned, about 3 to 4 minutes. Add beans and tomatoes; heat to boiling. Reduce heat and simmer, uncovered, until slightly thickened, 5 to 8 minutes. Season to taste with salt and pepper.

Yield: 4 servings

Each with: 299 g water; 325 calories (10% from fat, 33% from protein, 57% from carb); 27 g protein; 4 g total fat; 1 g saturated fat; 2 g monounsaturated fat; 1 g polyunsaturated fat; 47 g carb; 16 g fiber; 8 g sugar; 353 mg phosphorus; 163 mg calcium; 6 mg iron; 53 mg sodium; 1076 mg potassium; 631 IU vitamin A; 3 mg vitamin E; 31 mg vitamin C; 33 mg cholesterol

Chicken Chili Verde

Here is yet another chili variation. Called "green chili" in Spanish, it does not contain tomatoes and has chicken instead of the more traditional beef. If you can't find cannellini beans, which are an Italian white kidney bean, you can substitute any other white bean, such as navy or great northern beans.

3 cups (300 g) cooked cannellini beans, drained

1 cup (160 g) chopped onion

½ teaspoon minced garlic

4 ounces (115 g) chopped chiles

2 teaspoons oregano

1½ teaspoons cumin

¼ teaspoon ground cloves

¼ teaspoon cayenne

3 cups (420 g) cooked diced chicken

2 cups (470 ml) low-sodium chicken broth

Combine all ingredients in a large pot and simmer gently about 1 hour.

Yield: 6 servings

Each with: 146 g water; 259 calories (20% from fat, 44% from protein, 36% from carb); 28 g protein; 6 g total fat; 2 g saturated fat; 2 g monounsaturated fat; 1 g polyunsaturated fat; 24 g carb; 7 g fiber; 2 g sugar; 303 mg phosphorus; 91 mg calcium; 4 mg iron; 66 mg sodium; 637 mg potassium; 322 IU vitamin A; 11 mg vitamin E; 49 mg vitamin C; 62 mg cholesterol

Pork Chop and Bean Skillet

This makes a good dinner with fried potatoes.

6 center-cut pork chops

1 tablespoon (15 ml) olive oil

1 cup (160 g) chopped onion

½ teaspoon minced garlic

½ cup (120 ml) low-sodium chicken broth

½ cup (125 g) barbecue sauce

2 jalapeño peppers, chopped

4 cups (684 g) no-salt-added pinto beans, drained

TIP *You can either use canned no-salt-added beans or cook your own dried ones.*

In a large skillet, sear pork chops in oil until brown, about 5 minutes. Remove pork chops and place on plate. Add onion and garlic to skillet; cook 10 minutes. Stir in broth, barbecue sauce, jalapeños, and beans. Heat mixture to a boil. Return pork to skillet. Reduce heat. Cover and simmer 50 to 60 minutes, stirring sauce and turning chops occasionally until meat is fork-tender.

Yield: 6 servings

Each with: 171 g water; 401 calories (23% from fat, 33% from protein, 43% from carb); 34 g protein; 10 g total fat; 3 g saturated fat; 5 g monounsaturated fat; 1 g polyunsaturated fat; 43 g carb; 11 g fiber; 9 g sugar; 370 mg phosphorus; 76 mg calcium; 3 mg iron; 269 mg sodium; 874 mg potassium; 43 IU vitamin A; 1 mg vitamin E; 6 mg vitamin C; 63 mg cholesterol

Bean Balls

These are a vegetarian alternative to meatballs. If you are skeptical, you really should try these.

1½ cups (265 g) cooked great northern beans, drained

1 cup (115 g) whole wheat bread crumbs

1 tablespoon grated Parmesan cheese

2 eggs

2 tablespoons parsley

2 teaspoons onion powder

Mash beans and add rest of ingredients. Form into balls and steam for 20 minutes. Serve with spaghetti as a substitute for meatballs.

Yield: 6 servings

Each with: 62 g water; 180 calories (17% from fat, 22% from protein, 61% from carb); 10 g protein; 3 g total fat; 1 g saturated fat; 1 g monounsaturated fat; 1 g polyunsaturated fat; 28 g carb; 4 g fiber; 2 g sugar; 165 mg phosphorus; 94 mg calcium; 2 mg iron; 71 mg sodium; 306 mg potassium; 201 IU vitamin A; 27 mg vitamin E; 3 mg vitamin C; 80 mg cholesterol

Chickpea Sandwich Spread

Are you looking for something a little different for a sandwich? Try this along with lettuce and tomato on a whole grain bread.

1½ cups (246 g) cooked chickpeas, drained (save juice)

½ teaspoon onion powder

2/3 cup (30 g) chopped chives

1½ tablespoons (24 g) no-salt-added tomato paste

1/8 teaspoon lemon juice

Mash chickpeas and mix with rest of ingredients. Add 1/3 cup of the reserved juice and process in a blender or food processor. Use as sandwich spread.

Yield: 6 servings

Each with: 50 g water; 77 calories (8% from fat, 17% from protein, 75% from carb); 3 g protein; 1 g total fat; 0 g saturated fat; 0 g monounsaturated fat; 0 g polyunsaturated fat; 15 g carb; 3 g fiber; 1 g sugar; 61 mg phosphorus; 26 mg calcium; 1 mg iron; 184 mg sodium; 162 mg potassium; 309 IU vitamin A; 0 mg vitamin E; 6 mg vitamin C; 0 mg cholesterol

Italian Baked Beans

Here is an Italian-flavored version of baked beans.

1 pound (455 g) navy beans

8 cups (1.9 L) water

1 pound (455 g) hot Italian sausage links, sliced

1 cup (160 g) chopped onion

⅓ cup (50 g) green bell pepper, cut in 1-inch (2.5 cm) pieces

½ cup (35 g) halved mushrooms

2 bay leaves

⅓ cup (80 ml) ketchup

⅓ cup (113 g) molasses

1 tablespoon dry mustard

2 teaspoons crushed oregano

½ teaspoon black pepper

¼ teaspoon garlic salt

TIP

Serve over rice and top with a sprinkling of Parmesan cheese.

Rinse beans; place in large saucepan. Add water. Bring to boil; reduce heat and simmer, covered, for 1 hour. Transfer to bowl; cover and refrigerate overnight. Drain beans, reserving 1½ cups of the liquid. In slow cooker, combine drained beans, sausage, onion, bell pepper, mushrooms, and bay leaves. Blend reserved bean liquid with ketchup, molasses, mustard, oregano, pepper, and garlic salt; stir into bean mixture. Cover and cook on high heat for 6 hours or on low heat for 12 hours.

Yield: 8 servings

Each with: 310 g water; 452 calories (37% from fat, 17% from protein, 45% from carb); 20 g protein; 19 g total fat; 7 g saturated fat; 8 g monounsaturated fat; 3 g polyunsaturated fat; 52 g carb; 9 g fiber; 13 g sugar; 331 mg phosphorus; 142 mg calcium; 5 mg iron; 433 mg sodium; 1125 mg potassium; 141 IU vitamin A; 0 mg vitamin E; 11 mg vitamin C; 43 mg cholesterol

White Bean and Tuna Salad

This makes a great luncheon salad. It can also be a main dish in somewhat larger portions.

2 cups (200 g) cooked cannellini beans, drained and rinsed

13 ounces (368 g) tuna, drained

1 cup (180 g) seeded, diced tomato

½ cup (80 g) chopped red onion

2 tablespoons (30 ml) lemon juice

3 teaspoons (15 ml) Dijon mustard

⅓ cup (80 ml) olive oil

¼ cup chopped fresh basil

Combine beans, tuna, tomato, and onion in large bowl. Combine lemon juice and mustard in small bowl. Gradually whisk in olive oil. Add to salad. Mix in basil.

Yield: 4 servings

Each with: 192 g water; 406 calories (47% from fat, 29% from protein, 24% from carb); 30 g protein; 21 g total fat; 3 g saturated fat; 14 g monounsaturated fat; 3 g polyunsaturated fat; 24 g carb; 8 g fiber; 2 g sugar; 375 mg phosphorus; 129 mg calcium; 4 mg iron; 303 mg sodium; 769 mg potassium; 530 IU vitamin A; 6 mg vitamin E; 12 mg vitamin C; 39 mg cholesterol

TIP *Cannellini beans are large white beans like kidney beans. If you can't find them, you can substitute navy or pea beans.*

11

Main Dishes:
Grains

Main-dish recipes made up of mostly grains? Sure—just think of all the soups and casseroles you can make with barley, rice, or whole grain pasta. And while we're thinking about pasta, that opens another whole series of recipes.

Beef and Barley Stew

This hearty stew is a full meal in a bowl (although I prefer it with a slice of fresh hot bread).

1½ pounds (675 g) beef round steak

¼ cup (31 g) flour

2 tablespoons (28 ml) olive oil

1 cup (160 g) chopped onion

½ teaspoon crushed garlic

3 cups (710 ml) low-sodium beef broth

2 cups (260 g) sliced carrot

¼ cup (50 g) pearl barley

1 tablespoon (15 ml) soy sauce

½ teaspoon oregano

½ cup (50 g) chopped celery

½ teaspoon black pepper

Trim fat from meat and cut into bite-size cubes. Dust beef with flour. Using a heavy pot, brown beef in hot oil, browning all sides. Remove meat and set aside. Add onion and garlic to drippings and cook until onion is transparent. Return the meat to pot. Add broth, barley, soy sauce, and oregano. Cover and simmer for 45 minutes. Add carrot and simmer until meat is tender, about 40 minutes. Add water as needed. Season with pepper.

Yield: 6 servings

Each with: 257 g water; 352 calories (28% from fat, 52% from protein, 20% from carb); 45 g protein; 11 g total fat; 3 g saturated fat; 6 g monounsaturated fat; 1 g polyunsaturated fat; 17 g carb; 3 g fiber; 3 g sugar; 327 mg phosphorus; 42 mg calcium; 5 mg iron; 310 mg sodium; 693 mg potassium; 7222 IU vitamin A; 0 mg vitamin E; 5 mg vitamin C; 102 mg cholesterol

Beef Barley Skillet

This tasty and healthy family meal cooks in only one pan.

¾ pound (338 g) ground beef

½ cup (80 g) chopped onion

¼ cup (38 g) chopped green bell pepper

¼ cup (25 g) chopped celery

¼ teaspoon black pepper

½ teaspoon marjoram

1 teaspoon sugar

1 teaspoon Worcestershire sauce

2 cups (480 g) no-salt-added canned tomatoes, broken up

1½ cups (355 ml) water

¾ cup (150 g) pearl barley

Sauté meat, onion, green pepper, and celery in nonstick fry pan. Drain off excess fat; stir in remaining ingredients. Bring to a boil. Reduce heat to simmer; cover and cook about 1 hour.

Yield: 3 servings

Each with: 389 g water; 477 calories (21% from fat, 31% from protein, 48% from carb); 29 g protein; 9 g total fat; 3 g saturated fat; 3 g monounsaturated fat; 1 g polyunsaturated fat; 45 g carb; 10 g fiber; 7 g sugar; 326 mg phosphorus; 90 mg calcium; 6 mg iron; 129 mg sodium; 932 mg potassium; 292 IU vitamin A; 0 mg vitamin E; 30 mg vitamin C; 78 mg cholesterol

Stroganoff

Up the fiber in your stroganoff by using whole wheat noodles.

½ pound (225 g) ground beef, extra lean

½ cup (35 g) sliced mushrooms

1 packet onion soup mix

1 tablespoon whole wheat flour

1¾ cups (414 ml) water

8 ounces (225 g) whole wheat noodles, cooked and drained

8 tablespoons (120 g) plain fat-free yogurt

Brown beef and drain. Add mushrooms. Whisk dry soup mix and flour into water and heat. Stir until thickened. Combine thickened onion soup and cooked beef. Serve over whole wheat noodles. Garnish with a dollop of yogurt.

Yield: 4 servings

Each with: 178 g water; 360 calories (26% from fat, 23% from protein, 51% from carb); 21 g protein; 11 g total fat; 4 g saturated fat; 4 g monounsaturated fat; 1 g polyunsaturated fat; 48 g carb; 2 g fiber; 3 g sugar; 288 mg phosphorus; 95 mg calcium; 3 mg iron; 222 mg sodium; 397 mg potassium; 2 IU vitamin A; 1 mg vitamin E; 1 mg vitamin C; 40 mg cholesterol

Western Casserole

This simple beef-and-noodle casserole is updated to give you more fiber without sacrificing taste.

1 pound (455 g) beef stew meat, cut in cubes

¼ cup (30 g) whole wheat flour

¼ cup (60 ml) olive oil

6 ounces (170 g) no-salt-added tomato paste

½ cup (120 ml) dry red wine

1 cup (235 ml) water

1 teaspoon thyme

1 teaspoon oregano

1 cup (70 g) sliced mushrooms

1 cup (180 g) chopped tomato

4 ounces (115 g) whole wheat noodles, cooked and drained

1 cup (115 g) shredded Cheddar cheese

Coat meat with flour; brown in oil. Add all ingredients except noodles and cheese. Cover and simmer for 1 hour. Add noodles and cheese. Simmer 5 minutes more and serve.

Yield: 4 servings

Each with: 264 g water; 607 calories (47% from fat, 27% from protein, 26% from carb); 41 g protein; 31 g total fat; 11 g saturated fat; 15 g monounsaturated fat; 2 g polyunsaturated fat; 39 g carb; 3 g fiber; 6 g sugar; 563 mg phosphorus; 299 mg calcium; 6 mg iron; 341 mg sodium; 1114 mg potassium; 1239 IU vitamin A; 85 mg vitamin E; 20 mg vitamin C; 96 mg cholesterol

Chicken Barley Chowder

This simple, creamy soup of chicken and barley is perfect for a cold day.

2 tablespoons (28 ml) olive oil

½ cup (60 g) minced celery

¾ cup (120 g) minced onion

1 tablespoon flour

½ teaspoon black pepper

6 cups (1.4 L) low-sodium chicken broth

1 cup (200 g) pearl barley

1 pound (455 g) cooked boneless chicken breast, shredded

½ cup (120 ml) fat-free evaporated milk

Heat oil in heavy saucepan. Sauté celery and onion; sprinkle with flour and pepper. Gradually stir in broth and barley. Add chicken. Simmer covered for about an hour, stirring occasionally until barley is tender. Remove from heat and add milk.

Yield: 4 servings

Each with: 499 g water; 452 calories (23% from fat, 37% from protein, 41% from carb); 42 g protein; 12 g total fat; 2 g saturated fat; 6 g monounsaturated fat; 2 g polyunsaturated fat; 47 g carb; 9 g fiber; 6 g sugar; 528 mg phosphorus; 148 mg calcium; 4 mg iron; 236 mg sodium; 995 mg potassium; 218 IU vitamin A; 45 mg vitamin E; 4 mg vitamin C; 67 mg cholesterol

Chicken Barley Soup

This is a nice change from chicken and noodle or chicken and rice soup that features barley.

3 pound (1¼ kg) chicken, cut up

2 quarts (1.9 L) water

1½ cups (195 g) diced carrot

1 cup (120 g) diced celery

1 cup (200 g) pearl barley

½ cup (60 g) chopped onion

1 bay leaf

½ teaspoon poultry seasoning

½ teaspoon black pepper

½ teaspoon dried sage

Cook chicken in water until tender. Cool broth and skim off fat. Bone chicken and cut into bite-size pieces; return to kettle along with remaining ingredients. Return to heat and bring to a boil. Simmer covered for at least 1 hour until vegetables are tender and barley is done, adding more water if needed. Remove bay leaf and serve.

Yield: 6 servings

Each with: 546 g water; 400 calories (18% from fat, 54% from protein, 28% from carb); 53 g protein; 8 g total fat; 2 g saturated fat; 2 g monounsaturated fat; 2 g polyunsaturated fat; 27 g carb; 7 g fiber; 3 g sugar; 493 mg phosphorus; 69 mg calcium; 3 mg iron; 224 mg sodium; 829 mg potassium; 5595 IU vitamin A; 36 mg vitamin E; 9 mg vitamin C; 159 mg cholesterol

Chicken Chili with Barley

This is not your traditional chili. In fact, some might argue that it's not chili at all. But the flavor is great and it will be appreciated by anyone who likes Mexican or Tex-Mex cooking.

1 cup (160 g) chopped onion

½ teaspoon minced garlic

1 tablespoon (15 ml) olive oil

2 cups (475 ml) water

¾ cup (150 g) pearl barley

4 cups (1 kg) no-salt-added canned tomatoes

2 cups (475 ml) low-sodium chicken broth

6 ounces (170 g) frozen corn

1 can jalapeño peppers, chopped

1 tablespoon chili powder

½ teaspoon cumin

3 cups (420 g) cubed cooked chicken

In a Dutch oven, cook onion and garlic in the oil until onion is tender. Add remaining ingredients except chicken. Bring to a boil. Reduce heat, cover, and simmer 10 minutes, stirring occasionally. Add chicken and continue simmering an additional 5 to 10 minutes until chicken is heated through and barley is tender.

Yield: 9 servings

Each with: 267 g water; 210 calories (26% from fat, 34% from protein, 41% from carb); 18 g protein; 6 g total fat; 1 g saturated fat; 2 g monounsaturated fat; 2 g polyunsaturated fat; 22 g carb; 5 g fiber; 4 g sugar; 194 mg phosphorus; 57 mg calcium; 3 mg iron; 86 mg sodium; 529 mg potassium; 453 IU vitamin A; 7 mg vitamin E; 14 mg vitamin C; 42 mg cholesterol

Stir-Fried Chicken and Brown Rice

This is an Asian-style chicken stir-fry.

2 tablespoons (28 ml) olive oil, divided

8 ounces (225 g) boneless chicken breast sliced into strips

½ cup (75 g) chopped red bell pepper

½ cup (50 g) chopped scallions

3 cups (660 g) cooked, cooled brown rice

2 tablespoons (28 ml) soy sauce

1 tablespoon (15 ml) rice wine vinegar

1 cup (130 g) frozen peas, thawed

Heat large nonstick skillet over medium heat. Add 1 tablespoon oil. Add chicken, bell pepper, and scallions. Cook 5 minutes until chicken is cooked through. Remove to plate. Heat remaining oil in skillet. Add rice and cook 1 minute. Stir in soy sauce, vinegar, and peas; cook 1 minute. Stir in chicken and vegetable mixture.

Yield: 4 servings

Each with: 213 g water; 349 calories (26% from fat, 25% from protein, 49% from carb); 21 g protein; 10 g total fat; 2 g saturated fat; 6 g monounsaturated fat; 2 g polyunsaturated fat; 43 g carb; 6 g fiber; 3 g sugar; 313 mg phosphorus; 49 mg calcium; 2 mg iron; 177 mg sodium; 425 mg potassium; 1560 IU vitamin A; 3 mg vitamin E; 31 mg vitamin C; 33 mg cholesterol

Turkey and Wild Rice Bake

This is an easy and tasty casserole that uses leftover turkey.

6 ounces (170 g) wild and white rice mix

2⅓ cups (544 ml) water

½ cup (35 g) sliced mushrooms

14 ounces (400 g) artichoke hearts, quartered

2 ounces (55 g) pimento, drained and chopped

2 cups (350 g) cubed cooked turkey

1 cup (110 g) shredded Swiss cheese

Preheat oven to 350°F (180°C, gas mark 4). In 2-quart (2 L) casserole dish, combine rice and water. Stir in mushrooms, artichoke hearts, pimento, and turkey. Cover and bake about 1¼ hours or until liquid is absorbed. Top with cheese and bake uncovered for 5 to 10 minutes or until cheese is melted and golden brown.

Yield: 4 servings

Each with: 315 g water; 366 calories (11% from fat, 43% from protein, 46% from carb); 40 g protein; 5 g total fat; 2 g saturated fat; 1 g monounsaturated fat; 1 g polyunsaturated fat; 43 g carb; 8 g fiber; 3 g sugar; 599 mg phosphorus; 366 mg calcium; 3 mg iron; 195 mg sodium; 716 mg potassium; 597 IU vitamin A; 13 mg vitamin E; 17 mg vitamin C; 80 mg cholesterol

TIP *Chicken is just as good if you don't have turkey but are longing for this dish.*

Turkey Carcass Soup

This is a great use for the last of the Thanksgiving turkey. It's flavorful and full of healthy things.

1 turkey carcass, most meat removed

3 quarts (2.8 L) water

1 tablespoon peppercorns

1 cup (100 g) chopped celery

2 cups (320 g) chopped onion

4 cups (950 ml) chicken broth

1 cup (235 ml) dry red wine

1½ cups (195 g) chopped carrot

2 cups (300 g) chopped turnip

½ cup (97 g) rice

½ cup (100 g) pearl barley

In a large pot, barely cover turkey carcass with water. Add peppercorns and half of the chopped onion and celery. Simmer for 45 minutes. Drain, save liquid, and pick remaining meat from carcass. In saved liquid, add meat, chicken broth, and red wine; simmer 30 minutes. Add the rest of ingredients. Simmer until rice and barley are tender, at least 45 minutes and as much as 2 hours or more.

Yield: 6 servings

Each with: 856 g water; 302 calories (25% from fat, 33% from protein, 42% from carb); 23 g protein; 8 g total fat; 2 g saturated fat; 3 g monounsaturated fat; 2 g polyunsaturated fat; 28 g carb; 6 g fiber; 7 g sugar; 284 mg phosphorus; 90 mg calcium; 3 mg iron; 643 mg sodium; 790 mg potassium; 5468 IU vitaminA; 2 mg vitamin E; 16 mg vitamin C; 51 mg cholesterol

Linguine with Scallops

Seafood just seems to make any meal special. In this case, scallops turn an ordinary spaghetti dinner into something memorable.

1 tablespoon (15 ml) olive oil

1 tablespoon minced shallots

½ teaspoon crushed garlic

1 tablespoon minced fresh parsley

2 tablespoons minced fresh basil

¼ teaspoon crushed red pepper flakes

2 cups (480 g) no-salt-added canned tomatoes

½ cup (120 ml) dry white wine

2 tablespoons (32 g) no-salt-added tomato paste

1 pound (455 g) scallops

9 ounces (255 g) artichoke hearts, thawed

8 ounces (225 g) whole wheat linguine

2 tablespoons (18 g) pine nuts, toasted

In 3-quart (3 L) saucepan, heat oil over medium heat. Add shallots and garlic and sauté 3 minutes. Add parsley, basil, pepper flakes, tomatoes, wine, and tomato paste. Bring to boil and stir to break up tomatoes. Cover and simmer 20 minutes. Slice large scallops crosswise in half. Add scallops and artichoke hearts to tomato mixture. Cook until scallops are cooked and artichokes are hot, about 5 minutes. Cook linguine as package label directs; drain. On platter, toss pasta with scallop mixture and sprinkle with pine nuts. If desired, garnish with basil leaf.

Yield: 4 servings

Each with: 296 g water; 441 calories (17% from fat, 28% from protein, 54% from carb); 31 g protein; 8 g total fat; 1 g saturated fat; 3 g monounsaturated fat; 3 g polyunsaturated fat; 60 g carb; 5 g fiber; 5 g sugar; 500 mg phosphorus; 131 mg calcium; 5 mg iron; 247 mg sodium; 1058 mg potassium; 602 IU vitamin A; 17 mg vitamin E; 21 mg vitamin C; 37 mg cholesterol

Whole Wheat Linguine with White Clam Sauce

This recipe is simple to make and tastes great.

½ cup (120 ml) olive oil

1 cup (160 g) chopped onion

1 teaspoon minced garlic

6 ounces (170 g) minced clams, including liquid

6 ounces (170 g) whole clams, drained

½ cup (120 ml) water

1 tablespoon parsley

½ teaspoon oregano

¼ teaspoon black pepper

8 ounces (225 g) mushrooms, sliced

1 pound (455 g) whole wheat linguine, cooked and drained

Heat oil in skillet. Simmer onion and garlic until golden. Add clams, water, parsley, oregano, pepper, and mushrooms. Simmer for 15 minutes. Pour sauce over linguine.

Yield: 6 servings

Each with: 121 g water; 526 calories (34% from fat, 20% from protein, 47% from carb); 27 g protein; 20 g total fat; 3 g saturated fat; 13 g monounsaturated fat; 3 g polyunsaturated fat; 64 g carb; 1 g fiber; 2 g sugar; 428 mg phosphorus; 93 mg calcium; 19 mg iron; 74 mg sodium; 685 mg potassium; 386 IU vitamin A; 97 mg vitamin E; 16 mg vitamin C; 38 mg cholesterol

Linguine with Tuna

It's not scallops, but tuna can make a pretty fancy Italian meal too.

¾ cup (175 ml) olive oil, divided

1 cup (150 g) sliced green bell pepper

1 cup (150 g) sliced red bell pepper

1 cup (150 g) sliced yellow bell pepper

1 cup (70 g) sliced mushrooms

1 cup (160 g) thinly sliced onion

1 teaspoon crushed garlic

1 can solid white tuna

¾ cup (175 ml) dry white wine

4 ounces (115 g) romano cheese, grated

½ cup (30 g) chopped fresh parsley

1 pound (455 g) whole wheat linguine

Heat pan. Use enough olive oil to coat the bottom of the pan, about ¼ cup. Add pepper, mushrooms, onion, and garlic. Sauté until crisp-tender. Add remaining oil. Add the tuna and the wine. Stir. Add cheese and parsley. Serve over linguine cooked according to package directions.

Yield: 8 servings

Each with: 129 g water; 504 calories (46% from fat, 15% from protein, 39% from carb); 19 g protein; 26 g total fat; 6 g saturated fat; 16 g monounsaturated fat; 3 g polyunsaturated fat; 50 g carb; 1 g fiber; 3 g sugar; 335 mg phosphorus; 195 mg calcium; 3 mg iron; 192 mg sodium; 401 mg potassium; 1078 IU vitamin A; 14 mg vitamin E; 88 mg vitamin C; 24 mg cholesterol

Tuna and Pasta Salad

This is a great main dish salad for those hot summer days when you don't feel like doing much cooking.

8 ounces (225 g) whole wheat pasta

½ pound (225 g) pea pods

1 can tuna

6 ounces (170 g) artichoke hearts

½ cup (50 g) sliced green olives

½ pound (35 g) sliced fresh mushrooms

½ cup (120 ml) Italian dressing

½ teaspoon lemon pepper

¼ cup (25 g) grated Parmesan cheese

Cook pasta according to package directions; drain and let cool. Cook pea pods 1 minute in boiling water, remove, and let cool. Put pasta and pea pods into a bowl. Drain water from tuna and add to bowl with pea pods. Add artichokes and artichoke liquid, sliced olives, and sliced mushrooms. Combine with pasta and pour dressing over it all. Add lemon pepper and mix well. Sprinkle with Parmesan cheese.

Yield: 4 servings

Each with: 207 g water; 440 calories (28% from fat, 22% from protein, 49% from carb); 26 g protein; 15 g total fat; 3 g saturated fat; 4 g monounsaturated fat; 5 g polyunsaturated fat; 57 g carb; 9 g fiber; 6 g sugar; 394 mg phosphorus; 151 mg calcium; 5 mg iron; 782 mg sodium; 656 mg potassium; 801 IU vitamin A; 10 mg vitamin E; 38 mg vitamin C; 24 mg cholesterol

Tortellini Salad

This delightful Italian salad is based on packaged tortellini. It's delicious as either a main dish or a side dish.

7 ounces cheese tortellini

1 cup (71 g) broccoli florets

½ cup (30 g) finely chopped fresh parsley

1 tablespoon chopped pimento

6 ounces (170 g) marinated artichoke hearts, undrained

¼ cup (25 g) chopped scallions

2 ½ teaspoons chopped fresh basil

½ teaspoon garlic powder

½ cup (120 ml) Italian dressing

8 cherry tomatoes, halved

¼ cup (25 g) sliced ripe olives

¼ cup (25 g) grated Parmesan cheese

Cook tortellini according to package directions. Drain and cool. In large bowl combine all ingredients except tomatoes, olives, and cheese. Cover; refrigerate 4 to 6 hours. Just before serving, add tomatoes and mix lightly. Garnish with olives and sprinkle with Parmesan cheese.

Yield: 4 servings

Each with: 91 g water; 298 calories (41% from fat, 16% from protein, 42% from carb); 13 g protein; 14 g total fat; 4 g saturated fat; 4 g monounsaturated fat; 5 g polyunsaturated fat; 32 g carb; 5 g fiber; 3 g sugar; 108 mg phosphorus; 189 mg calcium; 3 mg iron; 898 mg sodium; 389 mg potassium; 1706 IU vitamin A; 7 mg vitamin E; 41 mg vitamin C; 39 mg cholesterol

Bean and Barley Stew

This is a hearty meatless stew with a whopping 11 grams of fiber.

2 tablespoons (28 ml) olive oil

1 cup (160 g) chopped onion

1 cup (130 g) sliced carrot

1½ cups (105 g) sliced mushrooms

4 cups (684 g) cooked pinto beans, drained

2 cups (480 g) no-salt-added canned tomatoes

⅛ teaspoon Cajun seasoning

¼ teaspoon basil

¼ teaspoon tarragon

¼ teaspoon oregano

¼ teaspoon celery seed

¼ teaspoon thyme

¼ teaspoon marjoram

¼ teaspoon sage

¼ teaspoon black pepper

2 tablespoons (28 ml) soy sauce

½ cup (95 g) brown rice

⅓ cup (65 g) pearl barley

6 cups (1.4 L) vegetable broth

Heat oil in a large kettle: Add onion, carrot, and mushrooms and sauté until softened, about 5 minutes. Add remaining ingredients. Bring to a boil. Reduce heat; simmer 1 to 2 hours until grains are tender.

Yield: 8 servings

Each with: 337 g water; 333 calories (23% from fat, 15% from protein, 62% from carb); 13 g protein; 9 g total fat; 2 g saturated fat; 5 g monounsaturated fat; 2 g polyunsaturated fat; 53 g carb; 11 g fiber; 4 g sugar; 265 mg phosphorus; 102 mg calcium; 4 mg iron; 1126 mg sodium; 753 mg potassium; 2773 IU vitamin A; 0 mg vitamin E; 12 mg vitamin C; 0 mg cholesterol

Broccoli Pasta Sauce

This vegetable-based pasta sauce features fresh broccoli, peppers, and tomatoes.

2 cups (142 g) broccoli florets

⅓ cup (80 ml) olive oil

1 teaspoon minced garlic

4 ounces (120 ml) dry white wine

1 cup (150 g) green bell pepper, chopped small

2 cups (360 g) fresh tomato, chopped small

1 teaspoon black pepper, fresh ground

3 tablespoons grated Parmesan cheese

½ teaspoon Italian seasoning

¾ cup (75 g) pitted, sliced black olives

½ pound (225 g) sliced mushrooms

TIP *To remove skin from tomatoes, place in boiling water for 30 seconds to 1 minute, then in cold water for a couple of minutes.*

Place broccoli in a pot of water; cover and let boil for 5 to 6 minutes. Drain water and set aside. Place oil and garlic in large skillet. Brown garlic on medium-low until light brown. Add wine and bell pepper and cook 6 to 7 minutes over medium heat. Add the tomato, black pepper, Parmesan cheese, and Italian seasoning. Cook 15 minutes uncovered on medium heat, stirring often. Add the broccoli, olives, and mushrooms. Cook 5 minutes on medium heat, covered. Stir often. Remove and serve over whole wheat pasta.

Yield: 6 servings

Each with: 157 g water; 185 calories (74% from fat, 9% from protein, 17% from carb); 4 g protein; 15 g total fat; 2 g saturated fat; 10 g monounsaturated fat; 2 g polyunsaturated fat; 8 g carb; 2 g fiber; 3 g sugar; 93 mg phosphorus; 75 mg calcium; 1 mg iron; 207 mg sodium; 385 mg potassium; 1304 IU vitamin A; 4 mg vitamin E; 50 mg vitamin C; 3 mg cholesterol

12

Main Dishes:
Vegetables and Fruits

Soups, stews, salads, casseroles . . . there are so many ways to incorporate vegetables into main dishes. Some recipes here would probably give you your five servings a day in one dish. Some of these are vegetarian, but there is also a great variety of beef, chicken, and seafood.

Beef Paprikash

The origin of this meal is Hungarian. It's the kind of slow-cooker meal that greets you with a wonderful aroma when you return home from work. Stick a loaf of bread in the bread machine on timed bake and you have an instant dinner.

2 pounds (900 g) round steak, cubed

6 potatoes, cut in ¾-inch (2 cm) pieces

1 cup frozen pearl onions

¼ cup (31 g) flour

1 tablespoon paprika

½ teaspoon black pepper

¼ teaspoon caraway seed

2 cups (475 ml) low-sodium beef broth

1 cup (130 g) no-salt-added frozen peas

½ cup (115 g) sour cream

Add beef, potatoes, onions, flour, and spices to slow cooker. Pour beef broth over. Cover and cook on low 7 to 8 hours. Stir in peas and sour cream. Cover and cook on low about 15 minutes longer, until peas are tender.

Yield: 6 servings

Each with: 472 g water; 590 calories (15% from fat, 36% from protein, 49% from carb); 52 g protein; 10 g total fat; 4 g saturated fat; 4 g monounsaturated fat; 1 g polyunsaturated fat; 72 g carb; 8 g fiber; 5 g sugar; 463 mg phosphorus; 76 mg calcium; 6 mg iron; 148 mg sodium; 1513 mg potassium; 1252 IU vitamin A; 20 mg vitamin E; 28 mg vitamin C; 96 mg cholesterol

Eggplant Stew

This recipe is a nice variation on the beef stew theme, with different vegetables and spices than you probably usually use.

1½ pounds (675 g) beef stew meat, cubed

2 tablespoons (28 ml) olive oil

2 cups (480 g) no-salt-added canned tomatoes

1 cup (160 g) chopped onion

2 tablespoons (32 g) no-salt-added tomato paste

½ teaspoon oregano

½ teaspoon basil

½ teaspoon cumin

¼ teaspoon red pepper flakes

½ teaspoon garlic powder

1 cup (235 ml) water

1 potato, peeled and cubed

1 cup (235 ml) white wine

1 eggplant, peeled and cubed

1 cup (70 g) sliced mushrooms

In a Dutch oven, brown half the beef at a time in the oil. Drain and return all meat to the pan. Add tomatoes, onion, tomato paste, and spices. Stir in water. Bring to a boil. Reduce heat and simmer, covered, for 45 minutes. Add potato and wine. Cover and simmer 10 minutes more. Stir in eggplant and mushrooms. Cover and simmer until meat and veggies are tender, 15 to 20 minutes.

Yield: 6 servings

Each with: 356 g water; 504 calories (50% from fat, 30% from protein, 19% from carb); 36 g protein; 27 g total fat; 9 g saturated fat; 13 g monounsaturated fat; 1 g polyunsaturated fat; 23 g carb; 5 g fiber; 7 g sugar; 283 mg phosphorus; 71 mg calcium; 4 mg iron; 78 mg sodium; 921 mg potassium; 217 IU vitamin A; 0 mg vitamin E; 17 mg vitamin C; 108 mg cholesterol

Italian Meat Sauce

Use this sauce over spaghetti or other pasta or as a cooking sauce for lasagna. The olives and artichokes give it more flavor than many Italian sauces, as well as a big increase in fiber.

1 pound (455 g) hamburger

1 tablespoon Italian seasoning

1 teaspoon minced garlic

1 teaspoon minced onion

1½ cups (105 g) sliced mushrooms

4 cups (1 kg) crushed tomatoes

¼ cup (25 g) sliced black olives

14 ounces (400 g) artichoke hearts, drained

Brown meat with seasoning, garlic, onion, and mushrooms. Drain grease. Add all other ingredients. Heat to boiling; simmer 30 minutes.

Yield: 4 servings

Each with: 321 g water; 447 calories (63% from fat, 21% from protein, 16% from carb); 24 g protein; 32 g total fat; 13 g saturated fat; 14 g monounsaturated fat; 2 g polyunsaturated fat; 18 g carb; 7 g fiber; 1 g sugar; 269 mg phosphorus; 59 mg calcium; 4 mg iron; 218 mg sodium; 952 mg potassium; 1177 IU vitamin A; 0 mg vitamin E; 45 mg vitamin C; 96 mg cholesterol

Pot Roast with Root Vegetables

This is a simple fall pot roast featuring root vegetables and not containing a lot of added ingredients. Cooking it in a covered roasting pan will ensure that the meat is very tender.

2 pound (900 g) beef bottom round roast

4 potatoes, quartered

4 turnips, peeled and cut into quarters

6 carrots, sliced

1 onion, peeled and quartered

1 parsnip, peeled and sliced

2 cups (475 ml) low-sodium beef broth

2 cups (480 g) no-salt-added canned tomatoes

Place all ingredients in large roasting pan. Cover and roast at 350°F (180°C, gas mark 4) until vegetables are done and meat is tender, about 2 hours.

Yield: 8 servings

Each with: 383 g water; 527 calories (38% from fat, 31% from protein, 31% from carb); 40 g protein; 22 g total fat; 9 g saturated fat; 9 g monounsaturated fat; 1 g polyunsaturated fat; 41 g carb; 6 g fiber; 6 g sugar; 370 mg phosphorus; 72 mg calcium; 5 mg iron; 209 mg sodium; 1492 mg potassium; 4280 IU vitamin A; 0 mg vitamin E; 35 mg vitamin C; 108 mg cholesterol

Irish Stew

This has become our traditional meal for St. Patrick's Day.

2 pounds (900 g) beef stew meat

½ teaspoon minced garlic

¼ teaspoon black pepper, fresh ground

1 cup (160 g) halved and sliced onion

12 ounces (355 ml) dark beer

2 cups (475 ml) low-sodium beef broth

3 tablespoons (48 g) no-salt-added tomato paste

2 cups (260 g) sliced carrot

4 potatoes, cut into quarters

2 turnips, cut into quarters

1 teaspoon rosemary

2 bay leaves

¼ cup (32 g) cornstarch

½ cup (120 ml) water

TIP *You could also use lamb in place of the beef if desired.*

Combine all ingredients except the cornstarch and water in a slow cooker and cook on low for 8 hours. Combine the cornstarch and water in a bowl and stir into the stew. Turn to high, cover the slow cooker, and allow the stew to cook an additional 30 minutes, until thickened slightly.

Yield: 8 servings

Each with: 420 g water; 461 calories (24% from fat, 38% from protein, 38% from carb); 43 g protein; 12 g total fat; 4 g saturated fat; 5 g monounsaturated fat; 1 g polyunsaturated fat; 43 g carb; 6 g fiber; 7 g sugar; 387 mg phosphorus; 64 mg calcium; 5 mg iron; 156 mg sodium; 1464 mg potassium; 5489 IU vitamin A; 0 mg vitamin E; 30 mg vitamin C; 127 mg cholesterol

Shepherd's Pie with Cornbread Crust

This is a meal in a pan. The cornbread on the bottom adds some substance to this while adding minimal fat and sodium.

1 pound (455 g) ground turkey

1 cup (160 g) chopped onion

12 ounces (340 g) mixed vegetables

3 cups (675 g) instant mashed potatoes, prepared according to package directions

4 ounces (113 g) shredded Cheddar cheese

Cornbread Crust

1 cup (120 g) whole wheat pastry flour

½ cup (70 g) cornmeal

1 tablespoon sugar

2 teaspoons baking powder

1 cup (235 ml) skim milk

1 egg

2 tablespoons (28 ml) canola oil

Sauté turkey and onion. Drain. Cook vegetables until almost done. Drain. To make crust, stir together flour, cornmeal, sugar, and baking powder. Combine milk, egg, and oil. Stir into dry ingredients until just mixed. Spread cornbread in the bottom of a 9 × 13-inch (23 × 33 cm) baking dish sprayed with nonstick vegetable oil spray. On top of cornbread, layer meat mixture, veggies, and potatoes. Sprinkle with cheese. Bake at 425°F (220°C, gas mark 7) for 20 minutes.

Yield: 8 servings

Each with: 131 g water; 417 calories (27% from fat, 27% from protein, 46% from carb); 28 g protein; 13 g total fat; 5 g saturated fat; 3 g monounsaturated fat; 3 g polyunsaturated fat; 48 g carb; 6 g fiber; 5 g sugar; 390 mg phosphorus; 258 mg calcium; 3 mg iron; 320 mg sodium; 672 mg potassium; 2091 IU vitamin A; 66 mg vitamin E; 21 mg vitamin C; 85 mg cholesterol

Taco Casserole

Call it Mexican lasagna if you wish, but in this case corn tortillas substitute for the noodles and are layered with beef and beans.

1 pound (455 g) ground beef

1 cup (160 g) chopped onion

1 cup (150 g) chopped green bell pepper

1 teaspoon minced garlic

8 ounces (225 g) no-salt-added tomato sauce

2 cups (480 g) no-salt-added canned tomatoes

1 tablespoon chili powder

½ teaspoon oregano

½ teaspoon cumin

12 corn tortillas

2 cups (512 g) no-salt-added kidney beans

¾ cup (90 g) shredded Cheddar cheese

In a skillet over medium heat, sauté the ground beef, onion, bell pepper, and garlic until the beef is done. Drain off excess fat. Add tomato sauce, tomatoes, and spices. Simmer mixture for 2 minutes. Place a layer of 4 tortillas in the bottom of a 9 × 13-inch (23 × 33 cm) baking pan that has been sprayed with nonstick vegetable oil spray. Place a layer of the beef mixture over top, then 4 more tortillas, the beans, the final 4 tortillas, and the rest of the beef mixture. Bake at 350°F (180°C, gas mark 4) for 30 minutes. Sprinkle with cheese and return to oven until cheese has melted.

Yield: 6 servings

Each with: 258 g water; 443 calories (33% from fat, 25% from protein, 42% from carb); 29 g protein; 17 g total fat; 7 g saturated fat; 6 g monounsaturated fat; 1 g polyunsaturated fat; 47 g carb; 11 g fiber; 5 g sugar; 465 mg phosphorus; 285 mg calcium; 5 mg iron; 374 mg sodium; 884 mg potassium; 863 IU vitamin A; 43 mg vitamin E; 34 mg vitamin C; 63 mg cholesterol

Italian Dinner Salad

This is a meal on a plate. It may be "only" a salad, but I guarantee you won't walk away from the table hungry.

4 cups (220 g) finely chopped romaine lettuce

2 cups (180 g) finely chopped cabbage

1 cup (150 g) chopped green bell pepper

1 cup (150 g) chopped red bell pepper

8 ounces (225 g) dry salami, cut up

2 cups (328 g) cooked chickpeas, drained

4 ounces (115 g) black olives

4 ounces (115 g) Swiss cheese, cut up

½ cup (50 g) thinly sliced celery

6 ounces (170 g) boneless chicken breast, cooked and chopped

Dressing

½ cup (160 ml) olive oil

2 tablespoons (28 ml) red wine vinegar

1 teaspoon (5 ml) balsamic vinegar

½ teaspoon minced garlic

1 teaspoon lemon juice

1 tablespoon (15 ml) Dijon mustard

1 teaspoon sugar

2 tablespoons Italian seasoning

⅛ teaspoon black pepper, fresh ground

Divide lettuce between 6 plates. Arrange other vegetables, meats, and cheese over lettuce. Shake dressing ingredients together in a jar with a screw-top lid and drizzle over salads.

Yield: 6 servings

Each with: 233 g water; 552 calories (61% from fat, 20% from protein, 20% from carb); 27 g protein; 38 g total fat; 11 g saturated fat; 22 g monounsaturated fat; 4 g polyunsaturated fat; 28 g carb; 7 g fiber; 4 g sugar; 347 mg phosphorus; 280 mg calcium; 4 mg iron; 1218 mg sodium; 638 mg potassium; 3092 IU vitamin A; 43 mg vitamin E; 75 mg vitamin C; 70 mg cholesterol

Asian Chicken Soup

This is an easy-to-make soup that can cook while you are running errands. It's a little different flavor than most soups, which can be a welcome change if you are tired of the same old thing. (Or am I the only one who gets bored?)

2 cups (140 g) sliced mushrooms

1½ cups sliced bok choy

1 cup (160 g) chopped onion

1 cup (130 g) sliced carrot

1 pound (455 g) boneless skinless chicken breasts, cut in 1-inch (2.5-cm) pieces

1 cup (190 g) brown rice

4 cups (950 ml) low-sodium chicken broth

¼ cup (60 ml) reduced-sodium soy sauce

1 tablespoon (15 ml) sesame oil

½ teaspoon garlic powder

1 teaspoon ground ginger

Place vegetables in bottom of slow cooker. Place chicken pieces on top. Sprinkle rice over top. Combine remaining ingredients and pour over. Cook on low for 8 to 10 hours or on high for 4 to 5 hours.

Yield: 6 servings

Each with: 322 g water; 199 calories (21% from fat, 47% from protein, 32% from carb); 24 g protein; 5 g total fat; 1 g saturated fat; 2 g monounsaturated fat; 2 g polyunsaturated fat; 16 g carb; 2 g fiber; 3 g sugar; 278 mg phosphorus; 53 mg calcium; 2 mg iron; 481 mg sodium; 596 mg potassium; 4385 IU vitamin A; 5 mg vitamin E; 13 mg vitamin C; 44 mg cholesterol

Chicken and Sausage Pie

This is an old-fashioned country-style dish with both chicken and sausage and a crispy cornmeal crust.

2 potatoes, cut in ½-inch (1-cm) pieces

½ pound (225 g) breakfast sausage

½ pound (225 g) boneless skinless chicken breasts

1 cup (160 g) diced onion

½ teaspoon garlic powder

½ cup (60 g) diced celery

½ cup (65 g) diced carrot

2 tablespoons (16 g) flour

¼ cup (60 ml) white wine

1½ cups (355 ml) low-sodium chicken broth

1 teaspoon thyme

1 teaspoon poultry seasoning

Cornmeal Crust

¾ cup (90 g) flour

½ cup (70 g) cornmeal

¼ cup (55 g) unsalted butter

2 tablespoons (28 ml) cold water

Boil potatoes until just soft. Drain. Crumble the sausage and place in a large, deep pan. Add the chicken. Cook over medium heat. Add onion, garlic powder, celery, and carrot and cook about 5 minutes or until vegetables are tender. Stir together flour, wine, and broth. Add to pan and bring to a boil. Turn heat to low, add thyme, poultry seasoning, and potatoes and cook until thickened and bubbly. Pour into 8 × 8-inch (20 × 20 cm) baking dish and set aside. To make the crust, mix flour and cornmeal in a large bowl. Cut in butter until texture resembles coarse meal. Sprinkle water over dough and knead with hands, adding only enough to make the dough form a ball. Refrigerate dough 30 minutes to 24 hours. Roll dough on a floured surface to ¼-inch (0.5 cm) thickness. Place dough over top of filling. Bake pie at 375°F (190°C, gas mark 5) for 30 minutes or until crust is lightly browned and filling is bubbly.

Yield: 6 servings

Each with: 204 g water; 344 calories (31% from fat, 11% from protein, 58% from carb); 9 g protein; 12 g total fat; 6 g saturated fat; 4 g monounsaturated fat; 1 g polyunsaturated fat; 50 g carb; 4 g fiber; 3 g sugar; 136 mg phosphorus; 38 mg calcium; 2 mg iron; 114 mg sodium; 568 mg potassium; 2113 IU vitamin A; 64 mg vitamin E; 11 mg vitamin C; 31 mg cholesterol

Chicken and Snow Peas

This is a fairly traditional Chinese-style recipe, similar to dishes like moo goo gai pan.

1 pound (455 g) boneless chicken breasts

2 tablespoons (16 g) cornstarch, divided

1 egg white

1 tablespoon sherry

½ teaspoon white pepper

8 ounces (225 g) mushrooms, sliced

1½ cups (355 ml) low-sodium chicken broth

1 tablespoon sliced gingerroot

2 tablespoons (28 ml) cold water

5 tablespoons (75 ml) olive oil, divided

¼ cup (25 g) sliced scallions

¼ cup (25 g) sliced celery

4 ounces (115 g) snow peas

¼ cup (31 g) sliced water chestnuts

1 cup (70 g) coarsely shredded napa cabbage

In a bowl, combine the chicken, 1 tablespoon of the cornstarch, the egg white, sherry, and pepper. Marinate at least 15 minutes. Simmer mushrooms in broth 15 minutes. Drain and reserve liquid. Simmer gingerroot in broth until ready to use. Mix remaining cornstarch with water. Shake well to thoroughly dissolve. Heat 3 tablespoons (45 ml) oil in a wok or heavy skillet. Add chicken and cook, stirring, just until pieces separate and chicken is no longer pink. Drain into a sieve over a bowl. Add remaining oil to wok. Add scallions, celery, snow peas, water chestnuts, mushrooms, and

(continued on page 224)

cabbage and stir-fry for 2 minutes. Remove ginger pieces from chicken broth. Add broth to wok. Bring to a boil. Return chicken to wok. Add water-cornstarch mixture. Cook, stirring, until thickened. Serve over steamed rice.

Yield: 4 servings

Each with: 235 g water; 251 calories (64% from fat, 16% from protein, 20% from carb); 10 g protein; 18 g total fat; 3 g saturated fat; 13 g monounsaturated fat; 2 g polyunsaturated fat; 13 g carb; 2 g fiber; 3 g sugar; 137 mg phosphorus; 38 mg calcium; 2 mg iron; 66 mg sodium; 474 mg potassium; 473 IU vitamin A; 1 mg vitamin E; 21 mg vitamin C; 11 mg cholesterol

Chicken Corn Chowder

This is a good soup for a cool fall day. Add bread and you will have a meal.

6 potatoes, peeled and diced

1½ cups (195 g) sliced carrot

1 cup (160 g) chopped onion

4 cups (950 ml) low-sodium chicken broth

12 ounces (340 g) frozen corn

2 cups (280 g) cooked, diced chicken

1 cup (235 ml) skim milk

¼ teaspoon garlic powder

½ teaspoon black pepper

1 cup (225 g) instant mashed potatoes

Cook potatoes, carrot, and onion in broth until soft. Add corn and chicken. Cook 5 minutes longer. Add milk, garlic powder, pepper, and mashed potatoes. Stir until potatoes are dissolved. Heat through.

Yield: 6 servings

Each with: 548 g water; 498 calories (10% from fat, 21% from protein, 69% from carb); 27 g protein; 6 g total fat; 2 g saturated fat; 2 g monounsaturated fat; 2 g polyunsaturated fat; 89 g carb; 9 g fiber; 8 g sugar; 391 mg phosphorus; 117 mg calcium; 2 mg iron; 169 mg sodium; 1716 mg potassium; 5617 IU vitamin A; 32 mg vitamin E; 39 mg vitamin C; 42 mg cholesterol

Chicken-Pasta Stir-Fry

This is an Asian-flavored use for leftover chicken that is quick and easy to make.

2 tablespoons (28 ml) olive oil

1 cup (160 g) coarsely chopped onion

1 cup (150 g) coarsely chopped bell pepper

2 cups (142 g) broccoli florets

1 teaspoon minced garlic

2 cups (280 g) cubed cooked chicken

8 ounces (225 g) whole wheat pasta, cooked

¼ cup (60 ml) soy sauce

3 tablespoons (45 ml) rice wine

1½ tablespoons (19 g) sugar

1½ tablespoons (25 ml) Worcestershire sauce

½ teaspoon ginger

Heat oil in wok or skillet. Sauté vegetables in hot oil until just tender. Stir in chicken and pasta. Mix together remaining ingredients and stir in until meat, pasta, and vegetables are well coated.

Yield: 4 servings

Each with: 128 g water; 343 calories (20% from fat, 13% from protein, 67% from carb); 11 g protein; 8 g total fat; 1 g saturated fat; 2 g monounsaturated fat; 4 g polyunsaturated fat; 59 g carb; 6 g fiber; 8 g sugar; 219 mg phosphorus; 57 mg calcium; 3 mg iron; 972 mg sodium; 470 mg potassium; 2238 IU vitamin A; 0 mg vitamin E; 94 mg vitamin C; 0 mg cholesterol

Chicken Polynesian

This variation of sweet-and-sour chicken is made different by the citrus fruit sections in the sauce.

2 chicken breasts, halved

4 chicken thighs

1 grapefruit

3 oranges

½ cup (120 ml) light corn syrup

¼ cup (60 ml) mustard

¼ cup (60 ml) cider vinegar

¼ teaspoon Tabasco sauce

⅛ teaspoon ginger

2 teaspoons cornstarch

1 tablespoon (15 ml) water

9 ounces (255 g) crushed pineapple

⅓ cup (36 g) slivered toasted almonds

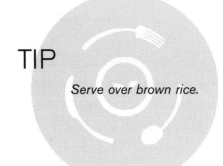

TIP

Serve over brown rice.

Place chicken skin side down in shallow baking dish. Section grapefruit, holding over bowl to catch juice. Measure juice. Section oranges, adding enough orange juice to grapefruit juice to make ½ cup (120 ml). In saucepan, blend corn syrup, mustard, vinegar, Tabasco, ginger, and fruit juices. Add cornstarch mixed with water; bring to boil. Boil 5 minutes, stirring constantly. Brush chicken with this mixture. Bake at 350°F (180°C, gas mark 4) for 1 hour, basting with sauce occasionally and turning once. Add crushed pineapple, orange and grapefruit sections, and almonds to remaining sauce. Heat; pour over chicken for last 5 minutes of baking time.

Yield: 8 servings

Each with: 159 g water; 223 calories (22% from fat, 19% from protein, 59% from carb); 11 g protein; 6 g total fat; 1 g saturated fat; 3 g monounsaturated fat; 1 g polyunsaturated fat; 34 g carb; 3 g fiber; 19 g sugar; 97 mg phosphorus; 62 mg calcium; 1 mg iron; 39 mg sodium; 341 mg potassium; 573 IU vitamin A; 4 mg vitamin E; 54 mg vitamin C; 26 mg cholesterol

Indian-Flavored Chicken

This is similar to the recipe for country captain soup, a curried chicken dish that supposedly came to England originally from India. The curry powder I use most often is a Blue Mountain brand from Jamaica that I get at a local Hispanic market. It's milder than most Asian curries, so if you can't find something similar, you may want to reduce the amount.

6 chicken thighs

2 cups (480 g) no-salt-added canned tomatoes

1 cup (160 g) chopped onion

½ teaspoon garlic powder

1 cup (130 g) frozen peas

1½ tablespoons curry powder

Place chicken in a 9 × 13-inch (23 × 33 cm) baking dish. Mix other ingredients together and pour over chicken. Bake at 350°F (180°C, gas mark 4) until chicken is done, about 45 minutes.

Yield: 6 servings

Each with: 152 g water; 100 calories (18% from fat, 41% from protein, 41% from carb); 11 g protein; 2 g total fat; 0 g saturated fat; 1 g monounsaturated fat; 1 g polyunsaturated fat; 11 g carb; 3 g fiber; 4 g sugar; 119 mg phosphorus; 49 mg calcium; 2 mg iron; 67 mg sodium; 340 mg potassium; 696 IU vitamin A; 8 mg vitamin E; 12 mg vitamin C; 34 mg cholesterol

Italian Chicken Soup

Here's one more cook-ahead meal for your slow cooker. This one is good either as a full meal or just to have on hand for lunches.

1 pound (455 g) boneless chicken breasts, cubed

4 cups (950 ml) low-sodium chicken broth

2 cups (480 g) low-sodium tomatoes

(continued on page 228)

4 ounces (115 g) mushrooms, sliced

½ cup (65 g) sliced carrot

½ cup (56 g) sliced zucchini

½ cup (62 g) frozen green beans

6 ounces (170 g) frozen spinach

½ teaspoon garlic powder

1 teaspoon basil

½ teaspoon oregano

Combine ingredients and place in slow cooker. Cover and cook on low 8 to 10 hours or on high 4 to 5 hours.

Yield: 6 servings

Each with: 305 g water; 78 calories (17% from fat, 40% from protein, 43% from carb); 9 g protein; 2 g total fat; 0 g saturated fat; 1 g monounsaturated fat; 0 g polyunsaturated fat; 10 g carb; 3 g fiber; 4 g sugar; 133 mg phosphorus; 73 mg calcium; 2 mg iron; 101 mg sodium; 568 mg potassium; 5706 IU vitamin A; 1 mg vitamin E; 23 mg vitamin C; 7 mg cholesterol

Moussaka

This variation of the typical Greek dish uses ground turkey rather than the more common lamb.

1½ pounds (675 g) eggplant, peeled and sliced

½ pound (225 g) ground turkey

1 cup (160 g) chopped onion

2 teaspoons minced garlic

½ teaspoon cinnamon

½ teaspoon oregano

1 cup (235 ml) low-sodium chicken broth

⅔ cup (110 g) cooked rice

8 ounces (225 g) no-salt-added tomato sauce

2 tablespoons (28 g) unsalted butter

¼ cup (30 g) whole wheat pastry flour

1½ cups (355 ml) skim milk

2 eggs, beaten

¼ teaspoon nutmeg

Coat a shallow 2-quart (2-L) baking dish with nonstick vegetable oil spray. Bring 3 cups (710 ml) water to boil in a large nonstick skillet. Add eggplant, cover, reduce heat, and simmer 10 minutes or until crisp-tender. Remove to paper towels to drain. Wipe skillet. Add turkey, onion, and garlic. Cook until turkey is no longer pink. Stir in cinnamon and oregano, then broth and rice. Cover and simmer 10 minutes, stirring 2 or 3 times. Stir in tomato sauce. Remove from heat. Melt butter in a 2-quart (2-L) saucepan. Whisk in flour and cook, stirring 1 to 2 minutes, without letting mixture brown. Gradually whisk in milk. Cook, whisking constantly, 4 to 5 minutes until thickened and smooth. Whisk about one-third of the hot mixture into beaten eggs and then whisk the egg mixture into the remaining sauce. Remove from heat; stir in nutmeg. Heat oven to 350°F (180°C, gas mark 4). To assemble: Cover bottom of prepared baking dish with half the eggplant slices. Spoon on all the filling and cover with remaining eggplant. Pour on sauce. Bake 20 to 25 minutes or until hot and bubbly and top is lightly golden.

Yield: 4 servings

Each with: 429 g water; 399 calories (25% from fat, 22% from protein, 53% from carb); 23 g protein; 11 g total fat; 5 g saturated fat; 3 g monounsaturated fat; 1 g polyunsaturated fat; 54 g carb; 9 g fiber; 9 g sugar; 378 mg phosphorus; 217 mg calcium; 4 mg iron; 434 mg sodium; 1072 mg potassium; 755 IU vitamin A; 143 mg vitamin E; 12 mg vitamin C; 155 mg cholesterol

Slow-Cooker Chicken Curry

I'm fond of curries. They make a particularly nice slow-cooker meal because they fill the house with such a great aroma for you to come home to. This one calls for a number of spices that are typical of curry powder.

5 medium potatoes, diced

1 cup (150 g) coarsely chopped green bell pepper

1 cup (160 g) coarsely chopped onion

1 pound (455 g) boneless chicken breasts, cubed

2 cups (480 g) no-salt-added canned tomatoes

1 tablespoon coriander

1½ tablespoons paprika

1 tablespoon ginger

¼ teaspoon red pepper flakes

½ teaspoon turmeric

¼ teaspoon cinnamon

⅛ teaspoon cloves

1 cup (235 ml) low-sodium chicken broth

2 tablespoons (28 ml) cold water

4 tablespoons (32 g) cornstarch

TIP *If you have a favorite curry powder on the shelf, you can substitute a couple of tablespoons of that for the other spices.*

Place potatoes, bell pepper, and onion in slow cooker. Place chicken on top. Mix together tomatoes, spices, and chicken broth. Pour over chicken. Cook on low 8 to 10 hours or on high 5 to 6 hours. Remove meat and vegetables. Turn heat to high. Stir cornstarch into water. Add to cooker. Cook until sauce is slightly thickened, about 15 to 20 minutes. Stir meat and vegetables into thickened sauce.

Yield: 5 servings

Each with: 440 g water; 351 calories (4% from fat, 12% from protein, 84% from carb); 11 g protein; 2 g total fat; 0 g saturated fat; 0 g monounsaturated fat; 1 g polyunsaturated fat; 76 g carb; 8 g fiber; 7 g sugar; 202 mg phosphorus; 78 mg calcium; 3 mg iron; 54 mg sodium; 1407 mg potassium; 1352 IU vitamin A; 1 mg vitamin E; 61 mg vitamin C; 9 mg cholesterol

Turkey Vegetable Sauté

This turkey and vegetable sauce has just a hint of Mexican flavor. I particularly like this one over whole wheat spaghetti, but it's also good over brown rice.

1 pound (455 g) ground turkey

1 cup (160 g) onion, cut in rings

1 cup (130 g) sliced carrot

½ cup (50 g) sliced celery

½ cup (75 g) chunked green bell pepper

4 ounces (115 g) mushrooms, sliced

½ teaspoon cumin

½ teaspoon garlic salt

1 cup (180 g) chopped tomato

15 black olives, halved

3 slices low-sodium bacon, cooked and broken into pieces (optional)

Brown turkey. Add onion, carrot, celery, bell pepper, and mushrooms; add cumin and garlic salt and cook over medium heat until vegetables are crisp-tender. Add tomatoes, olives, and bacon and heat through.

Yield: 6 servings

Each with: 161 g water; 197 calories (32% from fat, 52% from protein, 17% from carb); 25 g protein; 7 g total fat; 2 g saturated fat; 2 g monounsaturated fat; 1 g polyunsaturated fat; 8 g carb; 2 g fiber; 3 g sugar; 226 mg phosphorus; 50 mg calcium; 2 mg iron; 217 mg sodium; 521 mg potassium; 3873 IU vitamin A; 0 mg vitamin E; 20 mg vitamin C; 62 mg cholesterol

Chowder from the Sea

This one came about on a weekend when I didn't want to spend my day cooking and I knew everyone was going to be available for dinner at a different time. The answer...the slow cooker and a fish and shrimp soup that people could ladle up whenever they were ready.

½ pound (225 g) cod or other white fish, cubed

½ pound (225 g) shrimp, peeled

4 potatoes, shredded

1 cup (110 g) shredded carrot

½ cup (80 g) finely chopped onion

½ cup (75 g) finely chopped red bell pepper

½ cup (60 g) finely chopped celery

2 cups (475 ml) low-sodium chicken broth

1 cup (235 ml) skim milk

1 teaspoon seafood seasoning

Place fish and shrimp in slow cooker. Add vegetables. Pour broth over meat and vegetables. Add milk and seasoning. Stir to mix. Cook on low 8 to 10 hours.

Yield: 6 servings

Each with: 378 g water; 289 calories (5% from fat, 30% from protein, 65% from carb); 22 g protein; 2 g total fat; 0 g saturated fat; 0 g monounsaturated fat; 1 g polyunsaturated fat; 48 g carb; 5 g fiber; 4 g sugar; 295 mg phosphorus; 115 mg calcium; 2 mg iron; 186 mg sodium; 1161 mg potassium; 4209 IU vitamin A; 55 mg vitamin E; 35 mg vitamin C; 91 mg cholesterol

Niçoise Salad

This main-dish salad lets diners choose their ingredients from a central platter. The ingredients are typical of the type of salad served in Nice, France.

1 ounce (28 g) anchovies, minced

2 teaspoons Dijon mustard

3 tablespoons (45 ml) red wine vinegar

¼ cup (60 ml) olive oil

4 cups (20 g) butter lettuce

1 can tuna, drained

2 eggs, hard cooked and halved

1 large tomato, cut into wedges

2 medium potatoes, peeled, cooked, and sliced

½ cup (50 g) green beans, cooked, drained, and cooled

½ cup (75 g) sliced and slivered green bell pepper

½ cup (80 g) red onion, cut in rounds

½ cup (50 g) black olives, drained

½ cup (35 g) thinly sliced mushrooms

14 ounces (400 g) artichoke hearts, drained

½ cup (17 g) alfalfa sprouts

Combine first 4 ingredients to make dressing. Line a platter with butter lettuce. Place tuna in center. Arrange rest of ingredients in groups around tuna. Either serve as a salad or stuff pita bread halves with any ingredients from platter. Drizzle with dressing.

Yield: 4 servings

Each with: 465 g water; 459 calories (40% from fat, 21% from protein, 39% from carb); 25 g protein; 21 g total fat; 4 g saturated fat; 13 g monounsaturated fat; 3 g polyunsaturated fat; 47 g carb; 11 g fiber; 6 g sugar; 394 mg phosphorus; 130 mg calcium; 5 mg iron; 568 mg sodium; 1630 mg potassium; 2695 IU vitamin A; 42 mg vitamin E; 47 mg vitamin C; 143 mg cholesterol

Shrimp and Corn Chowder

This soup tastes richer than it is, with low fat and a nice dose of fiber.

2 slices low-sodium bacon, cut in ½-inch (1 cm) pieces

1 cup (160 g) chopped onion

¼ cup (25 g) sliced celery

6 potatoes, cut in ½-inch (1 cm) pieces

12 ounces (340 g) frozen corn

4 cups (950 ml) low-sodium chicken broth

¼ cup (30 g) whole wheat pastry flour

12 ounces (340 g) shrimp

¼ teaspoon white pepper

½ teaspoon thyme

2 cups (475 ml) skim milk

Cook bacon in Dutch oven, stirring frequently, until crisp. Stir in onion, celery, potatoes, and corn. Cook 5 to 6 minutes, stirring often, until onion and celery are soft. Beat in broth and flour with whisk. Heat to boiling, reduce heat, and simmer about 15 minutes, until potatoes are soft. Stir in remaining ingredients and cook 5 to 6 minutes longer, until shrimp are pink and firm.

Yield: 6 servings

Each with: 574 g water; 469 calories (8% from fat, 22% from protein, 70% from carb); 27 g protein; 4 g total fat; 1 g saturated fat; 1 g monounsaturated fat; 1 g polyunsaturated fat; 84 g carb; 8 g fiber; 6 g sugar; 467 mg phosphorus; 190 mg calcium; 3 mg iron; 236 mg sodium; 1614 mg potassium; 420 IU vitamin A; 81 mg vitamin E; 30 mg vitamin C; 91 mg cholesterol

Vegetable and Ham Chowder

It's kind of hard to describe the flavor of this filling soup. The cumin gives it a bit of a southwestern style, but then I like cumin and add it to all kinds of things.

1 tablespoon unsalted butter

1 cup (150 g) coarsely chopped red bell pepper

1 cup (160 g) chopped onion

16 ounces (455 g) frozen corn

1 cup (235 ml) low-sodium chicken broth

4 ounces (113 g) ham, cubed

½ teaspoon ground cumin

¼ teaspoon white pepper

3 cups (710 ml) fat-free evaporated milk, divided

⅓ cup (40 g) whole wheat pastry flour

⅛ teaspoon Tabasco sauce

In large saucepan, melt butter; sauté pepper and onion over medium heat for 5 minutes or until tender. Stir in corn, broth, ham, cumin, and white pepper. Cook for 5 more minutes, stirring occasionally, until corn is cooked. Pour ½ cup (120 ml) evaporated milk into bowl; whisk in flour until well blended. Add remaining evaporated milk; mix well. Slowly pour into saucepan. Increase heat to medium-high; cook, stirring constantly for 5 minutes until mixture comes to a boil and thickens. Boil for 1 minute; add Tabasco.

Yield: 6 servings

Each with: 258 g water; 260 calories (17% from fat, 27% from protein, 56% from carb); 18 g protein; 5 g total fat; 2 g saturated fat; 2 g monounsaturated fat; 1 g polyunsaturated fat; 38 g carb; 4 g fiber; 19 g sugar; 410 mg phosphorus; 388 mg calcium; 2 mg iron; 376 mg sodium; 852 mg potassium; 1503 IU vitamin A; 167 mg vitamin E; 40 mg vitamin C; 18 mg cholesterol

Borscht

Borscht is a traditional Russian or eastern European soup, but one you don't see that often in the United States. Which is a shame, because it tastes good and has a lot of good nutrition.

2 cups (140 g) finely shredded cabbage

½ cup (80 g) chopped onion

16-ounce (455 g) can of beets

3 cups (355 ml) low-sodium chicken broth

3 tablespoons (42 g) unsalted butter

2 teaspoons caraway seeds

1 teaspoon sugar

3 tablespoons (45 ml) lemon juice

Cook cabbage about 10 minutes in boiling water. Sauté onion in a soup pot a few minutes without browning. Drain and chop beets, reserving liquid. Add chicken broth to onion. When it comes to a boil, add cabbage and the water in which it cooked. Add chopped beets, butter, beet juice, and caraway seeds and simmer for 10 minutes. Add lemon juice. Serve with sour cream.

Yield: 6 servings

Each with: 231 g water; 113 calories (50% from fat, 13% from protein, 38% from carb); 4 g protein; 7 g total fat; 4 g saturated fat; 2 g monounsaturated fat; 0 g polyunsaturated fat; 12 g carb; 3 g fiber; 7 g sugar; 67 mg phosphorus; 38 mg calcium; 2 mg iron; 190 mg sodium; 306 mg potassium; 229 IU vitamin A; 48 mg vitamin E; 19 mg vitamin C; 15 mg cholesterol

Cream of Broccoli Soup

I suppose this really should be called cream of vegetable soup, but the broccoli seems to dominate.

20 ounces (560 g) frozen mixed vegetables

10 ounces (280 g) frozen broccoli, chopped fine

8 slices low-sodium bacon

¼ cup (40 g) chopped onion

¼ cup (30 g) whole wheat pastry flour

4 cups (950 ml) skim milk

Boil frozen mixed vegetables and broccoli. Set aside to drain. Fry bacon until crispy. Set aside bacon. Pour enough bacon grease in soup pan to cover bottom of pan. Simmer onion until clear. Mix in flour and then add milk. Stir well. Add vegetables and bacon. Simmer until soup is thickened. Add salt and pepper to taste. This soup has better flavor when eaten the next day.

Yield: 6 servings

Each with: 276 g water; 219 calories (21% from fat, 28% from protein, 51% from carb); 15 g protein; 5 g total fat; 2 g saturated fat; 2 g monounsaturated fat; 1 g polyunsaturated fat; 28 g carb; 6 g fiber; 4 g sugar; 331 mg phosphorus; 278 mg calcium; 2 mg iron; 363 mg sodium; 616 mg potassium; 4907 IU vitamin A; 101 mg vitamin E; 24 mg vitamin C; 15 mg cholesterol

Florentine Soup

This spinach soup is a creamy delight. Cream cheese makes it thicker and richer.

1 cup (70 g) sliced mushrooms

½ cup (80 g) chopped onion

1 tablespoon unsalted butter

1 tablespoon flour

2 cups (475 ml) skim milk

12 ounces (340 g) fresh spinach

¼ teaspoon garlic powder

8 ounces (225 g) cream cheese

Sauté mushrooms and onion in butter until onion is translucent. Stir in flour. Slowly add milk while stirring. Add spinach and garlic powder. Cook until spinach is tender. (Do not overcook!) Stir in cream cheese until melted and warm. You may want to thin with up to 1 cup more of milk. Serve warm.

Yield: 8 servings

Each with: 125 g water; 160 calories (63% from fat, 16% from protein, 20% from carb); 7 g protein; 12 g total fat; 7 g saturated fat; 3 g monounsaturated fat; 1 g polyunsaturated fat; 8 g carb; 2 g fiber; 1 g sugar; 132 mg phosphorus; 179 mg calcium; 1 mg iron; 163 mg sodium; 319 mg potassium; 5680 IU vitamin A; 151 mg vitamin E; 3 mg vitamin C; 36 mg cholesterol

Fresh Tomato Meat Sauce

This recipe is a little different variation of spaghetti sauce. It makes a large batch. You can freeze the leftovers if you like. As you might guess, this was developed when the tomatoes in the garden were producing in quantity.

1 pound (455 g) ground beef

½ pound (225 g) Italian sausage

1 onion, chopped

1 green bell pepper, chopped

½ pound (225 g) mushrooms, sliced

15 tomatoes

1 tablespoon minced garlic

2 tablespoons (28 ml) olive oil

6 cans no-salt-added tomato paste

2 tablespoons oregano

1 tablespoon basil

2 tablespoons parsley

½ cup (120 ml) red wine

Crumble beef and sausage into a large skillet. Add onion, pepper, and mushrooms. Cook until meat is done. Immerse tomatoes in boiling water for about 30 seconds. Drain, peel, and chop finely. In a large Dutch oven, sauté garlic in olive oil until lightly browned, about 2 minutes. Add tomatoes, tomato paste, spices, wine, and meat/veggie mixture. Simmer slowly until desired thickness, 1 to 2 hours.

Yield: 8 servings

Each with: 180 g water; 404 calories (48% from fat, 26% from protein, 26% from carb); 26 g protein; 22 g total fat; 7 g saturated fat; 10 g monounsaturated fat; 2 g polyunsaturated fat; 27 g carb; 6 g fiber; 16 g sugar; 299 mg phosphorus; 79 mg calcium; 6 mg iron; 1253 mg sodium; 1689 mg potassium; 2100 IU vitamin A; 0 mg vitamin E; 31 mg vitamin C; 70 mg cholesterol

Gazpacho

This light and refreshing cold soup is perfect for a summer evening.

48 ounces (1.4 L) tomato juice

1 cup (100 g) chopped celery

1 cup (180 g) chopped tomato

1 cup (135 g) chopped cucumber

1 cup (150 g) chopped green bell pepper

½ cup (80 g) finely chopped onion

½ cup (50 g) finely chopped scallions

¼ cup finely chopped fresh cilantro

¼ cup (60 ml) white wine vinegar

¼ cup (60 ml) lemon juice

2 teaspoons Tabasco sauce, to taste

1 tablespoon (15 ml) olive oil

Combine all of the above ingredients in large container. Serve ice cold with croutons and grated Parmesan cheese.

Yield: 4 servings

Each with: 500 g water; 130 calories (24% from fat, 11% from protein, 65% from carb); 4 g protein; 4 g total fat; 1 g saturated fat; 3 g monounsaturated fat; 1 g polyunsaturated fat; 24 g carb; 4 g fiber; 16 g sugar; 105 mg phosphorus; 74 mg calcium; 2 mg iron; 78 mg sodium; 1148 mg potassium; 2463 IU vitamin A; 0 mg vitamin E; 110 mg vitamin C; 0 mg cholesterol

New England Corn Chowder

This is a warming and filling soup. Add a nice slice of fresh-baked whole wheat bread and you couldn't ask for a better dinner.

3 slices low-sodium bacon, diced

$^2/_3$ cup (110 g) chopped onion

2 potatoes

3 cups (355 ml) skim milk

15 ounces (420 g) creamed corn

10 ounces (280 g) frozen corn

2 tablespoons (28 g) unsalted butter

Cook bacon pieces in large soup pot. Remove bacon and add onion. Sauté until translucent. Peel and dice potatoes. Bring to slow boil in separate pot for 20 minutes. Warm milk in separate pan. Add creamed corn to bacon and onion. Add corn and warm milk. Drain diced potatoes and add to soup.

Yield: 4 servings

Each with: 394 g water; 360 calories (24% from fat, 17% from protein, 60% from carb); 16 g protein; 10 g total fat; 5 g saturated fat; 3 g monounsaturated fat; 1 g polyunsaturated fat; 56 g carb; 6 g fiber; 5 g sugar; 424 mg phosphorus; 292 mg calcium; 2 mg iron; 194 mg sodium; 1441 mg potassium; 715 IU vitamin A; 161 mg vitamin E; 25 mg vitamin C; 26 mg cholesterol

Old-Fashioned Vegetable Soup

This is a summer vegetable soup full of good things from the garden.

2 cups (480 g) no-salt-added canned tomatoes

1 quart (946 ml) low-sodium chicken broth

½ cup (80 g) chopped onion

½ cup (50 g) chopped celery

2 bay leaves

2 ½ teaspoons basil, divided

½ teaspoon black pepper

2 cups (140 g) coarsely chopped cabbage

½ cup (50 g) cauliflower

1 teaspoon parsley flakes

1 cup corn

1 cup (130 g) sliced carrot

1 cup (113 g) sliced zucchini

2 potatoes, peeled and diced

Place tomatoes in a large pot with broth. Bring to a boil. Add onion and celery, bay leaves, 1½ teaspoons basil, and black pepper. Cover and simmer for 1 hour. Add cabbage, cauliflower, parsley, corn, carrot, zucchini, and potato. Cover and simmer until vegetables are tender, 45 to 60 minutes longer. Add remaining basil; simmer 5 minutes longer. Remove bay leaves before serving.

Yield: 8 servings

Each with: 312 g water; 130 calories (8% from fat, 17% from protein, 75% from carb); 6 g protein; 1 g total fat; 0 g saturated fat; 0 g monounsaturated fat; 0 g polyunsaturated fat; 27 g carb; 4 g fiber; 4 g sugar; 138 mg phosphorus; 44 mg calcium; 2 mg iron; 70 mg sodium; 816 mg potassium; 3030 IU vitamin A; 0 mg vitamin E; 35 mg vitamin C; 0 mg cholesterol

Pumpkin Soup

This soup can be sipped from a mug or packed in a travel mug and taken with you.

½ cup (80 g) chopped onion

½ teaspoon minced garlic

1 teaspoon (5 ml) olive oil

½ cup (90 g) chopped tomato

2 cups (490 g) pumpkin

2 cups (475 ml) low-sodium chicken broth

½ teaspoon paprika

1½ teaspoons curry powder

In a large saucepan, cook the onion and garlic in the oil until tender, 2 to 3 minutes. Stir in the remaining ingredients and heat to boiling. Reduce heat, cover, and simmer 10 minutes, stirring occasionally, until vegetables are tender. Place in blender and process until smooth.

Yield: 4 servings

Each with: 261 g water; 86 calories (22% from fat, 18% from protein, 60% from carb); 4 g protein; 2 g total fat; 1 g saturated fat; 1 g monounsaturated fat; 0 g polyunsaturated fat; 15 g carb; 4 g fiber; 6 g sugar; 93 mg phosphorus; 48 mg calcium; 2 mg iron; 44 mg sodium; 449 mg potassium; 19380 IU vitamin A; 0 mg vitamin E; 9 mg vitamin C; 0 mg cholesterol

Pumpkin Vegetable Soup

This easy soup has a lot of flavor, both from the vegetables and the curry powder. To make it vegetarian, substitute vegetable broth for the chicken and omit the chicken breast.

½ cup (80 g) chopped onion

½ teaspoon minced garlic

1 teaspoon (5 ml) olive oil

2 cups (310 g) mixed vegetables, frozen

1 can pumpkin

1 can no-salt-added canned tomatoes

½ cup (120 ml) water

1½ teaspoons curry powder

½ teaspoon paprika

2 cups (475 ml) low-sodium chicken broth

1 cup (140 g) chopped cooked chicken breast

In a large saucepan, cook the onion and garlic in the oil until tender, 2 to 3 minutes. Stir in the remaining ingredients and heat to boiling. Reduce heat, cover, and simmer 10 minutes, stirring occasionally, until vegetables are tender.

Yield: 4 servings

Each with: 261 g water; 158 calories (19% from fat, 42% from protein, 39% from carb); 16 g protein; 3 g total fat; 1 g saturated fat; 2 g monounsaturated fat; 1 g polyunsaturated fat; 15 g carb; 5 g fiber; 4 g sugar; 172 mg phosphorus; 43 mg calcium; 2 mg iron; 442 mg sodium; 396 mg potassium; 4059 IU vitamin A; 2 mg vitamin E; 5 mg vitamin C; 30 mg cholesterol

Tomato Vegetable Soup

This recipe starts with a cream of tomato-type soup and then adds to it to end up with a really good spicy vegetable soup.

1 cup (160 g) finely chopped onion

½ teaspoon finely chopped garlic

½ cup (75 g) finely chopped green bell pepper

1 cup (235 ml) low-sodium chicken broth

½ cup (115 g) canned corn

½ cup (113 g) canned peas

1 cup (105 g) macaroni

1 teaspoon low-sodium beef bouillon

2 cups (480 g) no-salt-added canned tomatoes

½ cup (34 g) nonfat dry milk powder

¼ teaspoon salt-free seasoning blend, such as Mrs. Dash

¼ teaspoon white pepper

1½ cups (355 ml) water

¼ cup (34 g) jalapeño peppers, roasted and minced

Sauté onion, garlic, and bell pepper until well cooked. Set aside. In a separate pot, combine chicken broth, juice from corn and peas, plus enough water to cook the macaroni (close to a quart). Bring to boil. Add macaroni. Cook for 12 minutes. Drain the macaroni and store broth for next time. Puree the bouillon, tomatoes, dry milk, seasonings, water, and sautéed onion, garlic, and bell pepper. Combined pureed sauce, macaroni, peas, corn, and minced jalapeños and simmer for 30 minutes.

Yield: 4 servings

Each with: 371 g water; 174 calories (6% from fat, 21% from protein, 73% from carb); 10 g protein; 1 g total fat; 0 g saturated fat; 0 g monounsaturated fat; 0 g polyunsaturated fat; 34 g carb; 5 g fiber; 12 g sugar; 196 mg phosphorus; 168 mg calcium; 2 mg iron; 108 mg sodium; 625 mg potassium; 926 IU vitamin A; 60 mg vitamin E; 36 mg vitamin C; 2 mg cholesterol

Vegetable Pasta Sauce

This pasta sauce can't be beat. It's low in calories, fat free, has 3 grams of fiber, and a great Italian flavor on top of all that.

1 cup (160 g) finely chopped onion

1 teaspoon crushed garlic

2 teaspoons basil

1½ teaspoons oregano

1 bay leaf

28 ounces (800 g) no-salt-added canned tomatoes

16 ounces (455 g) no-salt-added tomato sauce

¼ teaspoon black pepper, fresh ground

4 tablespoons (16 g) chopped fresh parsley

In a large pot, heat onion, garlic, basil, oregano, bay leaf, tomatoes, tomato sauce, pepper, and parsley. Mix well, mashing tomatoes with a fork. Bring to boiling, reduce heat, and simmer uncovered, stirring occasionally, for 1½ hours. Remove bay leaf. Serve over whole wheat pasta.

Yield: 6 servings

Each with: 218 g water; 64 calories (5% from fat, 14% from protein, 81% from carb); 2 g protein; 0 g total fat; 0 g saturated fat; 0 g monounsaturated fat; 0 g polyunsaturated fat; 14 g carb; 3 g fiber; 8 g sugar; 61 mg phosphorus; 71 mg calcium; 2 mg iron; 28 mg sodium; 597 mg potassium; 668 IU vitamin A; 0 mg vitamin E; 28 mg vitamin C; 0 mg cholesterol

13

Main Dishes:
Combinations

Combination dishes are a great way to up the fiber content. This chapter contains a number of soups, casseroles, pasta dishes, and salads. Many contain both legumes and vegetables, but there are also those that incorporate whole grains.

Beef, Bean, and Cabbage Stew

This is another recipe based on one sent in by a newsletter subscriber. It makes a great meal with cornbread and a salad.

1 pound (455 g) lean ground beef

½ cup (80 g) chopped onion

1 cup (70 g) cole slaw mix or shredded cabbage

2 cups (480 g) canned no-salt-added canned tomatoes

2 cups (342 g) cooked Mexican beans

1 cup (235 ml) water

Break beef up into fine pieces and brown with the chopped onion and slaw mix or cabbage until the vegetables become clear. Add tomatoes, beans, and water. Bring to boil and simmer 10 minutes to blend the flavors.

Yield: 5 servings

Each with: 265 g water; 345 calories (39% from fat, 35% from protein, 25% from carb); 30 g protein; 15 g total fat; 6 g saturated fat; 7 g monounsaturated fat; 1 g polyunsaturated fat; 22 g carb; 8 g fiber; 3 g sugar; 268 mg phosphorus; 95 mg calcium; 5 mg iron; 83 mg sodium; 818 mg potassium; 132 IU vitamin A; 0 mg vitamin E; 18 mg vitamin C; 73 mg cholesterol

Mexican Beef Salad

This is a kind of taco salad without the tortillas, this makes a great light dinner for a hot day.

1 pound (455 g) ground beef, extra lean

½ cup (80 g) chopped onion

1 tablespoon chili powder

2 teaspoons oregano

½ teaspoon cumin

1 cup (100 g) cooked kidney beans, drained and rinsed

1 pound (455 g) chickpeas, drained and rinsed

1 cup (180 g) diced tomato

2 cups (110 g) iceberg lettuce

½ cup (58 g) shredded Cheddar cheese

Cook ground beef and onion in a skillet over medium-high heat until beef is no longer pink, 10 to 12 minutes. Drain. Stir in chili powder, oregano, and cumin. Cook for 1 minute. Mix in beans, chickpeas, and tomato. Portion lettuce onto serving plates. Top with shredded cheese. Then top with beef mixture.

Yield: 4 servings

Each with: 263 g water; 601 calories (42% from fat, 27% from protein, 31% from carb); 41 g protein; 28 g total fat; 12 g saturated fat; 11 g monounsaturated fat; 3 g polyunsaturated fat; 47 g carb; 15 g fiber; 8 g sugar; 525 mg phosphorus; 242 mg calcium; 8 mg iron; 213 mg sodium; 1071 mg potassium; 1284 IU vitamin A; 43 mg vitamin E; 11 mg vitamin C; 96 mg cholesterol

Mexican Spaghetti Pie

This is a Mexican-flavored version of spaghetti pie. The kidney beans provide extra fiber as well as flavor.

12 ounces (342 g) whole wheat spaghetti

4 tablespoons (55 g) unsalted butter

¼ cup (25 g) grated Parmesan cheese

4 eggs, beaten

½ cup (80 g) chopped onion

1 pound (455 g) ground beef

2 cups (200 g) cooked kidney beans, drained

2 cups (480 g) no-salt-added canned tomatoes

6 ounces (170 g) no-salt-added tomato paste

4 ounces (115 g) canned green chiles, chopped

2 tablespoons chili powder

1 teaspoon cumin

½ cup (60 g) shredded Monterey Jack cheese

TIP *If you like things spicier, add some red pepper flakes along with the other spices.*

Cook and drain spaghetti and let cool slightly. Stir in butter, Parmesan cheese, and eggs. Spread into the bottom of a large baking dish coated with nonstick vegetable oil spray. Brown onion and ground beef. Stir in kidney beans, undrained tomatoes, and tomato paste. Add chopped green chiles, chili powder, and cumin. Simmer for 30 minutes. Pour meat mixture over pasta in baking dish. Top with the shredded cheese. Bake in a 350°F (180°C, gas mark 4) oven for 30 to 40 minutes or until brown.

Yield: 8 servings

Each with: 152 g water; 607 calories (27% from fat, 25% from protein, 48% from carb); 36 g protein; 17 g total fat; 8 g saturated fat; 5 g monounsaturated fat; 2 g polyunsaturated fat; 68 g carb; 17 g fiber; 6 g sugar; 530 mg phosphorus; 236 mg calcium;9 mg iron; 232 mg sodium; 1332 mg potassium; 1345 IU vitamin A; 106 mg vitamin E; 14 mg vitamin C; 183 mg cholesterol

Southwestern Vegetable Stew

This stew evokes not just the flavor of Mexico, but also that of the southwestern Native American tribes with the use of squash and corn. It's delicious with cornbread.

¾ cup (120 g) chopped onion

½ teaspoon finely chopped garlic

2 tablespoons (28 ml) vegetable oil

1 cup (150 g) red bell pepper, cut into strips

½ cup (72 g) poblano chiles, seeded and cut into strips

1 jalapeño pepper, seeded and chopped

1 cup (140 g) cubed acorn squash

4 cups (950 ml) low-sodium chicken broth

½ teaspoon black pepper

½ teaspoon ground coriander

1 cup (113 g) thinly sliced zucchini

1 cup (113 g) thinly sliced yellow squash

10 ounces (280 g) frozen corn

2 cups (342 g) cooked pinto beans, drained

Cook and stir onion and garlic in oil in 4-quart (4 L) Dutch oven over medium heat until onion is tender. Stir in bell pepper, poblano, and jalapeño. Cook 15 minutes. Stir in squash, broth, black pepper, and coriander. Heat to boiling; reduce heat. Cover and simmer until squash is tender, about 15 minutes. Stir in remaining ingredients. Cook uncovered, stirring occasionally, until zucchini is tender, about 10 minutes.

Yield: 6 servings

Each with: 336 g water; 220 calories (24% from fat, 19% from protein, 57% from carb); 11 g protein; 6 g total fat; 1 g saturated fat; 2 g monounsaturated fat; 3 g polyunsaturated fat; 34 g carb; 8 g fiber; 5 g sugar; 199 mg phosphorus; 58 mg calcium; 2 mg iron; 57 mg sodium; 759 mg potassium; 1001 IU vitamin A; 0 mg vitamin E; 54 mg vitamin C; 0 mg cholesterol

Italian Oven Chowder

This Italian dish, halfway between a soup and a casserole, cooks in the oven while you do other things. The cheese and cream make this very rich tasting.

1 cup (113 g) sliced zucchini

1½ cups (240 g) sliced onion

2 cups (328 g) cooked chickpeas

2 cups (480 g) no-salt-added canned tomatoes, chopped

1½ cups (355 ml) dry white wine

2 teaspoons minced garlic

1 teaspoon basil

1 bay leaf

2 ounces (55 g) shredded Monterey Jack cheese

2 ounces (55 g) grated Romano cheese

1 cup (235 ml) whipping cream

Combine zucchini, onion, chickpeas, tomatoes and their liquid, wine, garlic, basil, and bay leaf in 3-quart (3 L) baking dish. Cover and bake at 400°F (200°C, gas mark 6) for 1 hour, stirring once halfway through. Season to taste with salt and pepper. Stir in cheeses and cream. Bake 10 minutes longer. Remove bay leaf before serving.

Yield: 6 servings

Each with: 258 g water; 309 calories (42% from fat, 16% from protein, 42% from carb); 11 g protein; 13 g total fat; 7 g saturated fat; 4 g monounsaturated fat; 1 g polyunsaturated fat; 29 g carb; 5 g fiber; 5 g sugar; 245 mg phosphorus; 257 mg calcium; 2 mg iron; 427 mg sodium; 485 mg potassium; 480 IU vitamin A; 81 mg vitamin E; 17 mg vitamin C; 40 mg cholesterol

Taco Salad

This recipe is a meal in itself. And you couldn't ask for more flavor.

1 pound (455 g) ground beef

1 tablespoon taco seasoning

2 cups (110 g) shredded lettuce

6 ounces (170 g) corn chips

2 cups (504 g) refried beans

1 cup (180 g) chopped tomato

½ cup (80 g) chopped onion

½ cup (75 g) chopped green bell pepper

½ cup (115 g) sour cream

½ cup (130 g) salsa

Brown the ground beef with the taco seasoning. Drain. Layer lettuce, chips, beef, beans, tomato, onion, and pepper. Top with sour cream and salsa.

Yield: 4 servings

Each with: 318 g water; 523 calories (39% from fat, 25% from protein, 36% from carb); 33 g protein; 23 g total fat; 10 g saturated fat; 9 g monounsaturated fat; 2 g polyunsaturated fat; 48 g carb; 11 g fiber; 4 g sugar; 438 mg phosphorus; 183 mg calcium; 5 mg iron; 538 mg sodium; 1006 mg potassium; 842 IU vitamin A; 50 mg vitamin E; 31 mg vitamin C; 92 mg cholesterol

Texas Cornbread Skillet Meal

This makes a nice meal-in-a-pot sort of dinner. I've also made a meatless variation of it for lunch that was every bit as good.

1 pound (455 g) ground beef

1 cup (160 g) chopped onion

1 tablespoon minced garlic clove

2 cups (480 g) no-salt-added canned tomatoes

2 cups (344 g) cooked black-eyed peas, drained

1½ teaspoons Cajun seasoning

½ cup (70 g) cornmeal

½ cup (62 g) flour

1 tablespoon baking powder

1 egg

½ cup (120 ml) skim milk

In a large cast-iron or ovenproof skillet, brown ground beef, onion, and garlic. Add undrained tomatoes, black-eyed peas, and seasoning. Stir well. In a separate bowl, combine cornmeal, flour, and baking powder. Stir egg and milk together and then stir into dry ingredients. Top meat mixture with cornbread batter and cook in 425°F (220°C, gas mark 7) oven about 20 to 25 minutes or until cornbread is golden brown.

Yield: 4 servings

Each with: 311 g water; 608 calories (32% from fat, 28% from protein, 39% from carb); 43 g protein; 22 g total fat; 8 g saturated fat; 9 g monounsaturated fat; 2 g polyunsaturated fat; 60 g carb; 9 g fiber; 9 g sugar; 494 mg phosphorus; 334 mg calcium; 8 mg iron; 510 mg sodium; 1086 mg potassium; 394 IU vitamin A; 41 mg vitamin E; 17 mg vitamin C; 145 mg cholesterol

Chicken and Black Beans

This is a Mexican-flavored skillet meal featuring marinated chicken and black beans.

½ cup (120 ml) Italian dressing

½ teaspoon crushed garlic

¼ teaspoon red pepper flakes

12 ounces (340 g) boneless chicken breast, cut in 1-inch (2.5 cm) cubes

2 teaspoons (10 ml) olive oil

1 cup (150 g) chopped green bell pepper

¾ cup (120 g) chopped onion

¾ teaspoon oregano

¼ teaspoon black pepper, fresh ground

¼ teaspoon cumin

2 cups (344 g) cooked black beans, drained and rinsed

2 cups (480 g) no-salt-added canned tomatoes

¼ cup chopped fresh cilantro

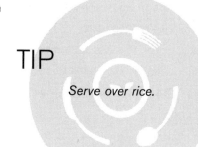

TIP

Serve over rice.

Combine dressing, garlic, and red pepper. Place chicken in large glass bowl, pour dressing over chicken, cover, and refrigerate 30 to 60 minutes (or overnight). Remove chicken from marinade, drain well, and discard marinade. Heat oil in large skillet over medium-high heat until hot. Add chicken, cook 5 to 7 minutes, stirring until chicken is slightly brown, spooning off any excess liquid. Add bell pepper, onion, oregano, pepper, and cumin. Cook, stirring, 4 to 5 minutes or until vegetables are tender. Add black beans and tomatoes. Cook 2 to 3 minutes more or until thoroughly heated. Garnish with cilantro; serve immediately.

Yield: 4 servings

Each with: 314 g water; 355 calories (31% from fat, 32% from protein, 37% from carb); 29 g protein; 12 g total fat; 2 g saturated fat; 4 g monounsaturated fat; 5 g polyunsaturated fat; 33 g carb; 10 g fiber; 7 g sugar; 332 mg phosphorus; 90 mg calcium; 4 mg iron; 562 mg sodium; 896 mg potassium; 550 IU vitamin A; 5 mg vitamin E; 46 mg vitamin C; 49 mg cholesterol

Chili-Chicken Stew

It may have a Mexican flavor, but make no mistake—this is real comfort food. It will raise your spirits even faster than Grandma's chicken noodle soup.

6 boneless chicken breasts, cut in 1-inch (2.5-cm) cubes

1 cup (160 g) chopped onion

1 cup (150 g) chopped green bell pepper

½ teaspoon minced garlic

1 tablespoon (15 ml) vegetable oil

4 cups (1 kg) no-salt-added stewed tomatoes, undrained and chopped

2 cups (342 g) cooked pinto beans, drained

⅔ (173 g) cup salsa

1 teaspoon ground cumin

2 tablespoons chili powder

¾ cup (180 g) fat-free sour cream

½ cup (50 g) sliced scallions

½ cup (58 g) shredded Cheddar cheese

1 avocado, diced

Cook chicken, onion, bell pepper, and garlic in hot oil in a Dutch oven until lightly browned. Add tomatoes, beans, salsa, cumin, and chili powder. Cover, reduce heat, and simmer 20 minutes. Top individual servings with remaining ingredients.

Yield: 6 servings

Each with: 214 g water; 338 calories (32% from fat, 35% from protein, 33% from carb); 27 g protein; 11 g total fat; 4 g saturated fat; 4 g monounsaturated fat; 2 g polyunsaturated fat; 26 g carb; 9 g fiber; 3 g sugar; 355 mg phosphorus; 181 mg calcium; 3 mg iron; 175 mg sodium; 840 mg potassium; 1276 IU vitamin A; 63 mg vitamin E; 29 mg vitamin C; 65 mg cholesterol

Mexican Chicken and Black Beans

This is a quick one-pan meal. All you need is a little leftover rice to have it on the table in less than a half-hour.

1 pound (455 g) boneless chicken breast, cut in 1-inch (2.5 cm) cubes

½ cup (80 g) chopped onion

1 teaspoon crushed garlic

2 cups (344 g) cooked black beans, rinsed and drained

1 cup (180 g) chopped tomato

3 tablespoons (48 g) salsa, mild or hot

½ cup (115 g) fat-free sour cream

1 cup (220 g) cooked brown rice

1 avocado, sliced

Spray large skillet with nonstick vegetable oil spray; heat over medium heat until hot. Sauté chicken, onion, and garlic until chicken is cooked, 5 to 8 minutes. Stir in beans, tomato, salsa, and sour cream. Cook until hot, 1 to 2 minutes. Season to taste with salt and pepper. Serve over rice, garnished with avocado.

Yield: 4 servings

Each with: 290 g water; 410 calories (25% from fat, 36% from protein, 39% from carb); 37 g protein; 11 g total fat; 4 g saturated fat; 5 g monounsaturated fat; 1 g polyunsaturated fat; 40 g carb; 12 g fiber; 2 g sugar; 450 mg phosphorus; 87 mg calcium; 3 mg iron; 125 mg sodium; 977 mg potassium; 459 IU vitamin A; 37 mg vitamin E; 16 mg vitamin C; 78 mg cholesterol

Mexican Chicken Soup

This is a flavorful Mexican chicken noodle soup. Serve it with cornmeal bread for a complete meal.

1½ pounds (675 g) boneless chicken breasts, cut in bite-size pieces

1 cup (150 g) green bell pepper, cut in strips

1 cup (160 g) diced onion

½ teaspoon minced garlic

2 cups (480 g) no-salt-added canned tomatoes

4 ounces (115 g) chopped green chiles

2 cups (475 ml) low-sodium chicken broth

2 tablespoons (28 ml) vinegar

1 teaspoon oregano

10 ounces (280 g) frozen corn

2 cups (342 g) cooked pinto beans, drained

2 ounces (55 g) egg noodles

Mix all ingredients together, except noodles, in Dutch oven. Simmer until chicken is cooked through and vegetables are tender, about 30 minutes. Add noodles and cook until they are done, about 10 minutes.

Yield: 6 servings

Each with: 385 g water; 304 calories (8% from fat, 46% from protein, 46% from carb); 36 g protein; 3 g total fat; 1 g saturated fat; 1 g monounsaturated fat; 1 g polyunsaturated fat; 36 g carb; 9 g fiber; 5 g sugar; 395 mg phosphorus; 88 mg calcium; 4 mg iron; 188 mg sodium; 940 mg potassium; 252 IU vitamin A; 7 mg vitamin E; 39 mg vitamin C; 66 mg cholesterol

Smoked Chicken Minestrone

Although not a very traditional minestrone, I was just looking for something with beans in it and a way to use up the last of a smoked chicken. If you don't have smoked chicken, regular chicken will also work.

½ pound (225 g) dry cannellini beans

½ pound (225 g) dry chickpeas

2 smoked chicken thighs

2 cups (475 ml) low-sodium chicken broth

¼ cup (40 g) chopped onion

⅓ cup (43 g) sliced carrot

1 cup (113 g) sliced zucchini

½ teaspoon garlic powder

1 teaspoon basil

1 teaspoon oregano

2 cups (480 g) no-salt-added canned tomatoes

¼ cup (25 g) Parmesan cheese

Soak beans and drain. Simmer chicken in broth and enough water to cover until meat separates from bones. Cool, skim off fat, and remove meat from bones. Return meat to broth. Add other ingredients and simmer 1 to 1½ hours, until beans are tender. Add additional water as needed. Garnish with Parmesan cheese.

Yield: 4 servings

Each with: 386 g water; 229 calories (8% from fat, 33% from protein, 59% from carb); 20 g protein; 2 g total fat; 1 g saturated fat; 1 g monounsaturated fat; 1 g polyunsaturated fat; 35 g carb; 9 g fiber; 5 g sugar; 353 mg phosphorus; 124 mg calcium; 4 mg iron; 781 mg sodium; 914 mg potassium; 2044 IU vitamin A; 0 mg vitamin E; 21 mg vitamin C; 17 mg cholesterol

Pork and Chickpea Stir-Fry

Here is another quick, tasty, nutritious dinner.

½ pound (225 g) boneless pork loin chops, cut into 1½-inch-thick (4-cm) strips

¼ cup (25 g) sliced scallions, with tops

½ teaspoon crushed garlic

2 teaspoons (10 ml) olive oil

1½ cups (106 g) broccoli florets

10 ounces (280 g) chickpeas, drained and rinsed

¼ cup (60 ml) low-sodium beef broth

¼ cup (60 ml) soy sauce

2 teaspoons cornstarch

1 cup (220 g) cooked brown rice

Stir-fry pork, scallions, and garlic in oil in wok or large skillet over high heat until pork is browned, 3 to 5 minutes. Add broccoli and stir-fry 2 to 3 minutes. Add chickpeas and cook, covered, over medium heat until broccoli is crisp-tender, 3 to 4 minutes. Combine broth, soy sauce, and cornstarch. Stir into mixture. Cook and stir until thickened. Serve over rice.

Yield: 4 servings

Each with: 176 g water; 287 calories (22% from fat, 30% from protein, 49% from carb); 21 g protein; 7 g total fat; 1 g saturated fat; 3 g monounsaturated fat; 2 g polyunsaturated fat; 35 g carb; 7 g fiber; 4 g sugar; 323 mg phosphorus; 69 mg calcium; 3 mg iron; 585 mg sodium; 579 mg potassium; 884 IU vitamin A; 1 mg vitamin E; 28 mg vitamin C; 36 mg cholesterol

Minestrone with Italian Sausage

1 cup (208 g) dried navy beans

4 cups (950 ml) low-sodium chicken broth

2 quarts (1.9 L) water

1 pound (455 g) sweet Italian sausage

1½ pounds (675 g) cabbage

1½ cups (195 g) sliced carrot

2 medium potatoes, diced

2 cups (480 g) no-salt-added canned tomatoes

¼ cup (60 ml) olive oil

1½ cups (240 g) diced onion

½ cup (60 g) diced celery

1 cup (113 g) sliced zucchini

½ teaspoon minced garlic

¼ teaspoon black pepper

¼ cup chopped fresh parsley

4 ounces (115 g) whole wheat pasta

½ cup (50 g) grated Parmesan cheese

1½ teaspoons Italian seasoning

Cover beans with cold water. Soak overnight. Drain. Pour chicken broth and water into an 8-quart (8 L) kettle. Add the beans. Bring to boiling. Reduce heat and simmer, covered, 1 hour. In medium skillet, simmer sausage gently in water to cover until cooked through, about 20 minutes. Drain well. Sauté over medium heat until browned all over. Slice sausage ¼ inch (0.5 cm) thick on the diagonal; set aside. Wash cabbage and quarter; remove core and slice ¼ inch (0.5 cm) thick. Add to soup along with carrot, potatoes, and tomatoes. Cover; cook 30 minutes longer. Heat oil in medium skillet. Sauté onion, stirring, about 5 minutes. Add celery, zucchini, garlic, and black pepper to skillet and sauté over low heat, stirring occasionally, 20 minutes. Add to bean mixture with parsley, pasta, and Italian seasoning. Cook slowly, covered and stirring occasionally, 30 minutes. Add sausage; heat through. Serve hot sprinkled with Parmesan cheese.

Yield: 10 servings

Each with: 558 g water; 320 calories (32% from fat, 22% from protein, 46% from carb); 18 g protein; 12 g total fat; 3 g saturated fat; 6 g monounsaturated fat; 1 g polyunsaturated fat; 39 g carb; 7 g fiber; 7 g sugar; 269 mg phosphorus; 163 mg calcium; 3 mg iron; 531 mg sodium; 974 mg potassium; 3566 IU vitamin A; 6 mg vitamin E; 43 mg vitamin C; 18 mg cholesterol

Sausage and Chickpea Soup

This is a hearty soup with Italian flavors.

1 pound (455 g) Italian sausage

½ teaspoon minced garlic

1 cup (160 g) chopped onion

⅓ cup (20 g) chopped fresh parsley

¾ cup (98 g) sliced carrot

1 cup (70 g) sliced mushrooms

2 cups (328 g) cooked chickpeas

3 cups (355 ml) low-sodium beef broth

½ teaspoon sage

½ teaspoon black pepper

Crumble sausage and cook in 3-quart (3 L) saucepan over medium-high heat, stirring often, until browned. Add garlic, onion, parsley, carrot, and mushrooms. Cook until limp. Add chickpeas and remaining ingredients. Bring to a boil and then lower heat and simmer covered, about 10 minutes. Skim off excess fat.

Yield: 4 servings

Each with: 395 g water; 581 calories (58% from fat, 18% from protein, 24% from carb); 26 g protein; 38 g total fat; 13 g saturated fat; 17 g monounsaturated fat; 5 g polyunsaturated fat; 35 g carb; 7 g fiber; 3 g sugar; 331 mg phosphorus; 97 mg calcium; 4 mg iron; 1315 mg sodium; 815 mg potassium; 4491 IU vitamin A; 0 mg vitamin E; 18 mg vitamin C; 86 mg cholesterol

Tuna Tacos

Looking for a quick lunch or dinner? These no-cook tacos are tasty and healthy, as well as being a snap to make.

6½ ounces (184 g) tuna, drained and flaked

⅓ cup (33 g) chopped scallions

¼ cup (65 g) salsa

2 cups (110 g) shredded lettuce

8 corn taco shells

1 cup (164 g) cooked chickpeas, drained

1 cup (180 g) chopped tomato

⅓ cup (33 g) ripe olives

TIP *Substitute 8 6-inch (15.2 cm) flour tortillas for the taco shells if soft tacos are preferred.*

In a medium bowl toss together tuna, scallions, and salsa until combined. To assemble tacos: Sprinkle lettuce into each taco shell. Divide tuna mixture among tacos, along with chickpeas, tomatoes, and olives. Garnish as desired with toppings.

Yield: 4 servings

Each with: 180 g water; 359 calories (30% from fat, 20% from protein, 50% from carb); 18 g protein; 12 g total fat; 2 g saturated fat; 6 g monounsaturated fat; 3 g polyunsaturated fat; 45 g carb; 6 g fiber; 2 g sugar; 274 mg phosphorus; 97 mg calcium; 3 mg iron; 509 mg sodium; 512 mg potassium; 620 IU vitamin A; 3 mg vitamin E; 15 mg vitamin C; 19 mg cholesterol

Mexican Pitas

Is this what they call "fusion" cooking . . . a mixing of cultures and tastes? Whatever you call it, these Mexican-flavored pocket sandwiches are a hit with everyone who tries them.

½ pound (225 g) ground turkey

½ cup (80 g) chopped onion

2 teaspoons taco seasoning

2 cups (342 g) cooked pinto beans, drained

½ cup (130 g) salsa

3 whole wheat pitas, halved

2 cups (110 g) shredded lettuce

1 cup (180 g) shredded tomato

½ cup (58 g) shredded Cheddar cheese

Brown turkey and onion in skillet. Drain. Add taco seasoning, beans, and salsa and heat. Spoon mixture into each pita pocket. Add lettuce, tomato, and cheese.

Yield: 3 servings

Each with: 304 g water; 591 calories (20% from fat, 30% from protein, 49% from carb); 46 g protein; 14 g total fat; 6 g saturated fat; 3 g monounsaturated fat; 2 g polyunsaturated fat; 74 g carb; 17 g fiber; 6 g sugar; 599 mg phosphorus; 271 mg calcium; 6 mg iron; 622 mg sodium; 1206 mg potassium; 1093 IU vitamin A; 57 mg vitamin E; 11 mg vitamin C; 81 mg cholesterol

Bean and Corn Burritos

Not only are these burritos delicious, but also they provide almost your whole day's fiber requirement in one dish.

½ cup (80 g) chopped onion

¼ cup (38 g) diced green bell pepper

1 teaspoon minced jalapeño pepper

½ teaspoon minced garlic

1 teaspoon ground cumin

⅛ teaspoon white pepper

2 cups (200 g) cooked kidney beans, drained and mashed

½ cup frozen corn, thawed and drained

4 flour tortillas

¾ cup (90 g) shredded Cheddar cheese

1 cup (260 g) salsa

¼ cup (60 g) fat-free sour cream

¼ cup chopped fresh cilantro

Spray a nonstick skillet with nonstick vegetable oil spray. Place over medium heat until hot. Add onion, bell pepper, jalapeño, and garlic. Sauté until tender. Stir in cumin and white pepper. Cook 1 minute, stirring constantly. Remove from heat; stir in mashed beans and corn. Spread ½ cup (50 g) bean mixture evenly over surface of each tortilla. Sprinkle 3 tablespoons cheese down center of each tortilla. Roll up tortillas and place seam side down on a baking sheet. Bake at 425°F (220°C, gas mark 7) for 7 to 8 minutes or until thoroughly heated. For each serving, top each burrito with ¼ cup (65 g) salsa and 1 tablespoon sour cream. Garnish with fresh cilantro.

Yield: 4 servings

Each with: 129 g water; 551 calories (19% from fat, 24% from protein, 57% from carb); 32 g protein; 12 g total fat; 6 g saturated fat; 4 g monounsaturated fat; 1 g polyunsaturated fat; 78 g carb; 26 g fiber; 6 g sugar; 585 mg phosphorus; 394 mg calcium; 9 mg iron; 414 mg sodium; 1646 mg potassium; 715 IU vitamin A; 79 mg vitamin E; 16 mg vitamin C; 32 mg cholesterol

Veggie Pizza with Whole Wheat Crust

There is nothing like hot pizza, fresh from the oven.

1 cup (120 g) whole wheat flour

1 teaspoon yeast

½ cup (120 ml) hot water

1 tablespoon (15 ml) olive oil

1 cup (160 g) minced onion

8 ounces (225 g) mushrooms, coarsely chopped

2 tablespoons (28 ml) olive oil

¼ teaspoon black pepper

½ teaspoon crumbled oregano

6 ounces (170 g) pizza sauce

4 ounces (115 g) shredded mozzarella cheese

2 cups (360 g) sliced tomato

2 ounces (55 g) grated Parmesan cheese

To make the crust: In a small bowl mix flour and yeast. With fork, stir in water and 1 tablespoon olive oil to form a soft dough. Cover lightly with plastic wrap. Let rise in warm place for about 30 minutes. Fit into a 12-inch (30 cm) pizza pan coated with nonstick vegetable oil spray, building up edges slightly. Bake at 425°F (220°C, gas mark 7) for 10 minutes. Sauté onion and mushrooms in oil in small skillet for 10 minutes or until mushroom liquid is evaporated. Sprinkle with pepper and oregano. Spread partially baked pizza shell with the pizza sauce. Distribute onion mixture evenly over sauce. Sprinkle with mozzarella. Top with sliced tomato. Sprinkle with Parmesan cheese. Bake at 425°F (220°C, gas mark 7) for 10 minutes or until hot and bubbly and crust is browned.

Yield: 4 servings

Each with: 245 g water; 403 calories (47% from fat, 19% from protein, 35% from carb); 19 g protein; 22 g total fat; 8 g saturated fat; 11 g monounsaturated fat; 2 g polyunsaturated fat; 36 g carb; 7 g fiber; 6 g sugar; 415 mg phosphorus; 335 mg calcium; 3 mg iron; 641 mg sodium; 758 mg potassium; 1075 IU vitamin A; 66 mg vitamin E; 29 mg vitamin C; 35 mg cholesterol

Ziti and Vegetables

Here's an updated version of baked ziti that still tastes as good but is healthier.

1 tablespoon (15 ml) olive oil

1 cup (130 g) thinly sliced carrot

1 cup (160 g) sliced onion

1 cup (113 g) sliced zucchini

1 cup (70 g) sliced mushrooms

1 cup (71 g) broccoli florets

4 ounces (115 g) shredded Muenster cheese, divided

1 cup (235 ml) tomato juice

1 cup (140 g) cooked whole wheat ziti

1 teaspoon chopped fresh basil

1 teaspoon chopped fresh parsley

1/8 teaspoon black pepper

In 10-inch (25 cm) skillet or a wok heat oil; add carrot and cook, stirring quickly and frequently, until carrot is tender, 1 to 2 minutes. Add onion, zucchini, mushrooms, and broccoli; continue stir-frying until vegetables are tender-crisp. Remove skillet (or wok) from heat and stir in 2 ounces (55 g) cheese, the tomato juice, ziti, basil, parsley, and pepper. Preheat oven to 350°F (180°C, gas mark 4). Transfer macaroni mixture to 2-quart (2 L) casserole dish and sprinkle with remaining cheese. Bake until cheese is melted and mixture is bubbly, about 20 minutes.

Yield: 4 servings

Each with: 197 g water; 279 calories (39% from fat, 18% from protein, 44% from carb); 13 g protein; 13 g total fat; 6 g saturated fat; 5 g monounsaturated fat; 1 g polyunsaturated fat; 32 g carb; 5 g fiber; 7 g sugar; 274 mg phosphorus; 258 mg calcium; 2 mg iron; 219 mg sodium; 598 mg potassium; 6578 IU vitamin A; 84 mg vitamin E; 39 mg vitamin C; 27 mg cholesterol

Pizza Primavera

Yes, you read that right—Not pasta, but pizza primavera. A white-sauce pizza with the traditional primavera vegetables. Try this the next time you really don't want pepperoni.

2 cups (142 g) broccoli florets

1 cup (130 g) julienned carrot

½ cup snow pea pods, halved crosswise

2 tablespoons (16 g) cornstarch

8 ounces (235 ml) fat-free evaporated milk

½ cup (50 g) grated Parmesan cheese, divided

¼ cup (60 ml) dry white wine

⅛ teaspoon garlic powder

⅓ cup (33 g) sliced scallions

2 tablespoons chopped fresh basil

½ cup (60 g) shredded provolone cheese

1 whole wheat pizza crust

Cook broccoli and carrot in boiling water 2 minutes. Add snow peas; cook 1 minute. Drain and rinse under cold running water; set aside. Combine cornstarch and milk in a large saucepan; stir well. Bring to a boil and cook 2 minutes or until thickened, stirring constantly. Remove from heat; stir in ¼ cup (25 g) Parmesan cheese and next 4 ingredients. Add broccoli mixture, scallions, and basil, tossing gently; set aside. Sprinkle provolone cheese over prepared crust, leaving a ½-inch (1 cm) border. Spoon vegetable mixture on top of cheese. Sprinkle with remaining Parmesan cheese. Bake at 500°F (250°C, gas mark 10) for 12 minutes on bottom rack of oven. Remove pizza to a cutting board; let stand 5 minutes.

Yield: 6 servings

Each with: 98 g water; 363 calories (22% from fat, 19% from protein, 59% from carb); 17 g protein; 9 g total fat; 4 g saturated fat; 3 g monounsaturated fat; 1 g polyunsaturated fat; 52 g carb; 2 g fiber; 6 g sugar; 224 mg phosphorus; 327 mg calcium; 1 mg iron; 841 mg sodium; 360 mg potassium; 4789 IU vitamin A; 80 mg vitamin E; 30 mg vitamin C; 16 mg cholesterol

Fettuccine with Vegetables

Fresh vegetables and Romano cheese make the pasta dish special.

½ pound (225 g) asparagus

2 tablespoons (28 g) unsalted butter

2 tablespoons (28 ml) olive oil

½ teaspoon minced garlic

1 cup (113 g) zucchini, seeds removed, diced small

¼ cup (25 g) thinly sliced scallions

½ cup (65 g) frozen peas, defrosted and drained

¼ teaspoon black pepper

8 ounces (225 g) whole wheat fettuccine

¼ cup minced fresh parsley

3 tablespoons minced fresh chives

2 ounces (55 g) grated Romano cheese

Cut the asparagus on the diagonal into ½-inch (1 cm) pieces. Bring a pan of water to a boil, add asparagus, and time for 2 minutes. Drain, rinse with cold water, and pat dry. In a large skillet, heat butter and oil over medium heat. Add garlic and sauté for 1 minute. Stir in zucchini and scallions, sautéing for 2 minutes. Add asparagus, peas, and pepper, heating for 2 minutes. After cooking fettuccine, drain it and put back into hot pan. Add vegetables, parsley, chives, and cheese, stirring to coat.

Yield: 4 servings

Each with: 119 g water; 402 calories (37% from fat, 15% from protein, 48% from carb); 16 g protein; 17 g total fat; 7 g saturated fat; 8 g monounsaturated fat; 1 g polyunsaturated fat; 50 g carb; 3 g fiber; 3 g sugar; 322 mg phosphorus; 211 mg calcium; 4 mg iron; 248 mg sodium; 413 mg potassium; 1623 IU vitamin A; 60 mg vitamin E; 18 mg vitamin C; 30 mg cholesterol

Mexican Topped Potatoes

These hot topped potatoes with a Mexican accent are sure to be a hit with the young people as well as adults.

2 baking potatoes

½ cup (115 g) low-fat cottage cheese

1 cup (171 g) cooked pinto beans, drained

½ cup (130 g) salsa

¼ cup (25 g) chopped scallions

½ cup (50 g) black olives

⅓ cup (50 g) sliced red bell pepper

½ cup (58 g) shredded Cheddar cheese

Bake potatoes. Slit open. Loosen pulp with fork. Spoon over each potato: cottage cheese, beans, salsa, scallions, olives, bell pepper, and shredded cheese. Return to microwave or oven to reheat and melt cheese.

Yield: 2 servings

Each with: 523 g water; 657 calories (22% from fat, 20% from protein, 58% from carb); 33 g protein; 17 g total fat; 8 g saturated fat; 6 g monounsaturated fat; 1 g polyunsaturated fat; 98 g carb; 19 g fiber; 7 g sugar; 622 mg phosphorus; 418 mg calcium; 7 mg iron; 791 mg sodium; 2295 mg potassium; 1609 IU vitamin A; 97 mg vitamin E; 109 mg vitamin C; 39 mg cholesterol

Asparagus Strata

This can be either breakfast or dinner—fancy enough to serve guests, but easy enough to make often for family.

1 pound (455 g) asparagus

6 slices whole wheat bread

2 cups (225 g) shredded Cheddar cheese, divided

1 cup (150 g) cubed ham

5 eggs

¾ teaspoon Worcestershire sauce

¼ teaspoon garlic powder

1¾ cups (410 ml) skim milk

2 tablespoons (20 g) minced onion

⅛ teaspoon cayenne

Cut asparagus into 1-inch (2.5 cm) pieces, drop into boiling, salted water and cook rapidly for 4 minutes. Drain. If using frozen asparagus, thaw and drain. Trim crusts from bread. Fit into 7 x 11-inch (28 cm) baking dish sprayed with nonstick vegetable oil spray. Sprinkle 1¼ cups (145 g) Cheddar cheese over the bread slices and distribute the asparagus and ham. Beat the remaining ingredients, except the reserved cheese, together until blended. Pour over the layered ingredients, cover, and refrigerate at least 8 hours or overnight. Bake uncovered in 350°F (180°C, gas mark 4) oven for 30 minutes. Top with remaining cheese and continue baking for 10 minutes until center is firm. Allow to stand for 5 minutes before cutting.

Yield: 8 servings

Each with: 158 g water; 303 calories (50% from fat, 29% from protein, 21% from carb); 22 g protein; 17 g total fat; 9 g saturated fat; 5 g monounsaturated fat; 1 g polyunsaturated fat; 16 g carb; 2 g fiber; 3 g sugar; 398 mg phosphorus; 378 mg calcium; 3 mg iron; 576 mg sodium; 413 mg potassium; 1051 IU vitamin A; 167 mg vitamin E; 6 mg vitamin C; 191 mg cholesterol

Artichoke Pie

This is a nice meatless meal with a kind of Italian flavor.

3 eggs

3 ounces (85 g) cream cheese with chives, softened

¾ teaspoon garlic powder

¼ teaspoon black pepper

1½ cups (225 g) shredded mozzarella cheese, divided

1 cup (250 g) ricotta cheese

½ cup (115 g) low-fat mayonnaise

1 can artichoke hearts

1 cup (164 g) cooked chickpeas

½ cup (50 g) sliced black olives

2 ounces (55 g) pimento, drained and diced

2 tablespoons fresh parsley

1 9-inch (23 cm) pie shell, unbaked

⅓ cup (33 g) grated Parmesan cheese

In a mixing bowl, beat eggs. Stir in cream cheese, garlic powder, and pepper. Stir in 1 cup (150 g) of the mozzarella, the ricotta, and mayonnaise. Quarter 2 artichoke hearts and set aside. Chop remaining artichoke hearts; fold into cheese mixture. Fold in chickpeas, olives, pimento, and parsley. Turn mixture into pastry shell. Bake in a 350°F (180°C, gas mark 4) oven for 30 minutes. Top with remaining mozzarella and the Parmesan cheese. Bake about 15 minutes more until set. Let stand for 10 minutes. Top with quartered artichokes.

Yield: 8 servings

Each with: 128 g water; 371 calories (56% from fat, 19% from protein, 26% from carb); 17 g protein; 22 g total fat; 8 g saturated fat; 7 g monounsaturated fat; 2 g polyunsaturated fat; 23 g carb; 3 g fiber; 2 g sugar; 283 mg phosphorus; 288 mg calcium; 2 mg iron; 697 mg sodium; 282 mg potassium; 841 IU vitamin A; 122 mg vitamin E; 10 mg vitamin C; 130 mg cholesterol

Fiber-Rich Casserole

This makes either a great side dish or a meatless meal. It serves 4 as a main dish and 6 as a side dish.

1½ cups (355 ml) chicken broth

1 cup (130 g) thinly sliced carrot

½ cup (100 g) pearl barley

2 cups (200 g) cooked kidney beans, drained

¼ cup (40 g) chopped onion

¼ cup fresh parsley

3 tablespoons (27 g) bulgur

⅛ teaspoon garlic powder

¼ cup (30 g) shredded Cheddar cheese

Mix all together except cheese. Put in 1-quart (1 L) dish. Bake covered at 350°F (180°C, gas mark 4) for 50 minutes. Uncover; sprinkle on cheese. Return to oven to melt cheese.

Yield: 4 servings

Each with: 143 g water; 477 calories (9% from fat, 24% from protein, 67% from carb); 30 g Protein; 5 g total fat; 2 g saturated fat; 1 g monounsaturated fat; 1 g polyunsaturated fat; 82 g carb; 29 g fiber; 5 g sugar; 541 mg phosphorus; 223 mg calcium; 9 mg iron; 388 mg sodium; 1649 mg potassium; 5784 IU vitamin a; 21 mg ATE vitamin e; 12 mg vitamin c; 9 mg cholesterol

Yield: 6 servings

Each with: 96 g water; 318 calories (9% from fat, 24% from protein, 67% from carb); 20 g protein; 3 g total fat; 1 g saturated fat; 1 g monounsaturated fat; 1 g polyunsaturated fat; 55 g carb; 20 g fiber; 3 g sugar; 360 mg phosphorus; 148 mg calcium; 6 mg iron; 259 mg sodium; 1099 mg potassium; 3856 IU vitamin A; 14 mg vitamin E; 8 mg vitamin C; 6 mg cholesterol

Brown Rice and Beans

This is a simple but filling and good-tasting dish.

½ cup (95 g) brown rice

1½ cups (355 ml) water

⅓ cup (33 g) sliced celery

⅓ cup (55 g) chopped onion

½ cup (75 g) chopped green bell pepper

14 ounces (400 g) canned kidney beans, drained

2 cups (480 g) no-salt-added canned tomatoes

¼ teaspoon garlic powder

⅛ teaspoon Tabasco sauce

Cook rice in water until water is absorbed. In a skillet, cook celery, onion, and bell pepper slowly over low heat about 10 minutes. Add beans, tomatoes, and seasoning. Bring to a boil and then simmer, uncovered, about 10 minutes. Add cooked rice and mix.

Yield: 4 servings

Each with: 324 g water; 182 calories (3% from fat, 23% from protein, 74% from carb); 11 g protein; 1 g total fat; 0 g saturated fat; 0 g monounsaturated fat; 0 g polyunsaturated fat; 35 g carb; 12 g fiber; 4 g sugar; 189 mg phosphorus; 116 mg calcium; 4 mg iron; 32 mg sodium; 729 mg potassium; 253 IU vitamin A; 0 mg vitamin E; 29 mg vitamin C; 0 mg cholesterol

Bulgur Cheese Bake

This makes a great side dish and can also be used as a full meatless meal. It has a vaguely Italian flavor and is good with tomato sauce.

2 cups (475 ml) water

1 cup (140 g) bulgur

1 tablespoon (15 ml) olive oil

1 cup (160 g) finely chopped onion

½ teaspoon finely chopped garlic

½ cup (90 g) chopped, seeded plum tomatoes

2 eggs

½ cup (120 ml) skim milk

6 ounces (170 g) shredded Cheddar cheese

10 ounces (280 g) frozen chopped spinach, thawed and well drained

Preheat oven to 350°F (180°C, gas mark 4). Spray a 1½-quart (1.5 L) casserole dish with nonstick vegetable oil spray. Bring water to boiling in a medium-size saucepan. Add bulgur, lower heat, and simmer, uncovered, 10 minutes or until liquid is absorbed. Set pan aside. Heat oil in a medium-size skillet over medium heat. Add the onion and the garlic to the skillet and sauté for 5 minutes. Stir in tomatoes and sauté for 5 minutes. Stir onion mixture into the bulgur. Beat together eggs and milk in large bowl. Stir together with cheese, spinach, and bulgur mixture until well mixed. Spoon into the casserole dish. Bake in preheated oven for 30 minutes. Remove casserole and let stand for 15 minutes before serving.

Yield: 4 servings

Each with: 302 g water; 416 calories (44% from fat, 21% from protein, 34% from carb); 23 g protein; 21 g total fat; 11 g saturated fat; 8 g monounsaturated fat; 2 g polyunsaturated fat; 37 g carb; 10 g fiber; 3 g sugar; 463 mg phosphorus; 501 mg calcium; 3 mg iron; 402 mg sodium; 598 mg potassium; 9332 IU vitamin A; 167 mg vitamin E; 7 mg vitamin C; 164 mg cholesterol

Caribbean Vegetable Curry

This is a moderately spicy vegetarian curry meal, but you can adjust the amount of cayenne to your taste.

1 tablespoon (15 ml) olive oil

1 cup (160 g) thinly sliced onion

¾ teaspoon crushed garlic

1 apple, peeled, cored, and chopped

1½ teaspoons curry powder

1½ teaspoons grated lemon peel

1 teaspoon ginger

1 teaspoon coriander

⅛ teaspoon turmeric

⅛ teaspoon cayenne pepper

2 cups (344 g) cooked black-eyed peas, drained

2 cups (200 g) cooked kidney beans,

⅓ cup (50 g) raisins

1 cup (230 g) plain fat-free yogurt

3 eggs, hard boiled and halved

3 cups (495 g) cooked rice

6 radishes, thinly sliced

¼ cup (25 g) sliced scallions

½ cup chopped fresh cilantro

¼ cup (37 g) chopped peanuts

Heat oil in skillet. Sauté onion, garlic, and apple until soft. Combine curry powder, lemon peel, ginger, coriander, turmeric, and cayenne pepper. Stir into onion mixture. Add black-eyed peas, undrained kidney beans, and raisins. Cover; simmer 5 minutes. Remove from heat, stir in yogurt. Place egg halves on rice. Spoon curry over. Top with radishes, scallions, cilantro, and peanuts.

Yield: 6 servings

Each with: 218 g water; 524 calories (12% from fat, 22% from protein, 66% from carb); 29 g protein; 7 g total fat; 2 g saturated fat; 3 g monounsaturated fat; 1 g polyunsaturated fat; 89 g carb; 22 g fiber; 16 g sugar; 513 mg phosphorus; 238 mg calcium; 9 mg iron; 119 mg sodium; 1465 mg potassium; 495 IU vitamin A; 40 mg vitamin E; 13 mg vitamin C; 119 mg cholesterol

Chunky Pea Soup

This is something a little more than most split pea soups, with turnips and lots of other vegetables adding more than the usual substance and flavor.

1 cup (225 g) dried yellow split peas

1 cup (225 g) dried green split peas

7 cups (1.6 L) cold water

2 cups (130 g) sliced carrot

2 cups (300 g) peeled, diced turnip

2 cups (320 g) peeled, chopped onion

1 cup (100 g) chopped celery

½ cup (97 g) rice

¾ pound (340 g) ham

Sort and rinse peas. Add cold water, bring to boil. Cook for 1 hour. Add vegetables and rice and cook for 1 additional hour. Cut ham into small cubes and add for last 20 minutes of cooking.

Yield: 6 servings

Each with: 471 g water; 388 calories (13% from fat, 30% from protein, 56% from carb); 30 g protein; 6 g total fat; 2 g saturated fat; 2 g monounsaturated fat; 1 g polyunsaturated fat; 56 g carb; 20 g fiber; 12 g sugar; 419 mg phosphorus; 97 mg calcium; 4 mg iron; 698 mg sodium; 1194 mg potassium; 7347 IU vitamin A; 0 mg vitamin E; 17 mg vitamin C; 23 mg cholesterol

Country Vegetable Soup

We made this up as a mix to give for Christmas one year, packaging all the dry ingredients in a quart jar. It's a very tasty vegetarian soup as is, but you could also add chicken or beef if you like.

½ cup (98 g) split green peas

½ cup (100 g) barley

½ cup (96 g) lentils

½ cup (95 g) brown rice

2 tablespoons parsley

2 tablespoons onion flakes

½ teaspoon lemon pepper

2 tablespoons sodium-free beef bouillon

¼ cup (23 g) alphabet noodles

1½ cups (157 g) macaroni

3 quarts (2.8 L) water

½ cup (50 g) chopped celery

½ cup (65 g) sliced carrot

1 cup (70 g) shredded cabbage

2 cups (480 g) low-sodium tomatoes

Combine all ingredients in a large soup pot and simmer until vegetables are tender, about 1 hour.

Yield: 8 servings

Each with: 472 g water; 187 calories (4% from fat, 18% from protein, 78% from carb); 8 g protein; 1 g total fat; 0 g saturated fat; 0 g monounsaturated fat; 0 g polyunsaturated fat; 38 g carb; 8 g fiber; 4 g sugar; 151 mg phosphorus; 49 mg calcium; 2 mg iron; 96 mg sodium; 462 mg potassium; 1819 IU vitamin A; 0 mg vitamin E; 22 mg vitamin C; 0 mg cholesterol

Curried Vegetable Soup

This is slightly spicy vegetarian soup, (Did I already mention I like curry?)

½ cup (80 g) chopped onion

½ teaspoon minced garlic

1 teaspoon (5 ml) olive oil

2 cups (310 g) broccoli, cauliflower, and carrot mix, frozen

1 large potato, cut into 1-inch (2.5 cm) cubes

2 cups (490 g) pumpkin

2 cups (480 g) no-salt-added canned tomatoes

½ cup (120 ml) water

1½ teaspoons curry powder

½ teaspoon paprika

2 cups (475 ml) low-sodium chicken broth

In a large saucepan, cook the onion and garlic in the oil until tender, 2 to 3 minutes. Stir in the remaining ingredients and heat to boiling. Reduce heat; cover and simmer 10 minutes, stirring occasionally, until vegetables are tender.

Yield: 4 servings

Each with: 504 g water; 225 calories (13% from fat, 35% from protein, 52% from carb); 21 g protein; 3 g total fat; 1 g saturated fat; 1 g monounsaturated fat; 1 g polyunsaturated fat; 31 g carb; 9 g fiber; 11 g sugar; 269 mg phosphorus; 113 mg calcium; 5 mg iron; 129 mg sodium; 929 mg potassium; 23269 IU vitamin A; 3 mg vitamin E; 22 mg vitamin C; 33 mg cholesterol

Fiber-Rich Vegetable Soup

This is a meatless soup that could be made vegetarian by substituting vegetable broth for the beef. This recipe makes a big pot of soup, but it freezes well if you don't need it all when you make it.

2 cups (300 g) chopped green bell pepper

2 cups (320 g) chopped onion

2 tablespoons (28 ml) olive oil

6 cups (1.4 L) water

4 cups (950 ml) low-sodium beef broth

4 cups (1 kg) no-salt-added canned tomatoes, with liquid

2 tablespoons (30 ml) lemon juice

2 cups (260 g) diced carrot

1 cup (164 g) corn

1 cup (90 g) chopped cabbage

2 cups (200 g) chopped celery

1 cup (113 g) diced yellow squash

1 large potato, diced

2 cups (200 g) green beans

1 bay leaf

2 teaspoons marjoram

1 teaspoon thyme

½ teaspoon black pepper

¼ teaspoon crushed red pepper

½ cup (30 g) minced parsley

1 cup (200 g) pearl barley

In large pot, sauté green pepper and onion in oil about 2 to 3 minutes. Add water, broth, tomatoes, lemon juice, all vegetables, and all spices. Bring to low boil, reduce to simmer. Cover and simmer 20 minutes. Add barley and simmer 40 to 50 minutes longer. Remove bay leaf before serving.

Yield: 8 servings

Each with: 632 g water; 247 calories (16% from fat, 13% from protein, 70% from carb); 9 g protein; 5 g total fat; 1 g saturated fat; 3 g monounsaturated fat; 1 g polyunsaturated fat; 46 g carb; 11 g fiber; 10 g sugar; 196 mg phosphorus; 123 mg calcium; 4 mg iron; 151 mg sodium; 1066 mg potassium; 6347 IU vitamin A; 0 mg vitamin E; 70 mg vitamin C; 0 mg cholesterol

Healthy Chili

This is a healthier version of chili that doesn't suffer at all in the taste department. It is low in fat, high in fiber, but still just as tasty.

1 pound (455 g) ground turkey

4 cups (684 g) cooked pinto beans, undrained

18 ounces (510 g) no-salt-added tomato sauce

6 ounces (170 g) no-salt-added tomato paste

2 cups (475 ml) vegetable juice, such as V8

2 tablespoons chili powder

1 teaspoon cumin

1 teaspoon cinnamon

½ cup (70 g) bulgur

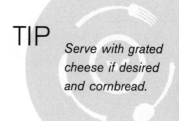

TIP

Serve with grated cheese if desired and cornbread.

Brown turkey and drain. Add remaining ingredients. Simmer 30 minutes. Stir often.

Yield: 6 servings

Each with: 295 g water; 410 calories (12% from fat, 35% from protein, 53% from carb); 37 g protein; 6 g total fat; 2 g saturated fat; 1 g monounsaturated fat; 2 g polyunsaturated fat; 56 g carb; 16 g fiber; 11 g sugar; 438 mg phosphorus; 120 mg calcium; 7 mg iron; 337 mg sodium; 1614 mg potassium; 1840 IU vitamin A; 0 mg vitamin E; 35 mg vitamin C; 57 mg cholesterol

Beer Vegetable Soup

This soup has a lot of flavor. It's good with just a simple bread like French or Italian.

1 pound (455 g) ground beef

1½ cups (195 g) sliced carrot

1 cup (100 g) sliced celery

1 tablespoon (15 ml) Worcestershire sauce

4 cups (1 kg) no-salt-added canned tomatoes, chopped

2 cups (475 ml) vegetable juice, such as V8

2 cans beer

1 teaspoon onion powder

½ teaspoon black pepper

½ cup (100 g) pearl barley

3 large potatoes, diced

In a Dutch oven, brown beef. Drain and return to pot. Add next 8 ingredients. Bring to a boil, reduce heat, and simmer 1 hour. Add barley and potatoes. Simmer until barley is tender, about another hour.

Yield: 8 servings

Each with: 435 g water; 354 calories (14% from fat, 24% from protein, 62% from carb); 17 g protein; 4 g total fat; 2 g saturated fat; 2 g monounsaturated fat; 0 g polyunsaturated fat; 44 g carb; 7 g fiber; 8 g sugar; 256 mg phosphorus; 83 mg calcium; 4 mg iron; 275 mg sodium; 1360 mg potassium; 4520 IU vitamin A; 0 mg vitamin E; 39 mg vitamin C; 39 mg cholesterol

Harvest Soup

This soup is full of flavor from the garden, with a fiber boost from canned beans. It cooks quickly, making it easy to prepare when you get home from work.

1 tablespoon (15 ml) olive oil

2 cups (320 g) chopped onion

1½ cups (195 g) thinly sliced carrot

1 cup (100 g) thinly sliced celery

1 teaspoon minced garlic

2 teaspoons Italian seasoning

6 cups (1.4 L) low-sodium chicken broth

3 cups (710 ml) vegetable juice, such as V8

¼ pound (115 g) green beans

1 bay leaf

⅛ teaspoon black pepper

2 cups (200 g) cooked kidney beans, drained

2 cups (364 g) cooked navy beans, drained

2 cups (226 g) coarsely chopped yellow squash

TIP *If you have other fresh vegetables like tomatoes or zucchini, they make a great addition.*

In 6-quart (6 L) Dutch oven over medium heat, in hot oil, cook onion, carrot, and celery with garlic and Italian seasoning until vegetables are tender. Stir in remaining ingredients except kidney beans, navy beans, and squash. Heat to boiling. Reduce heat to low; simmer 30 minutes. Add beans and squash; cook 5 minutes more or until squash is tender. Remove bay leaf before serving.

Yield: 8 servings

Each with: 379 g water; 427 calories (8% from fat, 24% from protein, 68% from carb); 27 g protein; 4 g total fat; 1 g saturated fat; 2 g monounsaturated fat; 1 g polyunsaturated fat; 75 g carb; 22 g fiber; 10 g sugar; 509 mg phosphorus; 195 mg calcium; 8 mg iron; 343 mg sodium; 1904 mg potassium; 4675 IU vitamin A; 0 mg vitamin E; 32 mg vitamin C; 0 mg cholesterol

Italian Garden Vegetable Soup

This is a vegetarian soup with Italian flavor.

2 tablespoons (28 ml) olive oil

1 cup (160 g) chopped onion

½ teaspoon minced garlic

½ cup (65 g) peeled and sliced carrot

½ cup (50 g) sliced celery

1 cup (113 g) sliced zucchini

2 cups (475 ml) low-sodium chicken broth

2 cups (480 g) no-salt-added canned tomatoes

2 cups (328 g) cooked chickpeas

½ teaspoon basil

½ teaspoon oregano

½ teaspoon black pepper

In large saucepan, heat oil. Add onion, cooking until soft. Add garlic; cook for 1 minute, stirring often. Add carrot, celery, and zucchini. Cook 3 minutes. Add broth, tomatoes, chickpeas, and spices. Stir. Cover and simmer for 10 minutes. Taste for seasonings. Serve with grated Parmesan cheese on top and croutons, if desired.

Yield: 6 servings

Each with: 269 g water; 182 calories (29% from fat, 15% from protein, 57% from carb); 7 g protein; 6 g total fat; 1 g saturated fat; 4 g monounsaturated fat; 1 g polyunsaturated fat; 27 g carb; 6 g fiber; 4 g sugar; 134 mg phosphorus; 74 mg calcium; 2 mg iron; 291 mg sodium; 513 mg potassium; 1998 IU vitamin A; 0 mg vitamin E; 17 mg vitamin C; 0 mg cholesterol

Italian Lentil Soup

This is a rich and hearty soup, full of flavor. Serve with Italian bread for a complete meal.

¾ cup (120 g) chopped onion

¾ cup (75 g) chopped celery

½ teaspoon minced garlic

2 tablespoons (28 ml) olive oil

4 cups (950 ml) vegetable broth

2 cups (475 ml) water

4 cups (1 kg) no-salt-added canned tomatoes

¾ cup (144 g) dry lentils, rinsed and drained

¾ cup (150 g) pearl barley

½ teaspoon dried rosemary, crushed

½ teaspoon dried oregano, crushed

¼ teaspoon black pepper

1 cup (130 g) thinly sliced carrot

In 4-quart (4 L) Dutch oven, cook onion, celery, and garlic in oil until tender. Add broth, water, tomatoes, lentils, barley, rosemary, oregano, and pepper. Bring to boil; reduce heat. Cover and simmer 45 minutes. Add carrot and simmer for 15 minutes or more until carrot is tender.

Yield: 5 servings

Each with: 547 g water; 321 calories (30% from fat, 12% from protein, 59% from carb); 10 g protein; 11 g total fat; 2 g saturated fat; 6 g monounsaturated fat; 2 g polyunsaturated fat; 49 g carb; 11 g fiber; 8 g sugar; 227 mg phosphorus; 125 mg calcium; 5 mg iron; 999 mg sodium; 834 mg potassium; 4616 IU vitamin A; 0 mg vitamin E; 25 mg vitamin C; 0 mg cholesterol

Italian Vegetable Soup

This hearty Italian-flavored soup is full of vegetables and beans.

1 pound (455 g) sweet Italian sausage

1 cup (160 g) diced onion

2 cups (480 g) no-salt-added canned tomatoes, chopped

8 ounces (225 g) no-salt-added tomato sauce

2 cups (475 ml) water

2 cups (475 ml) low-sodium beef broth

½ teaspoon basil

2 cups (328 g) cooked chickpeas

2 cups (200 g) cooked kidney beans

1½ cups (169 g) sliced zucchini

TIP

Serve with grated Parmesan cheese.

Brown sausage, breaking up into small pieces. Drain. Cook onion until transparent. Put sausage and onion in large kettle. Add tomatoes, water, broth, and basil. Drain beans and add to soup. Bring to boil. Simmer and cook 30 minutes. Add zucchini and cook another 15 minutes.

Yield: 6 servings

Each with: 436 g water; 461 calories (16% from fat, 28% from protein, 56% from carb); 33 g protein; 8 g total fat; 3 g saturated fat; 3 g monounsaturated fat; 1 g polyunsaturated fat; 66 g carb; 21 g fiber; 7 g sugar; 457 mg phosphorus; 181 mg calcium; 8 mg iron; 753 mg sodium; 1603 mg potassium; 313 IU vitamin A; 0 mg vitamin E; 26 mg vitamin C; 23 mg cholesterol

Winter Day Soup

This is just the kind of thing you need when you come in from shoveling snow. It's warm, filling, and delicious. Add a big slice of hot bread and you are set.

1 pound (455 g) ground beef

1½ cups (195 g) sliced carrot

1 cup (100 g) sliced celery

1 cup (160 g) diced onion

4 cups (1 kg) no-salt-added canned tomatoes, chopped

1 cup (200 g) pearl barley

4 cups (950 ml) low-sodium beef broth

½ teaspoon black pepper

2 tablespoons dried parsley

2 cups (475 ml) water

Brown ground beef in large soup pot. Skim off all fat. Add carrot, celery, and onion and sauté for a few minutes, until softened. Add tomatoes, barley, broth, pepper, parsley, and water. Simmer 1 hour until barley is fully cooked.

Yield: 4 servings

Each with: 759 g water; 526 calories (20% from fat, 31% from protein, 49% from carb); 33 g protein; 9 g total fat; 3 g saturated fat; 4 g monounsaturated fat; 1 g polyunsaturated fat; 53 g carb; 13 g fiber; 11 g sugar; 394 mg phosphorus; 153 mg calcium; 7 mg iron; 311 mg sodium; 1401 mg potassium; 8645 IU vitamin A; 0 mg vitamin E; 32 mg vitamin C; 78 mg cholesterol

Lentil and Barley Soup

Lentil and barley make a great combination, both in terms of flavor and nutrition. This hearty soup proves that, tasting great and packing 10 grams of fiber while remaining low in sodium and saturated fat.

¼ cup (60 ml) olive oil

½ teaspoon garlic

½ cup (80 g) diced onion

1 cup (110 g) shredded carrot

½ cup (50 g) sliced celery

1 teaspoon basil

3 quarts (2.8 L) water

1 pound (455 g) lentils

½ cup (100 g) pearl barley

½ teaspoon black pepper

¼ teaspoon garlic powder

¼ cup (60 ml) red wine

Heat oil in Dutch oven. Add garlic, onion, carrot, celery, and basil and cook until tender on low to medium heat, about 10 to 15 minutes. Add water, cover, and bring to boil. Add lentils, barley, pepper, garlic powder, and red wine. Reduce heat and simmer until beans are tender, about 1 hour.

Yield: 6 servings

Each with: 566 g water; 245 calories (36% from fat, 15% from protein, 49% from carb); 9 g protein; 10 g total fat; 1 g saturated fat; 7 g monounsaturated fat; 1 g polyunsaturated fat; 30 g carb; 10 g fiber; 3 g sugar; 192 mg phosphorus; 48 mg calcium; 3 mg iron; 34 mg sodium; 462 mg potassium; 3608 IU vitamin A; 0 mg vitamin E; 4 mg vitamin C; 0 mg cholesterol

Lentil Brown Rice Soup

This is a hearty soup of lentils and rice.

¾ cup (75 g) chopped celery

¾ cup (120 g) chopped onion

2 tablespoons (28 ml) olive oil

6 cups (1.4 L) water

¾ cup (144 g) lentils

4 cups (1 kg) no-salt-added canned tomatoes

½ teaspoon garlic powder

¼ teaspoon black pepper

¾ cup (142 g) brown rice

½ teaspoon rosemary

1 tablespoon (15 ml) Worcestershire sauce

½ cup (55 g) shredded carrot

Sauté celery and onion in oil in a Dutch oven. Add water and lentils. Cook 20 minutes. Add remaining ingredients, except carrot. Simmer 45 to 60 minutes. Add carrot. Cook 5 minutes more.

Yield: 6 servings

Each with: 447 g water; 199 calories (24% from fat, 11% from protein, 64% from carb); 6 g protein; 6 g total fat; 1 g saturated fat; 4 g monounsaturated fat; 1 g polyunsaturated fat; 33 g carb; 5 g fiber; 6 g sugar; 168 mg phosphorus; 80 mg calcium; 3 mg iron; 73 mg sodium; 566 mg potassium; 2048 IU vitamin A; 0 mg vitamin E; 22 mg vitamin C; 0 mg cholesterol

Russian Vegetable Soup

This soup has a little bit of everything in it, and that really gives it a spark of flavor.

1 pound (455 g) mixed dried beans

1 pound (455 g) ham hocks

3 quarts (2.8 L) water

2 tablespoons (28 ml) olive oil

1 cup (160 g) diced onion

1 cup (120 g) diced celery

½ cup (75 g) diced green bell pepper

1 teaspoon crushed garlic

2 cups (260 g) diced carrot

2 cups (300 g) diced rutabaga

2 cups (142 g) diced broccoli

1 cup (200 g) pearl barley

2 tablespoons dried parsley

1 tablespoon black pepper

1 teaspoon basil

1 teaspoon coriander

1 teaspoon nutmeg

Soak beans overnight. Drain and then add the beans, ham, and 3 quarts (2.8 L) of water to the pot. Bring to a boil and then let it simmer for an hour. (It can be refrigerated overnight at this point to skim off fat.) Remove meat from ham bones and return to pot. Heat oil in a skillet and sauté onion, celery, bell pepper, and garlic until softened, about 5 minutes. Add to pot. Simmer for another hour. Add carrot, rutabaga, broccoli, barley, and herbs. Simmer for another hour.

Yield: 8 servings

Each with: 522 g water; 421 calories (14% from fat, 29% from protein, 57% from carb); 32 g protein; 7 g total fat; 1 g saturated fat; 3 g monounsaturated fat; 1 g polyunsaturated fat; 62 g carb; 16 g fiber; 7 g sugar; 439 mg phosphorus; 215 mg calcium; 8 mg iron; 551 mg sodium; 1726 mg potassium; 5713 IU vitamin A; 0 mg vitamin E; 42 mg vitamin C; 35 mg cholesterol

Mexican Bean and Barley Soup

This is not quite chili and not quite bean soup, but it's definitely good. Cornbread is my personal choice of accompaniment.

½ cup (97 g) dried pinto beans

½ cup (125 g) dried kidney beans

½ cup (104 g) dried navy beans

½ cup (97 g) dried black beans

8 cups (1.9 L) water

½ cup (100 g) pearl barley

1 cup (160 g) chopped onion

2 bay leaves

2 teaspoons chili powder

2 teaspoons cumin

1 teaspoon oregano

½ teaspoon garlic powder

Rinse and pick over beans. Put into a 4- to 5-quart (4 to 5 L) heavy pot and cover with water. Let sit overnight. Drain. Add 8 cups (1.9 L) of water. Add barley, onion, and spices. Bring to a boil. Reduce heat to low. Cover and simmer for 2 hours, stirring occasionally, or until beans are tender but still firm. Uncover. Increase heat to medium-low and boil, gently stirring occasionally, 45 to 60 minutes, until soup is slightly thickened. Discard bay leaves before serving.

Yield: 6 servings

Each with: 363 g water; 220 calories (5% from fat, 21% from protein, 74% from carb); 12 g protein; 1 g total fat; 0 g saturated fat; 0 g monounsaturated fat; 1 g polyunsaturated fat; 42 g carb; 13 g fiber; 2 g sugar; 229 mg phosphorus; 90 mg calcium;4 mg iron; 27 mg sodium; 679 mg potassium; 272 IU vitamin A; 0 mg vitamin E; 4 mg vitamin C; 0 mg cholesterol

Pasta e Fagioli

In Italian, this means pasta and beans. It's a traditional Italian soup.

1½ cups (312 g) dried navy beans

6 cups (1.4 L) water

½ pound (225 g) whole wheat pasta

3 tablespoons (45 ml) olive oil

1 cup (160 g) chopped onion

1 cup (130 g) sliced carrot

1 cup (100 g) sliced celery

½ teaspoon crushed garlic

2 cups (360 g) tomato, peeled and diced

1 teaspoon dried sage

½ teaspoon dried oregano

¼ teaspoon black pepper

TIP *Serve garnished with parsley and Parmesan cheese.*

In large bowl, combine beans with 6 cups (1.4 L) cold water. Refrigerate overnight. Next day, pour beans and water into 6-quart (6 L) kettle. Bring to a boil, reduce heat, and simmer, covered, about 3 hours or until beans are tender. Stir several times during cooking; drain, reserving about 2 cups of liquid. Cook pasta. Heat oil in a large skillet. Sauté onion, carrot, celery, and garlic until soft (about 20 minutes). Do not brown. Add tomato, sage, oregano, and pepper. Cover and cook over medium heat, 15 minutes. In large saucepan or kettle, combine beans, pasta, and sautéed vegetables. Add 1½ cups (355 ml) of reserved bean liquid. Bring to a boil and cover; simmer 35 to 40 minutes, stirring several times and adding more liquid if needed.

Yield: 6 servings

Each with: 115 g water; 400 calories (18% from fat, 16% from protein, 66% from carb); 17 g protein; 8 g total fat; 1 g saturated fat; 5 g monounsaturated fat; 1 g polyunsaturated fat; 69 g carb; 13 g fiber; 6 g sugar; 341 mg phosphorus; 120 mg calcium; 5 mg iron; 38 mg sodium; 971 mg potassium; 4089 IU vitamin A; 0 mg vitamin E; 12 mg vitamin C; 0 mg cholesterol

Mixed Bean Soup

This is a good meal to feed a crowd, and also freezes well, so you can store some for later.

⅓ cup (69 g) dried navy beans

⅓ cup (83 g) dried red kidney beans

⅓ cup (67 g) dried baby lima beans

⅓ cup (67 g) dried chickpeas

⅓ cup (64 g) dried pinto beans

⅓ cup (75 g) dried split peas

⅓ cup (64 g) dried lentils

⅓ cup (56 g) dried black-eyed peas

⅓ cup (65 g) pearl barley

3½ quarts (3.3 L) water

½ teaspoon red pepper flakes

4 cups (1 kg) no-salt-added canned tomatoes

1½ cups (240 g) diced onion

¾ teaspoon minced garlic

½ cup (60 g) diced celery

1 cup (150 g) diced green bell pepper

2 tablespoons dried parsley

1 pound (455 g) boneless chicken breast, cut in 1-inch (2.5 cm) cubes

1 pound (455 g) smoked sausage, sliced

TIP *Packages of bean mixtures can be substituted for all different dried beans.*

Wash beans and barley; drain and add water to cover. Soak overnight and then drain. Add the 3½ quarts (3.3. L) water to the drained bean mixture. Cover and simmer until beans are tender, about 1½ hours. Add all other ingredients except the chicken and sausage. Simmer uncovered 1½ hours. Add chicken and sausage; simmer until chicken is done.

Yield: 10 servings

Each with: 556 g water; 280 calories (29% from fat, 33% from protein, 38% from carb); 23 g protein; 9 g total fat; 3 g saturated fat; 4 g monounsaturated fat; 2 g polyunsaturated fat; 27 g carb; 7 g fiber; 5 g sugar; 222 mg phosphorus; 79 mg calcium; 4 mg iron; 662 mg sodium; 648 mg potassium; 316 IU vitamin A; 3 mg vitamin E; 32 mg vitamin C; 58 mg cholesterol

Spinach Pesto Sauce

As a delicious variation on pesto, this makes a perfect sauce for whole wheat pasta.

10 ounces (280 g) frozen spinach, thawed and drained

½ teaspoon crushed garlic

¼ cup (25 g) grated Parmesan cheese

¼ cup (27 g) almonds

½ cup (30 g) fresh parsley

½ cup (120 ml) olive oil

¼ teaspoon black pepper, fresh ground

Process the above ingredients in food processor or blender. Serve over pasta.

Yield: 4 servings

Each with: 72 g water; 345 calories (85% from fat, 8% from protein, 7% from carb); 7 g protein; 34 g total fat; 5 g saturated fat; 23 g monounsaturated fat; 4 g polyunsaturated fat; 6 g carb; 4 g fiber; 1 g sugar; 130 mg phosphorus; 209 mg calcium; 2 mg iron; 172 mg sodium; 329 mg potassium; 9209 IU vitamin A; 7 mg vitamin E; 12 mg vitamin C; 6 mg cholesterol

14

Side Dishes and Salads:
Legumes

Just because something is a side dish doesn't mean it can't be a major contributor to the fiber in your diet. This is especially true if it contains legumes. Our barbecued baked beans contain 12 grams of fiber in one side-dish serving. This chapter not only contains enough variations on baked beans to keep you going a long time, but it also has some great salad ideas and some dishes with international flavors like curry.

Barbecued Baked Beans

This recipe starts with canned pork and beans but then expands on it to give it that homemade taste.

4 slices low-sodium bacon, diced

1 cup (160 g) chopped onion

⅓ cup (67 g) sugar

⅓ cup (75 g) packed brown sugar

¼ cup (60 ml) ketchup

¼ cup (60 ml) barbecue sauce

1 tablespoon (15 ml) mustard

½ teaspoon black pepper

½ teaspoon chili powder

16 ounces (455 g) pork and beans, undrained

16 ounces (455 g) kidney beans, rinsed and drained

16 ounces (455 g) great northern beans, rinsed and drained

In a large skillet, cook bacon and onion until meat is done and onion is tender. Drain any fat. Combine all remaining ingredients except beans. Add to meat mixture; mix well. Stir in beans. Place in a 2½-quart (2.5 L) casserole dish coated with nonstick vegetable oil spray. Bake, covered, at 350°F (180°C, gas mark 4) for 1 hour or until heated through.

Yield: 8 servings

Each with: 147 g water; 317 calories (8% from fat, 17% from protein, 74% from carb); 14 g protein; 3 g total fat; 1 g saturated fat; 1 g monounsaturated fat; 0 g polyunsaturated fat; 61 g carb; 12 g fiber; 23 g sugar; 248 mg phosphorus; 113 mg calcium; 4 mg iron; 446 mg sodium; 731 mg potassium; 127 IU vitamin A; 0 mg vitamin E; 6 mg vitamin C; 8 mg cholesterol

Brown Beans

This is a fairly traditional baked bean recipe, flavored with bacon and sweetened with both molasses and brown sugar.

2½ cups (483 g) dried pinto beans

4 ounces (115 g) bacon, cut up

1 cup (160 g) chopped onion

½ teaspoon minced garlic

⅛ teaspoon black pepper

2 tablespoons (40 g) molasses

1 teaspoon Worcestershire sauce

½ cup (120 ml) ketchup

1 tablespoon (15 ml) vinegar

½ cup (115 g) brown sugar

⅛ teaspoon dry mustard

1½ tablespoons cornstarch

1¼ cups (295 ml) cold water

Presoak beans in water to cover overnight. Bring to boiling; cover and simmer until tender. Drain. Mix remaining ingredients. Add mixture to cooked beans. Place in a 2½-quart (2.5 L) casserole dish coated with nonstick vegetable spray. Bake about 45 minutes.

Yield: 6 servings

Each with: 139 g water; 333 calories (22% from fat, 17% from protein, 61% from carb); 14 g protein; 8 g total fat; 3 g saturated fat; 4 g monounsaturated fat; 1 g polyunsaturated fat; 52 g carb; 7 g fiber; 27 g sugar; 228 mg phosphorus; 77 mg calcium; 3 mg iron; 462 mg sodium; 710 mg potassium; 195 IU vitamin A; 2 mg vitamin E; 7 mg vitamin C; 21 mg cholesterol

Chili Beans

These are good either by themselves or as an addition to chili or other dishes.

1 cup (194 g) dried black beans

1 cup (167 g) dried black-eyed peas

1 ham hock

3 cups (355 ml) low-sodium chicken broth

1½ tablespoons chili powder

1 tablespoon cumin

The night before, cover beans and peas with water and let stand to soften. Preheat oven to 275°F (140°C, gas mark 1). Combine beans, ham hock, broth, and spices in a heavy 2-quart (2 L) ovenproof pot over medium heat. Cover, bring to a boil, and place in the oven. Check the beans every 30 minutes and add ½ cup more broth each time if all the liquid has been absorbed. Cook for 1½ hours or until beans are soft.

Yield: 6 servings

Each with: 155 g water; 113 calories (17% from fat, 28% from protein, 55% from carb); 8 g protein; 2 g total fat; 1 g saturated fat; 1 g monounsaturated fat; 1 g polyunsaturated fat; 17 g carb; 5 g fiber; 2 g sugar; 127 mg phosphorus; 34 mg calcium; 2 mg iron; 102 mg sodium; 376 mg potassium; 592 IU vitamin A; 0 mg vitamin E; 2 mg vitamin C; 2 mg cholesterol

Cowboy Pinto Beans

4 cups (950 ml) water

2 cups (386 g) dried pinto beans

½ cup (80 g) chopped onion

1 teaspoon cumin

½ teaspoon crushed garlic

¼ cup (60 ml) olive oil

1 slice low-sodium bacon

Mix the water, beans, and onion in a 4-quart (4 L) Dutch oven. Cover and heat to boiling. Boil 2 minutes and remove from the heat; let stand for 1 hour. Add just enough water to the beans to cover. Stir in the remaining ingredients and heat to boiling. Cover and reduce the heat. Boil gently, stirring occasionally, until the beans are very tender, about 2 hours (add water during the cooking time if necessary); drain the beans.

Yield: 6 servings

Each with: 177 g water; 317 calories (29% from fat, 18% from protein, 52% from carb); 14 g protein; 10 g total fat; 2 g saturated fat; 7 g monounsaturated fat; 1 g polyunsaturated fat; 42 g carb; 10 g fiber; 2 g sugar; 277 mg phosphorus; 84 mg calcium; 4 mg iron; 28 mg sodium; 932 mg potassium; 5 IU vitamin A; 0 mg vitamin E; 5 mg vitamin C; 1 mg cholesterol

Creole Beans

These beans are a taste of New Orleans and are great with blackened chicken or fish.

¼ cup (25 g) sliced celery

¼ cup (40 g) coarsely chopped onion

¼ cup (38 g) chopped green bell pepper

1 teaspoon unsalted butter

2 cups (480 g) no-salt-added canned tomatoes

⅛ teaspoon garlic powder

⅛ teaspoon black pepper

1¼ cups (228 g) cooked navy beans

Cook celery, onion, and bell pepper in butter until tender, about 5 minutes. Break up large pieces of tomatoes. Add tomatoes and seasonings to cooked vegetables. Bring to a boil. Add beans and return to a boil. Reduce heat, cover, and simmer gently until flavors are blended and liquid is reduced, about 30 minutes. Stir occasionally to prevent sticking.

Yield: 2 servings

(continued on page 300)

Each with: 347 g water; 231 calories (11% from fat, 19% from protein, 70% from carb); 12 g protein; 3 g total fat; 1 g saturated fat; 1 g monounsaturated fat; 1 g polyunsaturated fat; 42 g carb; 15 g fiber; 8 g sugar; 223 mg phosphorus; 165 mg calcium; 5 mg iron; 43 mg sodium; 991 mg potassium; 472 IU vitamin A; 16 mg vitamin E; 39 mg vitamin C; 5 mg cholesterol

Italian Bean Bake

This is a really nice Italian side dish. If you can't find cannellini beans, which are a white kidney bean, you can substitute other white beans such as navy or great northern.

3 cups (300 g) cooked cannellini beans, drained

¾ cup (90 g) whole wheat bread crumbs

½ cup (80 g) chopped onion

2 tablespoons grated Romano cheese

1 teaspoon minced garlic

½ teaspoon basil

¼ teaspoon oregano

⅛ teaspoon thyme

⅛ teaspoon black pepper

3 tablespoons grated Parmesan cheese

Preheat oven to 350°F (180°C, gas mark 4). Coat a 2-quart (2 L) casserole dish with nonstick vegetable oil spray. In a bowl, combine all ingredients except Parmesan cheese. Pour into prepared dish. Cover and bake 30 minutes. Sprinkle with Parmesan cheese; cook uncovered 30 minutes more until cheese is melted.

Yield: 8 servings

Each with: 57 g water; 147 calories (15% from fat, 24% from protein, 61% from carb); 9 g protein; 2 g total fat; 1 g saturated fat; 1 g monounsaturated fat; 0 g polyunsaturated fat; 23 g carb; 5 g fiber; 1 g sugar; 174 mg phosphorus; 132 mg calcium; 2 mg iron; 94 mg sodium; 304 mg potassium; 33 IU vitamin A; 6 mg vitamin E; 2 mg vitamin C; 6 mg cholesterol

New England Baked Beans

These are traditional New England-style baked beans sweetened with maple syrup and slow cooked.

1 pound (455 g) navy beans

6 cups (1.4 L) water

2 slices bacon, cut in 1-inch (2.5-cm) cubes

1 cup (160 g) chopped onion

²/₃ cup (160 ml) maple syrup

3 tablespoons (60 g) molasses

Mix all ingredients in a bean pot or ovenproof casserole dish. Bake at 275°F (140°C, gas mark 1) for 5 hours.

Yield: 6 servings

Each with: 327 g water; 235 calories (6% from fat, 12% from protein, 83% from carb); 7 g protein; 2 g total fat; 0 g saturated fat; 1 g monounsaturated fat; 0 g polyunsaturated fat; 50 g carb; 4 g fiber; 29 g sugar; 127 mg phosphorus; 95 mg calcium; 2 mg iron; 416 mg sodium; 501 mg potassium; 2 IU vitamin A; 0 mg vitamin E; 3 mg vitamin C; 3 mg cholesterol

Rancher Beans

This is just the sort of thing you'd want for dinner after a day riding fences on the ranch—something hot, spicy, and filling.

8 slices bacon

2 jalapeño peppers, seeded and chopped

½ teaspoon chopped garlic

1 cup (160 g) chopped onion

¼ cup (60 ml) beer

1 tablespoon (15 ml) red wine vinegar

4 cups (684 g) cooked pinto beans, drained

6 ounces (170 g) no-salt-added tomato paste

(continued on page 302)

Heat the oven to 375°F (190°C, gas mark 5). Cook the bacon in a skillet until crisp and then stir in the jalapeños, garlic, and onion. Cook and stir until the onion is tender and then drain the excess fat. Mix the bacon mixture and remaining ingredients in a 2-quart (2 L) casserole dish coated with nonstick vegetable oil spray. Bake uncovered, stirring once, until the beans are hot and bubbly, about 45 minutes.

Yield: 6 servings

Each with: 134 g water; 261 calories (18% from fat, 24% from protein, 58% from carb); 16 g protein; 5 g total fat; 2 g saturated fat; 2 g monounsaturated fat; 1 g polyunsaturated fat; 39 g carb; 12 g fiber; 5 g sugar; 259 mg phosphorus; 71 mg calcium; 3 mg iron; 278 mg sodium; 898 mg potassium; 474 IU vitamin A; 1 mg vitamin E; 11 mg vitamin C; 12 mg cholesterol

Refried Beans

This makes a big batch of refried beans. The use of the slow cooker makes it easy to prepare. They freeze very nicely, so you can pack some away for the next time. The flavor is fairly traditional (despite the rather untraditional coffee in the ingredients) and not too spicy at all.

1 pound (455 g) pinto beans

4 cups (940 ml) water

1 cup (235 ml) coffee

1 teaspoon minced garlic

1 cup (160 g) diced onion

1 tablespoon cumin

2 teaspoons chili powder

1½ teaspoons oregano

Rinse beans and place in a large bowl covered with water overnight. Drain and place in slow cooker along with remaining ingredients. Stir well, cover, and cook 8 to 10 hours or until beans are tender. Use a potato masher or large spoon to mash the beans until desired consistency.

Yield: 12 servings

Each with: 114 g water; 121 calories (4% from fat, 24% from protein, 72% from carb); 7 g protein; 1 g total fat; 0 g saturated fat; 0 g monounsaturated fat; 0 g polyunsaturated fat; 22 g carb; 5 g fiber; 1 g sugar; 141 mg phosphorus; 50 mg calcium; 2 mg iron; 12 mg sodium; 502 mg potassium; 139 IU vitamin A; 0 mg vitamin E; 3 mg vitamin C; 0 mg cholesterol

Southwestern Beans

This is a quick and tasty bean dish with a little bit of a kick to it.

¼ cup (36 g) poblano chiles, roasted and peeled

½ pound (225 g) chorizo, bulk

1 cup (100 g) green beans, sliced

1 cup (180 g) chopped tomato

2 cans (16 ounces each) pinto beans

Heat the oven to 350°F (180°C, gas mark 4). Cook and stir the chiles and chorizo together until the chorizo is done. Drain off excess fat. Mix the chorizo mixture and remaining ingredients in an ungreased 2-quart (2 L) casserole dish. Drain one can of pinto beans and leave one undrained. Bake uncovered until hot and bubbly. Serve.

Yield: 4 servings

Each with: 85 g water; 275 calories (72% from fat, 21% from protein, 7% from carb); 15 g protein; 22 g total fat; 8 g saturated fat; 10 g monounsaturated fat; 2 g polyunsaturated fat; 5 g carb; 2 g fiber; 2 g sugar; 107 mg phosphorus; 20 mg calcium; 1 mg iron; 705 mg sodium; 391 mg potassium; 526 IU vitamin A; 0 mg vitamin E; 16 mg vitamin C; 50 mg cholesterol

Cowgirl Beans

I'm not quite sure why I decided these were cowgirl, rather than cowboy, beans, but whatever you call them they are good. The tomatoes add a little different texture and taste than typical baked beans, and the jalapeños add a little heat.

1¼ cups (241 g) dried pinto beans

6½ cups (1.5 L) water

¾ cup (120 g) finely chopped onion, divided

1 tablespoon (15 ml) olive oil

2 teaspoons jalapeño pepper, seeded and chopped

¾ cup (135 g) finely diced tomato

6 tablespoons chopped cilantro

Pick over the beans and wash them well. Put them in a kettle, add the water, bring to a boil, and simmer for 1 hour. Add half of the onion. Continue cooking uncovered 30 to 45 minutes longer. Heat the oil in a small skillet and add the remaining onion and the jalapeño. Cook briefly until the onion is wilted. Add the tomato and cilantro and cook, stirring, for 3 more minutes. Add the tomato mixture to the beans and continue to simmer, about 5 more minutes.

Yield: 6 servings

Each with: 299 g water; 172 calories (15% from fat, 21% from protein, 64% from carb); 9 g protein; 3 g total fat; 0 g saturated fat; 2 g monounsaturated fat; 0 g polyunsaturated fat; 28 g carb; 7 g fiber; 2 g sugar; 177 mg phosphorus; 61 mg calcium; 2 mg iron; 17 mg sodium; 649 mg potassium; 298 IU vitamin A; 0 mg vitamin E; 10 mg vitamin C; 0 mg cholesterol

Black-Eyed Peas and Lentils

This is a great side dish for chicken or pork, and a great fiber boost, having 10 grams per serving.

½ pound (225 g) black-eyed peas

½ pound (225 g) lentils

1 cup (160 g) chopped onion

2 cups (480 g) no-salt-added canned tomatoes

¼ teaspoon black pepper

½ teaspoon basil

Soak peas and lentils overnight or for several hours. Combine all ingredients in large pot and cover with water. Cook for approximately 1 hour, seasoning to taste.

Yield: 4 servings

Each with: 226 g water; 178 calories (4% from fat, 24% from protein, 72% from carb); 11 g protein; 1 g total fat; 0 g saturated fat; 0 g monounsaturated fat; 0 g polyunsaturated fat; 34 g carb; 10 g fiber; 8 g sugar; 206 mg phosphorus; 73 mg calcium; 4 mg iron; 21 mg sodium; 711 mg potassium; 197 IU vitamin A; 0 mg vitamin E; 17 mg vitamin C; 0 mg cholesterol

Curried Chickpeas

Try this with tandoori chicken for a real treat—it's a great curry-flavored side dish.

1 tablespoon mustard seeds

1 tablespoon (15 ml) olive oil

Dash red pepper flakes

½ cup (80 g) minced shallot

4 cups (656 g) cooked chickpeas

½ teaspoon turmeric

½ teaspoon cumin

(continued on page 306)

¼ teaspoon ginger

¼ cup chopped fresh cilantro

In a large saucepan, fry mustard seeds in oil until they begin to pop. Add red pepper flakes and shallot and sauté until shallots are soft. Add chickpeas, turmeric, cumin, ginger, and enough water to prevent sticking. Simmer for 15 minutes, sprinkle with cilantro, and serve.

Yield: 6 servings

Each with: 78 g water; 220 calories (23% from fat, 19% from protein, 59% from carb); 11 g protein; 6 g total fat; 1 g saturated fat; 3 g monounsaturated fat; 2 g polyunsaturated fat; 33 g carb; 9 g fiber; 5 g sugar; 210 mg phosphorus; 72 mg calcium; 4 mg iron; 11 mg sodium; 394 mg potassium; 309 IU vitamin A; 0 mg vitamin E; 3 mg vitamin C; 0 mg cholesterol

Dal

Dal is a traditional Indian food made with lentils or split peas.

1 cup (192 g) lentils

4 cups (950 ml) low-sodium chicken broth

2 tablespoons (16 g) grated gingerroot

¼ teaspoon turmeric

⅛ teaspoon cardamom

¼ teaspoon cayenne pepper

½ teaspoon cumin

2 tablespoons fresh cilantro

TIP

Serve with fresh, whole wheat flatbread.

Rinse the lentils and combine them in a medium-size saucepan with the broth. Bring the broth to a boil and then lower the heat and simmer for 1 hour. Add spices, continue to cook briefly.

Yield: 2 servings

Each with: 537 g water; 201 calories (15% from fat, 35% from protein, 51% from carb); 19 g protein; 4 g total fat; 1 g saturated fat; 1 g monounsaturated fat; 1 g polyunsaturated fat; 27 g carb; 8 g fiber; 3 g sugar; 330 mg phosphorus; 47 mg calcium; 5 mg iron; 149 mg sodium; 840 mg potassium; 282 IU vitamin A; 0 mg vitamin E; 3 mg vitamin C; 0 mg cholesterol

Dal with Tomato and Onion

This is another version of dal with added vegetables.

2 cups (384 g) lentils

1 cup (160 g) chopped onion

½ cup (90 g) chopped tomato

1 tablespoon grated gingerroot

1 teaspoon coriander

¾ teaspoon garam masala (an Indian spice blend)

2 tablespoons chopped fresh cilantro

Wash and pick through dry lentils. Soak for 2 hours. Drain water. Put lentils in a saucepan and add water to cover plus 1 inch (2.5 cm). Bring to a boil. Boil vigorously for 5 minutes. Drain water and rinse well. Add fresh water to lentils to cover plus 2 inches (5 cm). Bring to a boil and reduce to a simmer. Simmer until tender, about 30 minutes. While cooking, check constantly to make sure there is enough water to cover. If not, add some. Stir in remaining ingredients during last 30 minutes of cooking.

Yield: 4 servings

Each with: 125 g water; 136 calories (3% from fat, 27% from protein, 70% from carb); 10 g protein; 0 g total fat; 0 g saturated fat; 0 g monounsaturated fat; 0 g polyunsaturated fat; 25 g carb; 9 g fiber; 4 g sugar; 196 mg phosphorus; 33 mg calcium; 4 mg iron; 6 mg sodium; 488 mg potassium; 261 IU vitamin A; 0 mg vitamin E; 8 mg vitamin C; 0 mg cholesterol

Chickpea Loaf

This makes a nice but definitely different side dish. It also has plenty of protein and other good things to be used as a vegetarian main dish.

¾ cup (90 g) whole wheat bread crumbs

¼ cup (25 g) oat bran

1 egg white

½ cup (80 g) finely chopped onion

½ cup (55 g) grated carrot

¼ cup (25 g) finely chopped celery

2 cups (328 g) chickpeas, cooked and mashed

¼ teaspoon thyme

½ teaspoon savory

1 teaspoon basil

2 tablespoons chopped fresh parsley

Combine the bread crumbs and oat bran. Add the egg white and mix. Add the other ingredients. Put the mixture in a loaf pan or casserole dish, nonstick or sprayed with nonstick vegetable oil spray. Bake for 1 hour at 350°F (180°C, gas mark 4). Cut into slices to serve.

Yield: 6 servings

Each with: 88 g water; 170 calories (9% from fat, 16% from protein, 74% from carb); 7 g protein; 2 g total fat; 0 g saturated fat; 0 g monounsaturated fat; 1 g polyunsaturated fat; 32 g carb; 5 g fiber; 2 g sugar; 115 mg phosphorus; 68 mg calcium; 3 mg iron; 286 mg sodium; 257 mg potassium; 1968 IU vitamin A; 6 mg vitamin E; 7 mg vitamin C; 0 mg cholesterol

Pasta with Chickpeas

There was a time when eating pasta with beans just seemed strange to me, but not any more. If it still does to you, this might be a good recipe to start with to overcome that.

3 cups (492 g) cooked chickpeas

1 cup (160 g) chopped onion

½ teaspoon oregano

½ teaspoon garlic powder

¼ teaspoon black pepper, fresh ground

2 cups (480 g) no-salt-added canned tomatoes, chopped

½ teaspoon sugar

¼ cup (60 ml) dry red wine

3 cups (420 g) cooked whole wheat pasta

Combine the chickpeas and their liquid in a large saucepan with the onion, oregano, garlic powder, and pepper. Cook over medium heat for 10 minutes. Add the tomatoes, sugar, and wine. Bring to a boil; cover, reduce heat, and simmer for 30 minutes. Add the cooked pasta and stir well. Serve in soup bowls.

Yield: 6 servings

Each with: 195 g water; 361 calories (5% from fat, 16% from protein, 79% from carb); 15 g protein; 2 g total fat; 0 g saturated fat; 0 g monounsaturated fat; 1 g polyunsaturated fat; 73 g carb; 11 g fiber; 4 g sugar; 270 mg phosphorus; 93 mg calcium; 4 mg iron; 375 mg sodium; 526 mg potassium; 129 IU vitamin A; 0 mg vitamin E; 14 mg vitamin C; 0 mg cholesterol

Bean Patties

This is a tasty side dish made from leftover beans. It's great with a pork chop and some greens.

1½ cups (256 g) cooked pinto beans, drained

1 cup (160 g) finely chopped onion

½ cup (120 ml) fat-free evaporated milk

½ cup (62 g) flour

2 tablespoons (28 ml) olive oil

Mash pinto beans. Add onion and milk. Add enough flour to make patties. Heat oil in a heavy skillet. Spoon bean mixture into skillet, flattening into a pattie. Fry until brown, turning once.

Yield: 4 servings

TIP *You can substitute any other kind of leftover beans you have for the pinto beans.*

Each with: 103 g water; 249 calories (26% from fat, 16% from protein, 57% from carb); 10 g protein; 7 g total fat; 1 g saturated fat; 5 g monounsaturated fat; 1 g polyunsaturated fat; 36 g carb; 7 g fiber; 6 g sugar; 185 mg phosphorus; 134 mg calcium; 2 mg iron; 39 mg sodium; 461 mg potassium; 127 IU vitamin A; 38 mg vitamin E; 4 mg vitamin C; 1 mg cholesterol

Black-Eyed Pea Salad

This has become a traditional New Year's Day dish in our house. It's a way to get the black-eyed peas for luck that still goes with the roast beef dinner that we always have. Even children will usually eat a little of this, ensuring luck for the year.

1 teaspoon Dijon mustard

1½ teaspoons (8 ml) cider vinegar

1½ teaspoons (8 ml) olive oil

2 cups (344 g) cooked black-eyed peas

10 ounces (280 g) frozen corn, thawed

½ cup (75 g) finely chopped red bell pepper

¼ cup (40 g) finely chopped red onion

In a medium container, whisk the mustard, vinegar, and oil. Add all the vegetables. Toss to combine.

Yield: 4 servings

Each with: 139 g water; 198 calories (14% from fat, 19% from protein, 68% from carb); 10 g protein; 3 g total fat; 1 g saturated fat; 2 g monounsaturated fat; 1 g polyunsaturated fat; 36 g carb; 8 g fiber; 7 g sugar; 176 mg phosphorus; 25 mg calcium; 2 mg iron; 30 mg sodium; 567 mg potassium; 795 IU vitamin A; 0 mg vitamin E; 32 mg vitamin C; 0 mg cholesterol

Chickpea Salad

Here is something a little different, based on chickpeas. Serve it as a side dish or over lettuce as a salad.

14 ounces (397 g) artichoke hearts

¼ cup (60 ml) lemon juice

½ teaspoon black pepper

½ teaspoon minced garlic

2 cups (328 g) canned chickpeas, drained

16 cherry tomatoes, halved

3 eggs, hard cooked and cut in wedges

Drain artichoke hearts and reserve liquid. Make a dressing by combining artichoke liquid, lemon juice, pepper, and garlic. Set aside. In a bowl, place chopped artichoke hearts, the chickpeas, and the tomatoes. Pour the dressing over the mixture and refrigerate. Let marinate 6 to 12 hours. Before serving, top with chopped egg.

Yield: 4 servings

Each with: 215 g water; 267 calories (20% from fat, 21% from protein, 59% from carb); 15 g protein; 6 g total fat; 2 g saturated fat; 2 g monounsaturated fat; 1 g polyunsaturated fat; 41 g carb; 11 g fiber; 2 g sugar; 251 mg phosphorus; 88 mg calcium; 3 mg iron; 471 mg sodium; 699 mg potassium; 823 IU vitamin A; 58 mg vitamin E; 30 mg vitamin C; 178 mg cholesterol

Marinated Black-Eyed Peas

I've found that young people and others who say they don't like black-eyed peas don't seem to mind them at all if they're given a little extra flavor and made part of a salad. These peas are an easy way to meet that requirement.

4 cups (688 g) cooked black-eyed peas, drained

½ cup (120 ml) olive oil

⅓ cup (78 ml) white wine vinegar

¼ cup (40 g) chopped onion

1 teaspoon garlic powder

⅛ teaspoon black pepper

¼ teaspoon Tabasco sauce

Combine all ingredients in a large bowl, stirring well. Cover and marinate in refrigerator 3 days. Before serving, garnish with a few sliced onion rings and pepper rings, if desired.

Yield: 6 servings

Each with: 94 g water; 316 calories (53% from fat, 12% from protein, 35% from carb); 10 g protein; 19 g total fat; 3 g saturated fat; 13 g monounsaturated fat; 2 g polyunsaturated fat; 28 g carb; 7 g fiber; 6 g sugar; 143 mg phosphorus; 29 mg calcium; 3 mg iron; 8 mg sodium; 451 mg potassium; 88 IU vitamin A; 0 mg vitamin E; 4 mg vitamin C; 0 mg cholesterol

Mexican Bean Salad

This is a Mexican version of three bean salad, flavored with chili powder but without another dressing. Serve it as is as a side dish or as a salad drizzled with Italian or other dressing.

1 cup (160 g) sliced red onion

¼ cup (60 ml) water

1 tablespoon chili powder

1 cup (100 g) cooked green beans

1 cup (172 g) cooked black beans

1 cup (100 g) cooked kidney beans

1 cup (182 g) cooked navy beans

½ cup (82 g) frozen corn, thawed

2 tablespoons chopped cilantro

Place the onion in a saucepan with the water. Cook gently until the onion is soft and separated into rings, 4 to 5 minutes. Add the chili powder and stir until well mixed. Remove from heat. Combine all of the remaining ingredients in a large bowl and toss to mix well. Cover and chill for 1 to 2 hours to allow flavors to blend.

Yield: 6 servings

Each with: 88 g water; 289 calories (4% from fat, 24% from protein, 73% from carb); 18 g protein; 1 g total fat; 0 g saturated fat; 0 g monounsaturated fat; 1 g polyunsaturated fat; 54 g carb; 17 g fiber; 4 g sugar; 333 mg phosphorus; 120 mg calcium; 6 mg iron; 26 mg sodium; 1070 mg potassium; 559 IU vitamin A; 0 mg vitamin E; 9 mg vitamin C; 0 mg cholesterol

Pea Salad

Quick, how many kinds of peas can you name? This salad probably contains all of them.

1 cup (164 g) cooked chickpeas, drained and rinsed

1 cup (172 g) cooked black-eyed peas, drained

1 cup (130 g) frozen peas, cooked and cooled

½ cup (80 g) finely chopped onion

¾ cup (114 g) finely chopped green bell pepper

½ cup (100 g) sugar

⅓ cup (78 ml) cider vinegar

½ cup (120 ml) olive oil

¼ teaspoon black pepper

TIP *This may be served on lettuce and garnished with cherry tomatoes or pimento and sliced cucumbers.*

In a shallow container, stir together all ingredients. Cover tightly and chill.

Yield: 6 servings

Each with: 98 g water; 339 calories (50% from fat, 8% from protein, 43% from carb); 7 g protein; 19 g total fat; 3 g saturated fat; 13 g monounsaturated fat; 2 g polyunsaturated fat; 37 g carb; 6 g fiber; 22 g sugar; 113 mg phosphorus; 33 mg calcium; 2 mg iron; 92 mg sodium; 293 mg potassium; 662 IU vitamin A; 0 mg vitamin E; 20 mg vitamin C; 0 mg cholesterol

15

Side Dishes and Salads:
Grains

G rains are a natural for side dishes. Rice is probably the one you think of first, but don't ignore other choices such as barley and bulgur. We've included a number of recipes here to get you thinking about them.

Brown Rice Fritters

This is almost sweet enough to be a dessert, but it's also good as a side dish.

2 cups (440 g) cooked brown rice

3 eggs, beaten

¼ teaspoon vanilla extract

½ teaspoon nutmeg

¼ cup (50 g) sugar

6 tablespoons (48 g) flour

1 tablespoon baking powder

2 tablespoons (16 g) confectioners' sugar

Combine rice, eggs, vanilla, nutmeg, and sugar and mix well. Sift dry ingredients together and stir into rice mixture. Drop by spoonfuls into hot deep fat (360°F) and fry until brown. Drain on absorbent paper, sprinkle with confectioners' sugar, and serve hot.

Yield: 6 servings

Each with: 70 g water; 186 calories (18% from fat, 14% from protein, 68% from carb); 6 g protein; 4 g total fat; 1 g saturated fat; 1 g monounsaturated fat; 1 g polyunsaturated fat; 33 g carb; 1 g fiber; 11 g sugar; 167 mg phosphorus; 158 mg calcium; 1 mg iron; 286 mg sodium; 75 mg potassium; 137 IU vitamin A; 39 mg vitamin E; 0 mg vitamin C; 118 mg cholesterol

Mexican Rice

This family favorite is a quick and flavorful use for leftover rice.

1 cup (220 g) cooked brown rice

2 tablespoons (28 ml) olive oil

½ cup (80 g) chopped onion

¼ pound (113 g) shredded Cheddar cheese

1 jalapeño pepper, chopped

Brown rice in oil. Add remaining ingredients. Cover and simmer until heated through and cheese is melted.

Yield: 4 servings

Each with: 67 g water; 237 calories (63% from fat, 14% from protein, 23% from carb); 9 g protein; 17 g total fat; 7 g saturated fat; 8 g monounsaturated fat; 1 g polyunsaturated fat; 14 g carb; 1 g fiber; 1 g sugar; 192 mg phosphorus; 214 mg calcium; 1 mg iron; 179 mg sodium; 86 mg potassium; 312 IU vitamin A; 73 mg vitamin E; 3 mg vitamin C; 30 mg cholesterol

Tomato Pilaf

This makes a delicious side dish for any meal where you would normally have rice or noodles.

2 cups (480 g) no-salt-added canned tomatoes

2 teaspoons (10 ml) olive oil

½ cup (80 g) minced onion

1 cup (140 g) bulgur

½ cup (30 g) chopped fresh parsley

Drain tomatoes, reserving juice. Heat oil in a skillet and add onion. Sauté until tender. Add bulgur and brown for 1 minute until golden colored. Put in casserole dish. Add enough water to reserved tomato juice to make 2 cups (475 ml) liquid. Pour over wheat mixture along with parsley and tomatoes. Cover. Bake at 350°F (180°C, gas mark 4) for 45 minutes. Remove cover; stir and bake, uncovered, 5 minutes longer.

Yield: 4 servings

Each with: 141 g water; 171 calories (14% from fat, 12% from protein, 73% from carb); 6 g protein; 3 g total fat; 0 g saturated fat; 2 g monounsaturated fat; 1 g polyunsaturated fat; 34 g carb; 8 g fiber; 4 g sugar; 138 mg phosphorus; 64 mg calcium; 3 mg iron; 27 mg sodium; 440 mg potassium; 776 IU vitamin A; 0 mg vitamin E; 23 mg vitamin C; 0 mg cholesterol

Rice and Cheese Casserole

This cheesy rice side dish is a good use for leftover rice. And it is good enough that you may want to make sure some of it is left over.

2 cups (440 g) cooked brown rice

1 cup (115 g) shredded Cheddar cheese

2 tablespoons (20 g) chopped onion

3 eggs, slightly beaten

Place rice in a 1½-quart (1.5 L) baking dish. Combine remaining ingredients and pour over rice. Bake at 350°F (180°C, gas mark 4) for 25 minutes.

Yield: 4 servings

Each with: 120 g water; 303 calories (48% from fat, 21% from protein, 31% from carb); 16 g protein; 16 g total fat; 8 g saturated fat; 5 g monounsaturated fat; 1 g polyunsaturated fat; 24 g carb; 2 g fiber; 1 g sugar; 332 mg phosphorus; 271 mg calcium; 1 mg iron; 269 mg sodium; 138 mg potassium; 535 IU vitamin A; 144 mg vitamin E; 0 mg vitamin C; 212 mg cholesterol

Southern Rice Pilaf

This rice has lots of good things added to it.

2 cups (380 g) brown rice

4 tablespoons (55 g) unsalted butter, melted

½ teaspoon cumin seeds

¼ teaspoon cinnamon

2 whole cloves

1 cup (150 g) peas

3½ cups (830 ml) water

½ cup (80 g) finely sliced onion

¼ cup (27 g) slivered almonds

¼ cup (35 g) raisins

Wash rice, drain, and set aside for about 30 minutes. Put half the butter in a saucepan, add the cumin seeds, and heat. When cumin seeds turn slightly brown, add cinnamon and cloves and the peas. Fry for a minute and add the rice. Mix for another minute. Add the water and after it starts to boil, cover and put on low heat and cook until done, about 35 to 45 minutes. For garnish, take half the remaining butter and fry the onion until lightly brown and sprinkle on top of rice. With the rest of the butter, fry slivered almonds and raisins until lightly brown and sprinkle on top of the onion and rice. Serve hot.

Yield: 4 servings

Each with: 332 g water; 333 calories (45% from fat, 8% from protein, 47% from carb); 7 g protein; 17 g total fat; 8 g saturated fat; 6 g monounsaturated fat; 2 g polyunsaturated fat; 40 g carb; 6 g fiber; 10 g sugar; 180 mg phosphorus; 66 mg calcium; 2 mg iron; 144 mg sodium; 291 mg potassium; 1199 IU vitamin A; 95 mg vitamin E; 6 mg vitamin C; 31 mg cholesterol

Barley and Pine Nut Casserole

This is a simple but flavorful side dish with the additional crunch of pine nuts. It's good with any grilled meat, especially ones with Italian seasoning.

1 cup (200 g) pearl barley

½ cup (70 g) pine nuts, divided

3 tablespoons (42 g) unsalted butter, divided

1 cup (160 g) chopped onion

½ cup (30 g) minced fresh parsley

¼ cup (25 g) minced scallions

¼ teaspoon black pepper, freshly ground

3 cups (355 ml) low-sodium chicken broth, heated to boiling

(continued on page 320)

Preheat oven to 375°F (190°C, gas mark 5). Rinse and drain barley. Toast pine nuts in 1 table-spoon butter in a skillet. Remove nuts with slotted spoon and set aside. Add remaining butter to skillet with onion and barley and stir until toasted. Stir in nuts, parsley, scallions, and pepper. Spoon into a 1½-quart (1.5 L) casserole dish. Pour hot broth over casserole and mix well. Bake uncovered for 1 hour and 15 minutes.

Yield: 6 servings

Each with: 152 g water; 268 calories (48% from fat, 12% from protein, 41% from carb); 8 g protein; 15 g total fat; 5 g saturated fat; 4 g monounsaturated fat; 5 g polyunsaturated fat; 29 g carb; 6 g fiber; 2 g sugar; 196 mg phosphorus; 35 mg calcium; 2 mg iron; 45 mg sodium; 390 mg potassium; 651 IU vitamin A; 48 mg vitamin E; 10 mg vitamin C; 15 mg cholesterol

Barley Casserole

This barley casserole is flavored with beef broth, making it a great choice to have with steak or roast beef.

½ cup (80 g) chopped onion

2 tablespoons (28 ml) olive oil

2 cups (400 g) pearl barley

6 cups (1.4 L) low-sodium beef broth

¼ teaspoon black pepper

1 cup (235 ml) boiling water

Sauté onion in oil until transparent. Add barley and continue cooking until barley is lightly browned. Put in 2-quart (2 L) casserole dish that has been sprayed with nonstick vegetable oil spray. Just before baking, bring broth to a boil. Add broth, pepper, and water to barley and stir gently. Bake covered 1 hour or until barley is tender. Add more water or broth if necessary.

Yield: 8 servings

Each with: 218 g water; 200 calories (20% from fat, 15% from protein, 65% from carb); 8 g protein; 5 g total fat; 1 g saturated fat; 3 g monounsaturated fat; 1 g polyunsaturated fat; 35 g carb; 8 g fiber; 1 g sugar; 148 mg phosphorus; 29 mg calcium; 2 mg iron; 112 mg sodium; 320 mg potassium; 13 IU vitamin A; 0 mg vitamin E; 1 mg vitamin C; 0 mg cholesterol

Barley Mushroom Pilaf

This is a quick and easy way to give barley some extra flavor. We like this with chicken, but it would go with a number of meals.

2 teaspoons (10 ml) olive oil

½ cup (35 g) sliced mushrooms

1 cup (200 g) pearl barley

3 cups (710 ml) low-sodium chicken broth

2 tablespoons chopped scallions

¼ teaspoon rosemary

2 tablespoons grated Parmesan cheese

Heat olive oil in saucepan; add mushrooms and sauté until limp. Add barley, broth, scallions, and rosemary. Bring to a boil. Reduce heat to low, cover, and cook 45 minutes or until barley is tender and liquid is absorbed. Sprinkle Parmesan cheese over pilaf and serve.

Yield: 4 servings

Each with: 189 g water; 228 calories (20% from fat, 18% from protein, 62% from carb); 11 g protein; 5 g total fat; 1 g saturated fat; 3 g monounsaturated fat; 1 g polyunsaturated fat; 37 g carb; 8 g fiber; 1 g sugar; 207 mg phosphorus; 60 mg calcium; 2 mg iron; 108 mg sodium; 403 mg potassium; 56 IU vitamin A; 4 mg vitamin E; 1 mg vitamin C; 3 mg cholesterol

Barley Risotto

This is not exactly like traditional risotto, but it's still a delightful side dish.

½ cup (100 g) pearl barley

1 teaspoon (5 ml) olive oil

3 tablespoons (21 g) minced carrot

3 tablespoons (30 g) minced onion

3 tablespoons (24 g) minced celery

1 teaspoon rosemary

1 bay leaf

½ teaspoon black pepper

1½ cups (355 ml) vegetable broth

Put barley in heavy skillet over low heat and toast. Shake pan frequently. When barley turns light brown and smells nutty, about 15 to 20 minutes, remove from skillet. Heat oil in skillet, add minced vegetables, and sauté for 3 minutes. Add barley and stir to coat grains. Add herbs and broth. Simmer, covered, until barley is tender and liquid is absorbed, about 35 minutes. Remove bay leaf before serving.

Yield: 4 servings

Each with: 108 g water; 138 calories (24% from fat, 11% from protein, 65% from carb); 4 g protein; 4 g total fat; 1 g saturated fat; 2 g monounsaturated fat; 1 g polyunsaturated fat; 23 g carb; 5 g fiber; 1 g sugar; 87 mg phosphorus; 27 mg calcium; 1 mg iron; 450 mg sodium; 187 mg potassium; 1041 IU vitamin A; 0 mg vitamin E; 3 mg vitamin C; 0 mg cholesterol

Bulgur Pilaf

This simple dish can be used as a side dish similar to cooked rice.

2 tablespoons (28 ml) olive oil

½ cup (50 g) chopped celery

1 cup (160 g) chopped onion

1 cup (70 g) sliced mushrooms

1 cup (140 g) bulgur

½ teaspoon dried dill

¼ teaspoon dried oregano

¼ teaspoon black pepper, fresh ground

2 cups (475 ml) low-sodium chicken broth

Heat oil in a large skillet; add celery, onion, and mushrooms. Stir constantly until vegetables are tender. Add bulgur and cook until golden. Add seasonings and chicken broth. Cover and bring to a boil. Reduce heat and simmer 15 minutes.

Yield: 6 servings

Each with: 122 g water; 148 calories (31% from fat, 13% from protein, 56% from carb); 5 g protein; 5 g total fat; 1 g saturated fat; 4 g monounsaturated fat; 1 g polyunsaturated fat; 22 g carb; 5 g fiber; 2 g sugar; 114 mg phosphorus; 24 mg calcium; 1 mg iron; 37 mg sodium; 267 mg potassium; 49 IU vitamin A; 0 mg vitamin E; 3 mg vitamin C; 0 mg cholesterol

Bulgur Wheat with Squash

Sometimes grain side dishes can be pretty plain. This one gets it flavor from butternut squash, and it turns out to be a winning combination.

1½ tablespoons (21 g) unsalted butter

½ cup (80 g) chopped onion

1 cup (140 g) peeled and cubed butternut squash

½ cup (70 g) bulgur

2 whole cloves

2 cinnamon sticks

1 bay leaf

1 cup (235 ml) low-sodium chicken broth

Melt butter over medium heat. Add onion and squash. Cook until onion is soft. Add bulgur, cloves, cinnamon, and bay leaf. Stir until bulgur is brown. Stir in chicken broth. Cover and bring to a boil. Reduce heat and cook 15 minutes. Remove spices before serving.

Yield: 4 servings

Each with: 108 g water; 131 calories (32% from fat, 11% from protein, 57% from carb); 4 g protein; 5 g total fat; 3 g saturated fat; 1 g monounsaturated fat; 0 g polyunsaturated fat; 20 g carb; 4 g fiber; 2 g sugar; 89 mg phosphorus; 31 mg calcium; 1 mg iron; 24 mg sodium; 277 mg potassium; 3855 IU vitamin A; 36 mg vitamin E; 9 mg vitamin C; 11 mg cholesterol

Stuffed Tomatoes

Tomatoes stuffed with a rice/cheese/veggie mix make a nice side dish for just about any kind of meat.

6 medium tomatoes

2 tablespoons (28 ml) olive oil

⅓ cup (33 g) chopped celery

2 tablespoons (20 g) chopped onion

2 cups (440 g) cooked brown rice

¼ cup (25 g) grated Parmesan cheese

1 tablespoon chopped fresh parsley

1 teaspoon basil

⅛ teaspoon black pepper

⅛ teaspoon garlic powder

TIP *Use one lightly oiled custard cup for each tomato instead of a pie pan or baking dish, if desired.*

Cut a thin slice from the top of each tomato. Set tops aside. Scoop out center of tomatoes; chop pulp, and set aside. Place shells upside down on paper towels to drain. Lightly oil 9-inch (23 cm) pie plate or round baking dish. Place tomatoes in dish. Cover with aluminum foil. Preheat oven to 350°F (180°C, gas mark 4). Heat oil in medium saucepan. Add celery and onion. Sauté over moderate heat until celery is tender. Remove from heat. Add reserved tomato pulp, rice, cheese, parsley, basil, pepper, and garlic powder; mix well. Fill tomato shells with rice mixture. Replace tomato tops, if desired. Bake at 350°F (180°C, gas mark 4), 30 to 45 minutes or until tomatoes are tender.

Yield: 6 servings

Each with: 197 g water; 164 calories (36% from fat, 11% from protein, 53% from carb); 5 g protein; 7 g total fat; 2 g saturated fat; 4 g monounsaturated fat; 1 g polyunsaturated fat; 23 g carb; 3 g fiber; 1 g sugar; 124 mg phosphorus; 67 mg calcium; 1 mg iron; 86 mg sodium; 392 mg potassium; 1036 IU vitamin A; 5 mg vitamin E; 40 mg vitamin C; 4 mg cholesterol

Rigatoni with Artichoke Sauce

This is a nice pasta sauce flavored with marinated artichoke hearts.

1 pound (455 g) whole wheat rigatoni

6 ounces (170 g) artichoke hearts, drained

¼ cup (60 ml) olive oil

¾ teaspoon minced garlic

2 tablespoons chopped fresh parsley

3 cups (720 g) no-salt-added canned tomatoes, drained and chopped

⅛ teaspoon red pepper flakes

¼ cup (25 g) grated Parmesan cheese

¼ teaspoon black pepper, fresh ground

Cook pasta according to directions. Meanwhile, slice artichokes thinly. In large saucepan, heat oil and sauté garlic 2 minutes. Add artichoke hearts, parsley, tomatoes, and pepper flakes. Cook 20 minutes, stirring occasionally. Drain rigatoni and place in serving dish. Top pasta with sauce and sprinkle with Parmesan cheese and black pepper.

Yield: 6 servings

Each with: 145 g water; 395 calories (25% from fat, 14% from protein, 61% from carb); 15 g protein; 12 g total fat; 2 g saturated fat; 7 g monounsaturated fat; 2 g polyunsaturated fat; 65 g carb; 3 g fiber; 3 g sugar; 267 mg phosphorus; 123 mg calcium; 4 mg iron; 101 mg sodium; 478 mg potassium; 326 IU vitamin A; 5 mg vitamin E; 14 mg vitamin C; 4 mg cholesterol

Whole Wheat Pasta with Pesto

This is a quick and easy pasta meal with fresh pesto.

1 tablespoon (15 ml) olive oil

1 teaspoon (5 ml) water

⅛ teaspoon salt

½ teaspoon minced garlic

3 tablespoons minced fresh basil

3 tablespoons minced fresh parsley

¼ cup (25 g) grated Parmesan cheese

2 cups (210 g) whole wheat pasta, cooked

Combine oil, water, salt, garlic, basil, parsley, and Parmesan cheese in container of an electric blender. Cover and process until smooth pesto is formed. Combine pasta and pesto mixture in a medium bowl and toss gently.

Yield: 4 servings

Each with: 9 g water; 245 calories (21% from fat, 16% from protein, 63% from carb); 10 g protein; 6 g total fat; 2 g saturated fat; 3 g monounsaturated fat; 1 g polyunsaturated fat; 41 g carb; 5 g fiber; 0 g sugar; 191 mg phosphorus; 128 mg calcium; 3 mg iron; 176 mg sodium; 192 mg potassium; 412 IU vitamin A; 7 mg vitamin E; 5 mg vitamin C; 6 mg cholesterol

Better Than Stove Top

This do-it-yourself stuffing beats the boxed stuff both on taste and nutrition.

½ cup (80 g) chopped onion

¼ cup (25 g) sliced celery

¼ cup (55 g) unsalted butter, divided

1 tablespoon parsley flakes

½ teaspoon black pepper, fresh ground

½ teaspoon sage

½ teaspoon thyme

1 cup (235 ml) low-sodium chicken broth

2 cups (230 g) whole wheat bread crumbs

In a saucepan, sauté onion and celery in 1 tablespoon butter until tender. Stir in remaining ingredients, except bread, and simmer for 5 minutes. Add bread, cover, turn off heat, and allow to sit for 8 to 10 minutes.

Yield: 4 servings

Each with: 88 g water; 336 calories (39% from fat, 11% from protein, 50% from carb); 9 g protein; 15 g total fat; 8 g saturated fat; 4 g monounsaturated fat; 2 g polyunsaturated fat; 42 g carb; 3 g fiber; 4 g sugar; 120 mg phosphorus; 122 mg calcium; 3 mg iron; 102 mg sodium; 225 mg potassium; 431 IU vitamin A; 95 mg vitamin E; 2 mg vitamin C; 31 mg cholesterol

Sausage Stuffing

This stuffing is a little different, with sausage and cheese providing a flavor boost.

1 pound (455 g) whole wheat bread, day old

½ cup (120 ml) skim milk

10 ounces (280 g) frozen spinach

1 pound (455 g) breakfast sausage

1 cup (160 g) diced onion

1 cup (70 g) sliced mushrooms

1 teaspoon crushed garlic

1 tablespoon unsalted butter

1 cup (115 g) shredded Monterey Jack cheese

3 egg yolks

Discard ends of bread and tear remaining loaf into pieces; place in a bowl. Pour just enough milk over bread to cover; soak for 5 minutes. Strain out milk, squeeze bread dry, and set aside. Cook spinach per directions on package, cool, squeeze dry, and set aside. In a skillet, fry sausage, crumbling as you cook it. Drain grease; set aside. Sauté onion, mushrooms, and garlic in butter until onion becomes translucent. Add spinach and sausage to onion and garlic, mix well; set aside to cool. Combine bread and spinach mixture with cheese. Add egg yolks. Combine all ingredients into a 12 × 9 × 4-inch (30 × 23 × 10-cm) casserole dish coated with nonstick vegetable oil spray. Bake covered in 350°F (180°C, gas mark 4) oven for 35 to 45 minutes or until heated through.

Yield: 8 servings

Each with: 140 g water; 483 calories (54% from fat, 19% from protein, 27% from carb); 23 g protein; 29 g total fat; 12 g saturated fat; 12 g monounsaturated fat; 4 g polyunsaturated fat; 33 g carb; 4 g fiber; 5 g sugar; 327 mg phosphorus; 306 mg calcium; 4 mg iron; 878 mg sodium; 480 mg potassium; 4603 IU vitamin A; 86 mg vitamin E; 4 mg vitamin C; 141 mg cholesterol

Stuffing

Almost everyone has different herbs and additives they like in their stuffing. Feel free to change the seasonings with such ingredients as thyme and basil. You can also add other things like mushrooms or chopped turkey giblets if this is something you would normally do. The longer you let the bread cubes dry out before making the stuffing, the more broth you will need.

1 pound (455 g) whole wheat bread, cubed or crumbled

2 cups (475 ml) low-sodium chicken broth

1 cup (160 g) chopped onion

½ cup (50 g) chopped celery

2 teaspoons tarragon

1 teaspoon sage

1 teaspoon poultry seasoning

1½ teaspoons black pepper

Combine all ingredients and toss lightly. Place in a 9 × 13-inch (23 × 33 cm) baking dish coated with nonstick vegetable oil spray. Bake at 350°F (180°C, gas mark 4) until heated through, about 30 minutes.

Yield: 12 servings

Each with: 68 g water; 114 calories (13% from fat, 18% from protein, 69% from carb); 5 g protein; 2 g total fat; 0 g saturated fat; 0 g monounsaturated fat; 1 g polyunsaturated fat; 20 g carb; 2 g fiber; 3 g sugar; 77 mg phosphorus; 64 mg calcium; 2 mg iron; 213 mg sodium; 142 mg potassium; 31 IU vitamin A; 0 mg vitamin E; 1 mg vitamin C; 0 mg cholesterol

Curried Rice Salad

This spiced rice dish can be served either chilled or warm. The spices give a Middle Eastern or Indian sort of flavor.

1 cup (185 g) rice, long cooking

2 cups (475 ml) water

2 tablespoons (28 g) unsalted butter

½ cup (80 g) chopped onion

½ teaspoon minced garlic

½ teaspoon ginger

½ teaspoon cinnamon

1 bay leaf

¼ teaspoon ground coriander

¼ teaspoon ground black pepper

¼ teaspoon turmeric

¼ teaspoon ground cumin

⅛ teaspoon cayenne pepper

¼ cup (35 g) golden raisins

¼ cup (27 g) slivered almonds, toasted

½ cup (82 g) cooked chickpeas, drained

½ cup (75 g) fresh peas or defrosted frozen peas

Place the rice in a colander and rinse under cold running water. Place the rinsed rice in a large bowl and cover with 2 cups (475 ml) of water. Let soak 30 minutes. Drain and reserve the water for cooking. In a large pot, heat the butter over medium-high heat. Add the onion and cook, stirring, for 3 minutes. Add the garlic and ginger and cook, stirring, for 45 seconds. Add the cinnamon, bay leaf, coriander, pepper, turmeric, cumin, and cayenne and cook, stirring, until fragrant, about 45 seconds. Add the rice and cook, stirring, for 2 minutes. Add the reserved soaking liquid and raisins and bring to a boil. Reduce the heat to low, stir, cover, and simmer until the water is absorbed and the rice is tender, 20 minutes. Remove from the heat and let sit covered for 15 minutes. Fluff the rice with a fork and transfer to a large bowl. Combine with the remaining ingredients. Remove bay leaf. Serve warm or chilled.

Yield: 4 servings

Each with: 54 g water; 368 calories (28% from fat, 10% from protein, 62% from carb); 9 g protein; 12 g total fat; 4 g saturated fat; 5 g monounsaturated fat; 2 g polyunsaturated fat; 58 g carb; 6 g fiber; 9 g sugar; 187 mg phosphorus; 82 mg calcium; 4 mg iron; 21 mg sodium; 355 mg potassium; 631 IU vitamin A; 48 mg vitamin E; 5 mg vitamin C; 15 mg cholesterol

Mediterranean Rice Salad

This is another one of those salads that I'm always glad makes a lot so I have some left over for lunch the next day.

2½ cups (550 g) cooked, cooled brown rice

½ cup (50 g) chopped celery

½ cup (75 g) chopped green bell pepper

¼ cup (48 g) chopped pimento

¼ cup (25 g) chopped scallions

Dressing

6 ounces (170 g) artichoke hearts, undrained and chopped

1 cup (225 g) mayonnaise

1 teaspoon oregano

Mix ingredients well. Combine dressing ingredients, pour over rice mixture, and stir to blend.

Yield: 6 servings

Each with: 120 g water; 374 calories (70% from fat, 4% from protein, 26% from carb); 4 g protein; 30 g total fat; 5 g saturated fat; 7 g monounsaturated fat; 16 g polyunsaturated fat; 24 g carb; 3 g fiber; 1 g sugar; 103 mg phosphorus; 31 mg calcium; 1 mg iron; 237 mg sodium; 193 mg potassium; 499 IU vitamin A; 29 mg vitamin E; 19 mg vitamin C; 14 mg cholesterol

Sicilian-Style Pasta Salad

This is an Italian pasta salad with a deeper set of flavors than the usual one.

12 ounces (340 g) whole wheat pasta

⅓ cup (80 ml) olive oil

½ teaspoon finely minced garlic

1 cup (160 g) chopped onion

1 tablespoon chopped fresh parsley

1 tablespoon (16 g) no-salt-added tomato paste

¼ cup (60 ml) water

¼ cup (60 ml) dry white wine

1 teaspoon basil

¼ teaspoon ground rosemary

⅛ teaspoon ground marjoram

⅛ teaspoon black pepper

⅛ teaspoon ground thyme

⅛ teaspoon ground oregano

½ cup (75 g) chopped green bell pepper

½ cup (75 g) chopped red bell pepper

6 ounces (170 g) black olives

Cook pasta according to package directions. In a large skillet simmer oil, garlic, onion, and parsley until tender. Combine tomato paste and water. Add the tomato mixture, wine, and seasonings. Continue to simmer 5 to 7 minutes. Add bell peppers. Simmer an additional 2 minutes until tender. Pour over pasta and blend. Garnish with black olives. Chill approximately 1 to 2 hours. Serve cold.

Yield: 6 servings

Each with: 95 g water; 364 calories (38% from fat, 10% from protein, 52% from carb); 9 g protein; 16 g total fat; 2 g saturated fat; 11 g monounsaturated fat; 2 g polyunsaturated fat; 49 g carb; 7 g fiber; 2 g sugar; 166 mg phosphorus; 63 mg calcium; 3 mg iron; 258 mg sodium; 256 mg potassium; 659 IU vitamin A; 0 mg vitamin E; 30 mg vitamin C; 0 mg cholesterol

Vegetable Bulgur Salad

This healthy salad is full of the goodness of whole wheat and vegetables.

1 cup (70 g) bulgur

1 cup (235 ml) boiling water

½ cup (65 g) coarsely chopped carrot

½ cup (80 g) green sliced onion

½ cup (75 g) chopped green bell pepper

¼ cup (25 g) sliced celery

¼ cup (60 ml) lemon juice

⅓ cup (80 ml) olive oil

½ teaspoon pressed garlic

1½ teaspoons basil

½ teaspoon dry mustard

½ teaspoon black pepper, fresh ground

Cover bulgur with boiling water and let stand 1 hour. Cool; then add vegetables. Mix remaining ingredients to make dressing. Add dressing, cover, and let stand 4 hours.

Yield: 4 servings

Each with: 125 g water; 300 calories (53% from fat, 6% from protein, 40% from carb); 5 g protein; 19 g total fat; 3 g saturated fat; 13 g monounsaturated fat; 2 g polyunsaturated fat; 32 g carb; 8 g fiber; 2 g sugar; 124 mg phosphorus; 42 mg calcium; 1 mg iron; 27 mg sodium; 313 mg potassium; 2944 IU vitamin A; 0 mg vitamin E; 26 mg vitamin C; 0 mg cholesterol

Warm Rice Salad

This is a good side salad, but I also like it as a meal in itself, with maybe a little leftover chicken added on top.

1 tablespoon unsalted butter

½ cup (72 g) almonds

3 cups (355 ml) low-sodium chicken broth

½ cup (95 g) brown rice

½ cup (100 g) pearl barley

½ cup (75 g) raisins

2 tablespoons chopped fresh parsley

Vinaigrette

1 tablespoon (15 ml) red wine vinegar

½ teaspoon Dijon mustard

⅛ teaspoon black pepper

4 teaspoons (20 ml) olive oil

In a pie pan, microwave butter until melted. Stir in almonds; microwave on high for 2 minutes or until browned, stirring often. Chop and set aside. In a 1-quart (1 L) casserole dish, microwave broth, rice, and barley on high for 8 minutes or until boiling; stir. Cover and microwave at medium (50%) power for 45 minutes or until tender; stir in raisins. Let stand for 10 minutes. Make the vinaigrette: Combine vinegar, mustard, and pepper; whisk in oil. Stir into casserole; add parsley. Mound onto lettuce-lined plate; garnish with almonds.

Yield: 4 servings

Each with: 203 g water; 371 calories (42% from fat, 12% from protein, 46% from carb); 12 g protein; 19 g total fat; 4 g saturated fat; 11 g monounsaturated fat; 3 g polyunsaturated fat; 45 g carb; 7 g fiber; 14 g sugar; 246 mg phosphorus; 71 mg calcium; 3 mg iron; 74 mg sodium; 563 mg potassium; 254 IU vitamin A; 24 mg vitamin E; 3 mg vitamin C; 8 mg cholesterol

Whole Wheat Pasta Salad

This is an updated version of pasta salad, with more fiber and great taste.

8 ounces (225 g) whole wheat pasta

½ cup (30 g) finely chopped fresh parsley

¼ cup (25 g) chopped scallions

¼ cup (25 g) halved cherry tomatoes

½ cup (90 g) diced tomato, peeled and seeded

¼ cup (38 g) chopped green bell pepper

¼ cup (60 ml) lemon juice

¼ cup (60 ml) olive oil

½ teaspoon black pepper, fresh ground

Cook pasta in boiling water until tender. Drain and rinse under cold water. Drain thoroughly. Turn pasta into large bowl. Stir in parsley, scallions, tomato, and bell pepper. In separate bowl, mix lemon juice, oil, and black pepper. Pour over pasta mixture, mixing well. Cover and chill. To serve, garnish with lettuce leaves and tomato wedges or lemon and lime slices if desired.

Yield: 4 servings

Each with: 57 g water; 331 calories (37% from fat, 10% from protein, 53% from carb); 9 g protein; 14 g total fat; 2 g saturated fat; 10 g monounsaturated fat; 2 g polyunsaturated fat; 46 g carb; 6 g fiber; 1 g sugar; 161 mg phosphorus; 43 mg calcium; 3 mg iron; 11 mg sodium; 264 mg potassium; 887 IU vitamin A; 0 mg vitamin E; 28 mg vitamin C; 0 mg cholesterol

Barley Salad

This is a cool and crunchy salad. Serve it over lettuce leaves with grilled meat for a summer treat.

½ cup (78 g) cooked pearl barley

½ cup (62 g) water chestnuts, drained and sliced

1 cup (100 g) chopped celery

¼ cup (38 g) chopped green bell pepper

⅓ cup (58 g) pimentos

¼ cup (40 g) chopped onion

1 cup (150 g) cubed ham

1 tablespoon Italian seasoning

⅓ cup (67 g) sugar

¼ cup (60 ml) olive oil

¼ cup (60 ml) red wine vinegar

Mix together barley, water chestnuts, celery, bell pepper, pimentos, onion, and ham. Cover and chill. In a screw-top jar, combine remaining ingredients. Cover and shake well. Pour over salad and stir to mix just before serving.

Yield: 4 servings

Each with: 108 g water; 358 calories (43% from fat, 12% from protein, 45% from carb); 11 g protein; 17 g total fat; 3 g saturated fat; 11 g monounsaturated fat; 2 g polyunsaturated fat; 41 g carb; 6 g fiber; 19 g sugar; 164 mg phosphorus; 39 mg calcium; 2 mg iron; 404 mg sodium; 458 mg potassium; 630 IU vitamin A; 0 mg vitamin E; 24 mg vitamin C; 14 mg cholesterol

16

Side Dishes and Salads:
Vegetables and Fruits

Vegetables are a traditional side dish, and the good news is they'll provide a significant fiber boost right out of the garden or freezer. But that doesn't mean they have to be boring. This chapter contains a number of recipes to help you keep the vegetable options as fresh as the vegetables themselves.

Avocado-Stuffed Tomatoes

This is particularly good as an appetizer or as a side dish for a Mexican meal.

4 tomatoes

1 avocado

¼ teaspoon lemon juice

½ teaspoon chili powder

¼ cup (38 g) chopped green bell pepper

1 teaspoon parsley

¼ teaspoon coriander

Cut the tops off tomatoes and scoop out insides. Save insides for another dish. Mash avocado and mix with the rest of the ingredients. Stuff into the tomato shells.

Yield: 4 servings

Each with: 174 g water; 91 calories (51% from fat, 8% from protein, 41% from carb); 2 g protein; 6 g total fat; 1 g saturated fat; 3 g monounsaturated fat; 1 g polyunsaturated fat; 11 g carb; 4 g fiber; 0 g sugar; 57 mg phosphorus; 15 mg calcium; 1 mg iron; 20 mg sodium; 529 mg potassium; 1134 IU vitamin A; 0 mg vitamin E; 50 mg vitamin C; 0 mg cholesterol

Brussels Sprouts with Tarragon Mustard Butter

I suppose this is a also a newsletter subscriber recipe, technically speaking. It came from my daughter, who is a subscriber. She's also a brussels sprouts fan who wishes we had them more often, so she went searching online for recipes. This is a variation of one she found, and it's a winner.

1 pound (455 g) brussels sprouts

½ cup (120 ml) water

4 tablespoons (55 g) unsalted butter

(continued on page 340)

2 tablespoons (28 ml) Dijon mustard

1 teaspoon dried tarragon

¼ teaspoon black pepper

Cook the brussels sprouts in the water in a covered saucepan just until a knife tip inserted in the center meets no resistance. Drain. Melt butter in a skillet over medium heat. Whisk in mustard until smooth. Stir in the tarragon. Cook until bubbly, about 30 seconds. Stir in brussels sprouts, stirring to coat evenly. Continue cooking just until heated through. Sprinkle with pepper.

Yield: 4 servings

Each with: 137 g water; 155 calories (65% from fat, 11% from protein, 24% from carb); 5 g protein; 12 g total fat; 7 g saturated fat; 3 g monounsaturated fat; 1 g polyunsaturated fat; 10 g carb; 5 g fiber; 2 g sugar; 76 mg phosphorus; 40 mg calcium; 1 mg iron; 105 mg sodium; 349 mg potassium; 1417 IU vitamin A; 95 mg vitamin E; 52 mg vitamin C; 31 mg cholesterol

Cranberry Yam Bake

Here's a nice combination of traditional holiday flavors, but it's good at any time of the year.

3 cups (330 g) sliced sweet potatoes

½ cup (60 g) whole wheat pastry flour

½ cup (115 g) brown sugar

½ cup (40 g) quick-cooking oats

½ teaspoon cinnamon

⅓ cup (75 g) unsalted butter

2 cups (200 g) cranberries

2 tablespoons (26 g) sugar

Peel sweet potatoes, slice, and cook until soft. Drain. Combine flour, brown sugar, oats, and cinnamon. Cut in butter until crumbly. Sprinkle cranberries with sugar. In a 2-quart (2 L) casserole dish coated with nonstick vegetable oil spray, layer half the potatoes, half the cranberries, and half the crumbs. Repeat the layers. Bake at 250°F (120°C, gas mark ½) for 35 minutes.

Yield: 8 servings

Each with: 126 g water; 301 calories (25% from fat, 6% from protein, 69% from carb); 5 g protein; 9 g total fat; 2 g saturated fat; 4 g monounsaturated fat; 3 g polyunsaturated fat; 54 g carb; 6 g fiber; 25 g sugar; 124 mg phosphorus; 58 mg calcium; 2 mg iron; 40 mg sodium; 429 mg potassium; 19714 IU vitamin A; 72 mg vitamin E; 19 mg vitamin C; 0 mg cholesterol

Creamed Celery and Peas

Here's another recipe with a different-than-usual combination of ingredients.

⅓ cup (78 ml) water

2 cups (200 g) sliced celery

10 ounces (280 g) frozen peas

½ cup (115 g) sour cream

½ teaspoon rosemary

⅛ teaspoon garlic powder

¼ cup (27 g) slivered almonds

In a saucepan, bring water to boil. Add celery, cover, and cook for 8 minutes. Add peas; return to boil. Cover and cook 3 minutes more. Drain. Combine sour cream and spices; mix well. Place vegetables in a serving bowl. Top with sour cream mixture. Sprinkle with almonds.

Yield: 6 servings

Each with: 101 g water; 266 calories (60% from fat, 16% from protein, 24% from carb); 11 g protein; 17 g total fat; 1 g saturated fat; 11 g monounsaturated fat; 4 g polyunsaturated fat; 15 g carb; 7 g fiber; 5 g sugar; 232 mg phosphorus; 120 mg calcium; 2 mg iron; 198 mg sodium; 427 mg potassium; 1223 IU vitamin A; 20 mg vitamin E; 6 mg vitamin C; 8 mg cholesterol

Green Beans with Caramelized Pearl Onions

This makes a nice alternative to the usual green bean casserole. It's easier to make and lower in sodium, and the sweet flavor goes well with many different meals.

2 pounds (910 g) fresh green beans
1 pound (455 g) pearl onions
⅓ cup (75 g) unsalted butter
½ cup (115 g) brown sugar

Arrange beans in a steamer basket over boiling water. Cover and steam 15 minutes; set aside. Place onions in boiling water for 3 minutes. Drain and rinse with cold water. Cut off root ends of onions and peel. Arrange onions in steamer basket over boiling water. Cover and steam 5 minutes. Set onions aside. Melt butter in a heavy skillet over medium heat. Add sugar, and cook, stirring constantly, until bubbly. Add onions; cook 3 minutes, stirring constantly. Add beans and cook, stirring constantly, until thoroughly heated.

Yield: 8 servings

Each with: 155 g water; 177 calories (37% from fat, 6% from protein, 57% from carb); 3 g protein; 8 g total fat; 1 g saturated fat; 3 g monounsaturated fat; 2 g polyunsaturated fat; 27 g carb; 5 g fiber; 17 g sugar; 64 mg phosphorus; 68 mg calcium; 2 mg iron; 15 mg sodium; 370 mg potassium; 1120 IU vitamin A; 72 mg vitamin E; 23 mg vitamin C; 0 mg cholesterol

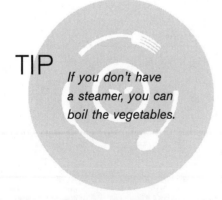

TIP *If you don't have a steamer, you can boil the vegetables.*

Sesame Green Beans

These beans are a perfect side dish. They taste great and are low in fat and calories and high in fiber. What more could you ask?

1 teaspoon sesame seeds

1 pound (455 g) green beans, thawed if frozen

½ cup (120 ml) low-sodium chicken broth

2 teaspoons (10 ml) lemon juice

Toast sesame seeds in a heavy nonstick skillet over medium heat, about 3 minutes, shaking pan constantly until seeds are browned and have popped. Add green beans and broth. Cover skillet and cook 7 to 8 minutes or until green beans are tender and liquid is evaporated. Remove from heat. Stir in lemon juice before serving.

Yield: 4 servings

Each with: 134 g water; 45 calories (12% from fat, 21% from protein, 67% from carb); 3 g protein; 1 g total fat; 0 g saturated fat; 0 g monounsaturated fat; 0 g polyunsaturated fat; 9 g carb; 4 g fiber; 2 g sugar; 57 mg phosphorus; 51 mg calcium; 1 mg iron; 16 mg sodium; 269 mg potassium; 783 IU vitamin A; 0 mg vitamin E; 20 mg vitamin C; 0 mg cholesterol

Spicy Limas

This recipe comes from a newsletter subscriber, who provided options for baking or cooking in the slow cooker. It's great as a stand-alone dish serving about 8 people or serve over brown rice, whole grain pasta, or vegetable pasta.

2 cups (404 g) dried lima beans

4 cups (940 ml) water

2 teaspoons Mrs. Dash extra spicy

½ teaspoon crushed garlic

1 cup (160 g) chopped onion

(continued on page 344)

½ cup (75 g) chopped green bell pepper

2 cups (480 g) no-salt-added canned tomatoes

1 tablespoon (20 g) honey

1 teaspoon basil

¼ cup thyme

Cook dried lima beans according to package directions. Mix all ingredients except lima beans together. Carefully stir in lima beans. Place in 2- to 4-quart (2 to 4 L) covered baking dish. Cover and bake at 350°F (180°C, gas mark 4) for 1 ½ hours or until liquid is absorbed and vegetables are tender.
Slow cooker option: Soak lima beans 6 to 8 hours in enough water to cover sufficiently and drain. Cook beans in covered slow cooker on low overnight (6 to 8 hours) and drain. Mix all other ingredients into slow cooker, cover, and cook on high for 1 hour or until vegetables are tender. Carefully stir in lima beans. Cook on low until liquid is absorbed.

Yield: 8 servings

Each with: 206 g water; 183 calories (3% from fat, 22% from protein, 76% from carb); 10 g protein; 1 g total fat; 0 g saturated fat; 0 g monounsaturated fat; 0 g polyunsaturated fat; 36 g carb; 10 g fiber; 8 g sugar; 194 mg phosphorus; 94 mg calcium; 6 mg iron; 21 mg sodium; 944 mg potassium; 170 IU vitamin A; 0 mg vitamin E; 15 mg vitamin C; 0 mg cholesterol

Asian Eggplant

Asian eggplant is usually long and thin, but what I had an abundance of from the garden was the more traditional American round ones, so that's what I used for this Japanese-flavored recipe.

1 eggplant, peeled and cubed

1 tablespoon (15 g) brown sugar

3 tablespoons (45 ml) reduced-sodium soy sauce

1 tablespoon ginger

1 tablespoon (15 ml) rice vinegar

½ teaspoon sesame oil

½ teaspoon minced garlic

Peel and cut eggplant into cubes of about ½ inch (1 cm). Spray a skillet with nonstick vegetable oil spray. Sauté eggplant in skillet until starting to become softened. Mix together remaining ingredients. Stir into eggplant. Cook and stir until eggplant is soft and evenly coated with sauce.

Yield: 4 servings

Each with: 119 g water; 54 calories (12% from fat, 12% from protein, 76% from carb); 2 g protein; 1 g total fat; 0 g saturated fat; 0 g monounsaturated fat; 0 g polyunsaturated fat; 11 g carb; 4 g fiber; 6 g sugar; 44 mg phosphorus; 16 mg calcium; 1 mg iron; 402 mg sodium; 307 mg potassium; 31 IU vitamin A; 0 mg vitamin E; 3 mg vitamin C; 0 mg cholesterol

Grilled Eggplant

If you are grilling almost any kind of meat, sprinkle it with Italian seasoning and grill this eggplant at the same time to accompany it.

1 eggplant

⅓ cup (80 ml) olive oil

½ teaspoon garlic powder

½ teaspoon Italian seasoning

⅛ teaspoon black pepper

Peel the eggplant and then cut into ¾-inch (2 cm) slices. Combine oil, garlic, and Italian seasoning; stir well. Brush eggplant slices with oil mixture and sprinkle with pepper. Place eggplant about 3 to 4 inches (10 cm) from coals. Grill over medium coals 10 minutes or until tender, turning and basting occasionally.

Yield: 6 servings

Each with: 71 g water; 125 calories (84% from fat, 3% from protein, 14% from carb); 1 g protein; 12 g total fat; 2 g saturated fat; 9 g monounsaturated fat; 1 g polyunsaturated fat; 5 g carb; 3 g fiber; 2 g sugar; 20 mg phosphorus; 8 mg calcium; 0 mg iron; 2 mg sodium; 180 mg potassium; 28 IU vitamin A; 0 mg vitamin E; 2 mg vitamin C; 0 mg cholesterol

Grilled Vegetable Stacks

Serve these as a side dish or add a portobello mushroom at the bottom of the stack to turn them into a vegetarian main dish.

½ teaspoon minced garlic

¼ cup (60 ml) balsamic vinegar

¼ cup (60 ml) olive oil

1 teaspoon basil

4 slices eggplant

1 cup (180 g) sliced tomato

4 slices red onion

1 cup (113 g) sliced zucchini

4 ounces (115 g) Swiss cheese

Combine garlic, vinegar, oil, and basil. In a large resealable plastic bag or bowl, pour marinade over all vegetables except tomato. Let sit for about 30 minutes. Remove vegetables from marinade and grill for 10 to 15 minutes or until browned and tender. To assemble stacks, layer eggplant, tomato, cheese, onion slices, and zucchini. Insert a metal or wooden skewer through the center of each stack from top to bottom. Return to grill for about 5 minutes or until cheese is melted. Carefully transfer stacks to serving plate and pull out skewers.

Yield: 4 servings

Each with: 546 g water; 308 calories (44% from fat, 17% from protein, 40% from carb); 14 g protein; 16 g total fat; 3 g saturated fat; 10 g monounsaturated fat; 2 g polyunsaturated fat; 33 g carb; 17 g fiber; 14 g sugar; 318 mg phosphorus; 334 mg calcium; 2 mg iron; 90 mg sodium; 1317 mg potassium; 556 IU vitamin A; 11 mg vitamin E; 23 mg vitamin C; 10 mg cholesterol

Harvest Vegetable Curry

This flavorful curry contains a variety of vegetables. Feel free to substitute, depending on availability and your taste.

1 cup (130 g) sliced carrot

2 cups (280 g) cubed butternut squash

2 cups (142 g) broccoli florets

1 cup (150 g) red bell pepper, cut in strips

1 cup (113 g) zucchini, cut in wedges

1 cup (160 g) red onion, quartered

1 cup (164 g) cooked chickpeas, drained

1 tablespoon (15 ml) olive oil

1 tablespoon curry powder

2 tablespoons minced gingerroot

1 teaspoon cumin

1 teaspoon minced garlic

¼ teaspoon red pepper flakes

¼ cup (60 ml) low-sodium chicken broth

2 tablespoons (30 ml) lemon juice

3 cups (660 g) cooked brown rice

2 tablespoons chopped fresh cilantro

Steam carrot and squash for 5 minutes. Add broccoli, bell pepper, zucchini, and red onion and steam for 5 minutes. Add chickpeas; steam for 3 to 5 minutes or until all vegetables are tender-crisp. Meanwhile, in a small saucepan, heat oil over medium heat and cook curry powder, ginger-root, cumin, garlic, and red pepper flakes, stirring often, for 2 minutes. Add broth and lemon juice and simmer uncovered for 2 minutes. Toss vegetables with sauce. Serve over hot rice or couscous. Sprinkle with cilantro.

Yield: 6 servings

Each with: 201 g water; 477 calories (11% from fat, 10% from protein, 79% from carb); 12 g protein; 6 g total fat; 1 g saturated fat; 3 g monounsaturated fat; 2 g polyunsaturated fat; 96 g carb; 8 g fiber; 6 g sugar; 415 mg phosphorus; 97 mg calcium; 3 mg iron; 158 mg sodium; 784 mg potassium; 10191 IU vitamin A; 0 mg vitamin E; 75 mg vitamin C; 0 mg cholesterol

Roasted Vegetables

This is a simple but tasty way to cook vegetables.

3 potatoes, cubed

3 turnips, cubed

1 cup (130 g) carrot, sliced 1 inch (2.5 cm) long

½ cup (75 g) green bell pepper, cut in chunks

½ cup (75 g) red bell pepper, cut in chunks

4 ounces (115 g) mushrooms

½ teaspoon onion powder

¼ teaspoon garlic powder

½ teaspoon thyme

Place vegetables in a single layer in a roasting pan. Spray with nonstick olive oil spray. Sprinkle with spices. Roast at 350°F (180°C, gas mark 4) until done, about 30 minutes, turning once.

Yield: 6 servings

Each with: 239 g water; 158 calories (3% from fat, 12% from protein, 86% from carb); 5 g protein; 0 g total fat; 0 g saturated fat; 0 g monounsaturated fat; 0 g polyunsaturated fat; 36 g carb; 5 g fiber; 5 g sugar; 152 mg phosphorus; 40 mg calcium; 2 mg iron; 50 mg sodium; 1082 mg potassium; 4037 IU vitamin A; 0 mg vitamin E; 50 mg vitamin C; 0 mg cholesterol

Potato and Carrot Bake

Looking for a different side dish for beef? Instead of boiled potatoes and carrots, try this.

6 potatoes, peeled and finely grated

1 cup (110 g) peeled, finely grated carrot

1 cup (160 g) finely chopped onion

3 eggs, beaten

6 tablespoons (45 g) whole wheat flour

2 tablespoons chopped parsley

½ teaspoon black pepper, fresh ground

1 teaspoon paprika

Preheat oven to 375°F (190°C, gas mark 5). In a large bowl, blend potato, carrot, and onion. Stir in eggs until well mixed. Stir in flour, parsley, and black pepper. Pour into a 9 x 13-inch (23 x 33 cm) pan coated with nonstick vegetable oil spray, filling to the top (it will shrink), and sprinkle with paprika. Bake 1 hour or until browned.

Yield: 8 servings

Each with: 273 g water; 259 calories (9% from fat, 14% from protein, 77% from carb); 9 g protein; 3 g total fat; 1 g saturated fat; 1 g monounsaturated fat; 1 g polyunsaturated fat; 52 g carb; 6 g fiber; 5 g sugar; 242 mg phosphorus; 53 mg calcium; 3 mg iron; 59 mg sodium; 1404 mg potassium; 3043 IU vitamin A; 29 mg vitamin E; 28 mg vitamin C; 89 mg cholesterol

Spinach Casserole

This is sort of an onion-flavored version of creamed spinach. It's good with steak or chicken.

20 ounces (560 g) frozen spinach, cooked and drained

½ packet onion soup mix

8 ounces (225 g) sour cream

1 teaspoon lemon juice

½ cup (58 g) shredded Cheddar cheese

Combine all ingredients except cheese in casserole dish coated with nonstick vegetable oil spray. Top with cheese. Bake at 325°F (170°C, gas mark 3) for 20 to 30 minutes.

Yield: 4 servings

Each with: 179 g water; 191 calories (57% from fat, 22% from protein, 21% from carb); 12 g protein; 13 g total fat; 8 g saturated fat; 4 g monounsaturated fat; 1 g polyunsaturated fat; 11 g carb; 5 g fiber; 1 g sugar; 209 mg phosphorus; 397 mg calcium; 3 mg iron; 339 mg sodium; 519 mg potassium; 17473 IU vitamin A; 99 mg vitamin E; 4 mg vitamin C; 39 mg cholesterol

Zucchini Casserole

Here's another use for the excess zucchini that I seem to have late each summer. This side dish goes well with chicken or fish.

3 cups (339 g) thinly sliced zucchini

1 cup (160 g) finely chopped red onion

2 tablespoons (28 ml) olive oil

4 ounces (115 g) chopped green chiles

6 tablespoons (45 g) whole wheat flour

¼ cup chopped fresh parsley

¼ teaspoon black pepper

3 cups (450 g) grated Monterey Jack cheese

2 eggs, lightly beaten

2 cups (450 g) cottage cheese

1 cup (100 g) grated Parmesan cheese

Sauté zucchini and onion in oil and place in large casserole dish. Cover with chiles, flour, parsley, and pepper. Sprinkle Monterey Jack cheese on top. Mix eggs and cottage cheese in bowl and spoon evenly over top of casserole. Sprinkle with Parmesan cheese. Bake at 350°F (180°C, gas mark 4) for 35 minutes.

Yield: 8 servings

Each with: 140 g water; 358 calories (59% from fat, 30% from protein, 11% from carb); 27 g protein; 24 g total fat; 13 g saturated fat; 8 g monounsaturated fat; 1 g polyunsaturated fat; 10 g carb; 2 g fiber; 3 g sugar; 421 mg phosphorus; 548 mg calcium; 2 mg iron; 544 mg sodium; 287 mg potassium; 785 IU vitamin A; 132 mg vitamin E; 17 mg vitamin C; 117 mg cholesterol

Mixed Vegetable Casserole

This creamy vegetable bake is good with fish or chicken.

10 ounces (280 g) frozen lima beans

10 ounces (280 g) frozen peas

10 ounces (280 g) frozen green beans

½ cup (80 g) diced onion

1 tablespoon (15 ml) olive oil

½ cup (115 g) mayonnaise

½ cup (115 g) sour cream

¼ cup (25 g) grated Parmesan cheese

Cook frozen vegetables according to package directions. Drain vegetables. Sauté onion in oil until tender. Stir in mayonnaise and sour cream. Fold in vegetables. Put in 2-quart (2 L) casserole dish coated with nonstick vegetable oil spray. Top with Parmesan cheese. Cook 20 minutes at 350°F (180°C, gas mark 4).

Yield: 6 servings

Each with: 146 g water; 303 calories (60% from fat, 12% from protein, 29% from carb); 9 g protein; 21 g total fat; 5 g saturated fat; 6 g monounsaturated fat; 8 g polyunsaturated fat; 22 g carb; 7 g fiber; 4 g sugar; 172 mg phosphorus; 116 mg calcium; 2 mg iron; 346 mg sodium; 429 mg potassium; 1542 IU vitamin A; 40 mg vitamin E; 16 mg vitamin C; 19 mg cholesterol

Spinach Artichoke Casserole

This can be used as an appetizer spread on crackers or bread or as a side dish with a meal.

1 can artichoke hearts

30 ounces (840 g) frozen spinach, drained and squeezed

8 ounces (225 g) fat-free cream cheese, softened

6 tablespoons (90 ml) skim milk

2 tablespoons (28 g) mayonnaise

¼ teaspoon black pepper

⅓ cup (33 g) grated Parmesan cheese

Spray 2-quart (2-L) ovenproof bowl with nonstick vegetable oil spray. Put artichoke hearts in bowl and then spinach. Mix cream cheese, milk, mayonnaise, and pepper. Pour over spinach and press spinach into the liquid. Sprinkle Parmesan cheese on top and bake at 375°F (190°C, gas mark 5) for 40 minutes.

Yield: 6 servings

Each with: 200 g water; 214 calories (35% from fat, 31% from protein, 34% from carb); 14 g protein; 7 g total fat; 2 g saturated fat; 2 g monounsaturated fat; 3 g polyunsaturated fat; 15 g carb; 7 g fiber; 1 g sugar; 210 mg phosphorus; 352 mg calcium;4 mg iron; 391 mg sodium; 634 mg potassium; 17488 IU vitamin A; 88 mg vitamin E; 5 mg vitamin C; 28 mg cholesterol

Summer Squash Casserole

Here's a good way to use up extra zucchini or yellow squash from the garden. I take whatever leftover ends of homemade bread there are, grind them into bread crumbs, and store them in the freezer for just this kind of recipe.

4 zucchini or yellow squash, sliced

1 cup (160 g) sliced onion

1 tablespoon unsalted butter, melted

¼ cup (60 g) sour cream

⅛ teaspoon paprika

2 tablespoons chopped chives

2 cups (230 g) whole wheat bread crumbs

Cook squash and onion until almost tender. Stir together butter, sour cream, paprika, and chives. Add drained squash. Place in 1 ½-quart (1.5 L) baking dish sprayed with nonstick vegetable oil spray. Top with bread crumbs. Bake at 350°F (180°C, gas mark 4) for 20 minutes.

Yield: 6 servings

Each with: 34 g water; 191 calories (28% from fat, 11% from protein, 61% from carb); 5 g protein; 6 g total fat; 3 g saturated fat; 1 g monounsaturated fat; 1 g polyunsaturated fat; 29 g carb; 2 g fiber; 3 g sugar; 77 mg phosphorus; 85 mg calcium; 2 mg iron; 56 mg sodium; 128 mg potassium; 191 IU vitamin A; 33 mg vitamin E; 3 mg vitamin C; 9 mg cholesterol

Vegetable Medley

Here's a good way to come up with a veggie side dish on those days when the garden didn't yield enough of any one thing. Feel free to use your imagination (and refrigerator veggie drawer contents) when deciding what ingredients to use.

½ pound (225 g) green beans

1 cup (180 g) chopped tomato

1 cup (113 g) cubed zucchini

¼ teaspoon garlic powder

1 teaspoon basil

Wash, trim, and cook beans until almost tender. Drain. Return to pan with other ingredients and cook to desired doneness.

Yield: 4 servings

Each with: 116 g water; 30 calories (5% from fat, 20% from protein, 75% from carb); 2 g protein; 0 g total fat; 0 g saturated fat; 0 g monounsaturated fat; 0 g polyunsaturated fat; 7 g carb; 3 g fiber; 2 g sugar; 44 mg phosphorus; 33 mg calcium; 1 mg iron; 8 mg sodium; 296 mg potassium; 780 IU vitamin A; 0 mg vitamin E; 19 mg vitamin C; 0 mg cholesterol

Twice-Baked Sweet Potatoes

Sweet potatoes are almost always boiled. Take a tip from restaurants like the Lone Star Steakhouse and bake them instead. They are an excellent source of vitamins A and C.

4 sweet potatoes

¼ cup (60 g) brown sugar

1 teaspoon cinnamon

2 tablespoons (28 g) unsalted butter

Scrub potatoes and score the skin with a knife to allow the steam to escape. Bake at 375°F (190°C, gas mark 5) until done, about 45 minutes. Or microwave until tender, about 10 minutes. Scoop out centers and mix with remaining ingredients. Place mixture in each potato skin. Bake at 350°F (180°C, gas mark 6) until heated through, about 10 to 15 minutes.

Yield: 4 servings

Each with: 123 g water; 219 calories (24% from fat, 4% from protein, 72% from carb); 2 g protein; 6 g total fat; 4 g saturated fat; 1 g monounsaturated fat; 0 g polyunsaturated fat; 41 g carb; 4 g fiber; 22 g sugar; 53 mg phosphorus; 61 mg calcium; 2 mg iron; 47 mg sodium; 399 mg potassium; 23946 IU vitamin A; 48 mg vitamin E; 19 mg vitamin C; 15 mg cholesterol

Two-Tone Twice-Baked Potatoes

This is one of those ideas that make you wonder why you never thought of it before. We had it as part of our Christmas dinner, and everyone thought it was a great idea.

3 baking potatoes

3 sweet potatoes

⅓ cup (77 g) sour cream

3 tablespoons (45 ml) skim milk

4 tablespoons chives

Pierce potatoes with a fork. Bake at 400°F (200°C, gas mark 6) until tender, 60 to 70 minutes. Cut a slice off the top of each baking potato. Scoop out the pulp, leaving the skin intact. Place in a bowl and mix together with half the sour cream, milk, and chives. Repeat with the sweet potatoes. Place sweet potato mixture in one end of each potato skin and baking potato mixture in the other end. Bake at 350°F (180°C, gas mark 4) until heated through, about 10 to 15 minutes.

Yield: 6 servings

Each with: 190 g water; 227 calories (12% from fat, 9% from protein, 79% from carb); 6 g protein; 3 g total fat; 2 g saturated fat; 1 g monounsaturated fat; 0 g polyunsaturated fat; 46 g carb; 5 g fiber; 6 g sugar; 149 mg phosphorus; 70 mg calcium; 2 mg iron; 47 mg sodium; 1012 mg potassium; 12084 IU vitamin A; 27 mg vitamin E; 25 mg vitamin C; 6 mg cholesterol

Twice-Baked Potatoes

With the addition of ground beef, these potatoes can become a whole meal. The microwave also makes it a quick meal.

4 medium potatoes

8 ounces (225 g) ground beef, extra lean

1 cup (71 g) finely chopped broccoli florets

1 cup (235 ml) water

1 cup (115 g) shredded Cheddar cheese, divided

½ cup (115 g) sour cream

¼ teaspoon black pepper, fresh ground

¼ cup (25 g) sliced scallions

Pierce potatoes all over with a fork. Place in the microwave and cook, turning once or twice, until the potatoes are soft, about 10 minutes. Meanwhile, brown meat in a large skillet over medium-high heat, stirring often, about 3 minutes. Transfer to a large bowl. Increase heat to high, add broccoli and water to the skillet, cover, and cook until tender, 4 to 5 minutes. Drain the broccoli; add to the meat. Carefully cut off the top third of the cooked potatoes; reserve the tops for another use. Scoop the insides out into a medium bowl. Place the potato shells in a small baking dish. Add ½

(continued on page 356)

cup (58 g) Cheddar cheese, sour cream, and pepper to the potato pulp and mash with a fork or potato masher. Add scallions and the potato mixture to the broccoli and meat; stir to combine. Evenly divide the potato mixture among the potato shells and top with the remaining Cheddar cheese. Microwave on high until the filling is hot and the cheese is melted, 2 to 4 minutes.

Yield: 4 servings

Each with: 452 g water; 572 calories (39% from fat, 19% from protein, 43% from carb); 27 g protein; 25 g total fat; 13 g saturated fat; 8 g monounsaturated fat; 1 g polyunsaturated fat; 62 g carb; 6 g fiber; 4 g sugar; 517 mg phosphorus; 326 mg calcium; 4 mg iron; 285 mg sodium; 1989 mg potassium; 1064 IU vitamin A; 115 mg vitamin E; 50 mg vitamin C; 86 mg cholesterol

Garlic Fried Potatoes

This is a nice flavorful side dish to use with a simple grilled piece of meat.

1 pound (455 g) red potatoes, cubed

1 cup (235 ml) low-sodium chicken broth

1 tablespoon (15 ml) olive oil

¾ teaspoon crushed garlic

Wash potatoes and cut into ½-inch (1 cm) cubes; do not peel. Heat chicken broth in a nonstick skillet just large enough to hold the potatoes in 1 layer. Add potatoes, cover, and simmer 5 minutes. Chicken broth will evaporate. Add olive oil and garlic. Toss for 5 minutes over medium heat. Add black pepper to taste.

Yield: 4 servings

Each with: 112 g water; 265 calories (13% from fat, 9% from protein, 78% from carb); 6 g protein; 4 g total fat; 1 g saturated fat; 3 g monounsaturated fat; 0 g polyunsaturated fat; 53 g carb; 9 g fiber; 2 g sugar; 133 mg phosphorus; 42 mg calcium; 8 mg iron; 42 mg sodium; 704 mg potassium; 11 IU vitamin A; 0 mg vitamin E; 15 mg vitamin C; 0 mg cholesterol

Spicy Oven-Baked French Fries

Southwestern flavors blend with spicy mustard for a zippy alternative to deep-fried fries. Feel free to increase the cayenne, red pepper, and chili powder if you like them spicier. You won't want to let the ketchup bottle near the table!

3 tablespoons (45 ml) olive oil

2 tablespoons (28 ml) lime juice

½ teaspoon minced garlic

½ teaspoon red pepper flakes

¼ teaspoon cayenne pepper

1 teaspoon chili powder

2 tablespoons (28 ml) Dijon mustard

½ teaspoon black pepper

4 potatoes, peeled and cut into ¼-inch-thick (0.5 cm) fries

Preheat the oven to 400°F (200°C, gas mark 6). In a large bowl, stir together the olive oil, lime juice, garlic, red pepper flakes, cayenne pepper, chili powder, mustard, and pepper. Add the potato slices and stir until evenly coated. Arrange fries in a single layer on a large baking sheet. Bake for 20 minutes in the preheated oven. Then turn the fries over and continue to bake for 10 to 15 more minutes, until crispy and browned.

Yield: 6 servings

Each with: 164 g water; 239 calories (27% from fat, 6% from protein, 67% from carb); 4 g protein; 7 g total fat; 1 g saturated fat; 5 g monounsaturated fat; 1 g polyunsaturated fat; 41 g carb; 4 g fiber; 2 g sugar; 88 mg phosphorus; 22 mg calcium; 1 mg iron; 71 mg sodium; 684 mg potassium; 228 IU vitamin A; 0 mg vitamin E; 17 mg vitamin C; 0 mg cholesterol

Home Fried Potatoes

This is a traditional breakfast kind of dish, but it also works just as well as a side dish at dinner.

4 potatoes

1 cup (160 g) chopped onion

4 tablespoons (55 g) unsalted butter

½ teaspoon black pepper, fresh ground

Boil potatoes until almost done through. Drain. Coarsely chop potatoes and onion. Melt butter in a heavy skillet. Add potatoes and onion. Grind pepper over. Fry until browned, turning frequently.

Yield: 4 servings

Each with: 270 g water; 376 calories (28% from fat, 6% from protein, 66% from carb); 6 g protein; 12 g total fat; 7 g saturated fat; 3 g monounsaturated fat; 1 g polyunsaturated fat; 64 g carb; 6 g fiber; 4 g sugar; 135 mg phosphorus; 38 mg calcium; 1 mg iron; 18 mg sodium; 1048 mg potassium; 365 IU vitamin A; 95 mg vitamin E; 25 mg vitamin C; 31 mg cholesterol

Potato Dumplings

Try these with sauerbraten or just plain grilled pork chops.

4 potatoes

1 egg, beaten

3 tablespoons (24 g) cornstarch

1 cup (115 g) whole wheat bread crumbs

¼ teaspoon black pepper

¼ cup (31 g) flour

Peel potatoes and boil in salted water until soft. Drain and mash until smooth. Blend in eggs, cornstarch, bread crumbs, and pepper. Mix thoroughly and shape into dumplings. You may need to add flour to make dumplings hold together. Roll each dumpling in flour and drop into rapidly boiling water. Cover and cook for about 15 or 20 minutes.

Yield: 6 servings

Each with: 163 g water; 271 calories (7% from fat, 10% from protein, 83% from carb); 7 g protein; 2 g total fat; 1 g saturated fat; 1 g monounsaturated fat; 1 g polyunsaturated fat; 57 g carb; 4 g fiber; 3 g sugar; 128 mg phosphorus; 54 mg calcium; 2 mg iron; 48 mg sodium; 703 mg potassium; 51 IU vitamin A; 13 mg vitamin E; 15 mg vitamin C; 39 mg cholesterol

Potato and Vegetable Hash

Adding vegetables makes hash-browned potatoes a more complete side dish, but they are still good for breakfast this way too. Depending on the meal, a number of different herbs could be added. We sprinkle them with a little garlic powder and basil just before turning.

2 potatoes, shredded

½ cup (80 g) shredded onion

¼ cup (38 g) shredded red bell pepper

¼ cup (38 g) shredded green bell pepper

¼ cup (28 g) shredded zucchini

⅓ cup (60 g) finely chopped tomato

2 tablespoons (28 ml) olive oil

Shred all vegetables except tomato. Mix together. Heat oil in a large skillet. Add vegetables and spread to an even layer. Cook until lightly browned. Turn over and add chopped tomato on top. Cover and cook until tender. Cut in wedges to serve.

Yield: 6 servings

Each with: 114 g water; 136 calories (30% from fat, 6% from protein, 64% from carb); 2 g protein; 5 g total fat; 1 g saturated fat; 3 g monounsaturated fat; 1 g polyunsaturated fat; 22 g carb; 2 g fiber; 2 g sugar; 51 mg phosphorus; 14 mg calcium; 0 mg iron; 7 mg sodium; 404 mg potassium; 300 IU vitamin A; 0 mg vitamin E; 23 mg vitamin C; 0 mg cholesterol

Avocado and Crabmeat Salad

This is another of those "fancy" salads that are good when you have guests. But go ahead and treat yourself even if there is no one but family. This makes enough that it could be a whole meal in itself.

1 cup (230 g) fat-free sour cream

4 tablespoons (64 g) low-fat mayonnaise

1 teaspoon Worcestershire sauce

1 avocado

1 cup asparagus, cut in 1-inch (2.5 cm) pieces

¼ cup (25 g) sliced black olives

1 pound (455 g) crabmeat

1 can artichoke hearts, quartered

TIP

Serve on lettuce and garnish with cherry tomatoes.

Combine sour cream, mayonnaise, and Worcestershire to make sauce. Peel and coarsely chop avocado. Combine asparagus, black olives, crabmeat, artichoke, and avocado. Pour sauce over salad and mix.

Yield: 8 servings

Each with: 130 g water; 172 calories (42% from fat, 38% from protein, 20% from carb); 14 g protein; 7 g total fat; 1 g saturated fat; 2 g monounsaturated fat; 1 g polyunsaturated fat; 7 g carb; 3 g fiber; 1 g sugar; 229 mg phosphorus; 82 mg calcium; 1 mg iron; 740 mg sodium; 396 mg potassium; 361 IU vitamin A; 35 mg vitamin E; 10 mg vitamin C; 44 mg cholesterol

Broccoli and Tomato Salad

As pretty as it is tasty, this salad is great with a piece of grilled meat or an egg dish like quiche.

1 pound (455 g) broccoli

¼ pound (115 g) mushrooms

¾ cup (75 g) olives, drained

8 ounces (225 g) cherry tomatoes

Dressing

⅓ cup (80 ml) olive oil

1 tablespoon (15 ml) white wine vinegar

1 tablespoon (15 ml) lemon juice

2 tablespoons chopped fresh parsley

¼ cup (25 g) minced scallions

¼ teaspoon minced garlic

¼ teaspoon black pepper, fresh ground

TIP *This is a colorful salad to serve in a glass bowl.*

Trim florets from broccoli, you should have about 1 quart (1 L). Reserve stems for another use. Drop broccoli florets into boiling water for 1 minute or just until they turn bright green; drain. Trim mushroom stems to ½ inch (1 cm). Combine broccoli, mushrooms, olives, and cherry tomatoes in bowl. Measure oil, vinegar, lemon juice, parsley, scallions, garlic, and pepper into small bowl. Whisk until blended. Pour dressing over vegetable mixture. Turn gently to coat vegetables. Cover and refrigerate 3 hours or more until ready to serve.

Yield: 4 servings

Each with: 162 g water; 249 calories (72% from fat, 7% from protein, 20% from carb); 5 g protein; 21 g total fat; 3 g saturated fat; 15 g monounsaturated fat; 2 g polyunsaturated fat; 13 g carb; 5 g fiber; 3 g sugar; 104 mg phosphorus; 88 mg calcium; 2 mg iron; 261 mg sodium; 603 mg potassium; 1351 IU vitamin A; 0 mg vitamin E; 117 mg vitamin C; 0 mg cholesterol

Broccoli Cauliflower Salad

This simple salad is good with grilled meat or any of a number of other meals.

1 pound (455 g) broccoli, cut in florets

1 pound (455 g) cauliflower, cut in florets

1 cup (160 g) thinly sliced red onion

½ cup (115 g) mayonnaise

¼ cup (60 ml) vinegar

¼ cup (50 g) sugar

¼ cup (60 ml) salad oil

3 tablespoons (45 ml) mustard

Mix broccoli and cauliflower florets. Add onion and combine other ingredients. Pour over vegetables. Refrigerate 2 hours before serving.

Yield: 6 servings

Each with: 174 g water; 307 calories (69% from fat, 6% from protein, 25% from carb); 4 g protein; 24 g total fat; 4 g saturated fat; 10 g monounsaturated fat; 9 g polyunsaturated fat; 20 g carb; 4 g fiber; 13 g sugar; 88 mg phosphorus; 63 mg calcium; 1 mg iron; 143 mg sodium; 413 mg potassium; 538 IU vitamin A; 15 mg vitamin E; 103 mg vitamin C; 7 mg cholesterol

Cabbage Fruit Salad

This is a great dish for fall when cabbage and apples are in season. It features a sweet creamy dressing.

2 cups (140 g) raw, shredded cabbage

1 medium apple, diced and unpeeled

1 tablespoon (15 ml) lemon juice

½ cup (75 g) raisins

¼ cup (60 ml) pineapple juice

1 ½ teaspoons lemon juice

1 tablespoon sugar

½ cup (115 g) sour cream

Prepare cabbage and apple. Use lemon juice to wet apple to prevent darkening. Toss cabbage, raisins, and apple. Mix fruit juices and sugar. Add sour cream and stir until smooth; add to salad and chill.

Yield: 4 servings

Each with: 102 g water; 169 calories (31% from fat, 5% from protein, 64% from carb); 2 g protein; 6 g total fat; 4 g saturated fat; 2 g monounsaturated fat; 0 g polyunsaturated fat; 29 g carb; 2 g fiber; 20 g sugar; 58 mg phosphorus; 64 mg calcium; 1 mg iron; 24 mg sodium; 338 mg potassium; 244 IU vitamin A; 50 mg vitamin E; 24 mg vitamin C; 13 mg cholesterol

Corn Salad

Because it is slightly sweet from the apple and very crunchy, this salad is great with barbecued meats.

1 cup (150 g) diced green bell pepper

1 avocado, cubed

1 cup (150 g) chopped apple

2 cups (328 g) corn, cooked and cooled

1 teaspoon Dijon mustard

1 tablespoon (15 ml) red wine vinegar

3 tablespoons (45 ml) olive oil

TIP *For a Mexican salad, omit the apple and add a teaspoon of ground cumin to the dressing.*

Place pepper, avocado, apple, and corn in salad bowl. Stir to mix. Combine remaining ingredients and pour over salad, tossing lightly.

Yield: 4 servings

Each with: 151 g water; 234 calories (56% from fat, 5% from protein, 38% from carb); 3 g protein; 16 g total fat; 2 g saturated fat; 11 g monounsaturated fat; 2 g polyunsaturated fat; 24 g carb; 5 g fiber; 6 g sugar; 77 mg phosphorus; 14 mg calcium; 1 mg iron; 23 mg sodium; 386 mg potassium; 201 IU vitamin A; 0 mg vitamin E; 37 mg vitamin C; 0 mg cholesterol

Date Apple Waldorf Salad

Here's another fruity, sweet dessert or salad. This is the kind of thing that kids love (and older people too).

1 orange

2 cups (300 g) diced unpeeled apple

½ cup (75 g) dates, snipped

½ cup (50 g) chopped celery

⅓ cup (40 g) chopped walnuts

¼ cup (60 g) mayonnaise

1 tablespoon sugar

¾ cup (56 g) whipped dessert topping (such as Cool Whip), thawed

Peel orange; section over bowl to catch juices. Halve sections and reserve 1 tablespoon juice. In medium bowl, combine apple, dates, celery, walnuts, and orange sections. Blend together mayonnaise, sugar, and reserved orange juice. Fold in the whipped dessert topping; combine with date mixture.

Yield: 6 servings

Each with: 76 g water; 211 calories (53% from fat, 5% from protein, 42% from carb); 3 g protein; 13 g total fat; 2 g saturated fat; 3 g monounsaturated fat; 6 g polyunsaturated fat; 24 g carb; 3 g fiber; 19 g sugar; 64 mg phosphorus; 37 mg calcium; 0 mg iron; 69 mg sodium; 258 mg potassium; 202 IU vitamin A; 21 mg vitamin E; 18 mg vitamin C; 9 mg cholesterol

Fiesta Salad

This simple but flavorful main-dish salad is good for those warmer spring evenings.

2 tablespoons (28 ml) olive oil

2 tablespoons (28 ml) lime juice

1 tablespoon (15 ml) lemon juice

¼ teaspoon garlic powder

½ teaspoon cumin

¼ teaspoon oregano

1 boneless chicken breast

4 cups (220 g) romaine lettuce

16 cherry tomatoes

1 avocado, peeled and sliced

¼ cup (27 g) shredded Swiss cheese

½ cup (36 g) crumbled tortilla chips

2 tablespoons (30 g) fat-free sour cream

¼ cup (65 g) salsa

Combine first 6 ingredients in a resealable plastic bag. Add chicken breast and marinate at least 2 hours, turning occasionally. Grill or sauté chicken breast until no longer pink. Cut into ½-inch-thick (1 cm) slices. Divide lettuce between two plates. Top with tomatoes, avocado, and chicken. Sprinkle with cheese and tortilla chips. Combine sour cream and salsa and pour over salad.

Yield: 2 servings

Each with: 236 g water; 457 calories (55% from fat, 16% from protein, 28% from carb); 19 g protein; 28 g total fat; 4 g saturated fat; 18 g monounsaturated fat; 4 g polyunsaturated fat; 32 g carb; 10 g fiber; 3 g sugar; 315 mg phosphorus; 268 mg calcium; 3 mg iron; 263 mg sodium; 1187 mg potassium; 6614 IU vitamin A; 24 mg vitamin E; 64 mg vitamin C; 33 mg cholesterol

Grapefruit, Avocado, and Spinach Salad

This is a great salad. I like to make a double batch of the dressing and use half to marinate boneless chicken breasts to grill as an accompaniment.

1½ pounds (680 g) fresh spinach

3 red grapefruit

2 avocados

¼ cup (60 ml) orange juice

2 tablespoons (30 ml) lemon juice

1 teaspoon sugar

2 tablespoons (28 ml) white wine vinegar

½ cup (120 ml) olive oil

Remove stems from spinach. Wash spinach thoroughly and dry. Tear leaves into bite-size pieces. Wrap gently in paper towels and refrigerate in plastic bags until ready to toss salad. Peel and section grapefruit. Slice avocados into quarters and then cut each slice into 2-inch (5 cm) chunks. Combine remaining ingredients for dressing. At serving time, toss spinach with dressing. Add grapefruit and avocados and gently toss again. Or arrange grapefruit and avocado slices on bed of dressed spinach on individual serving plates. Pass additional dressing, if desired.

Yield: 6 servings

Each with: 240 g water; 422 calories (52% from fat, 7% from protein, 41% from carb); 8 g protein; 26 g total fat; 4 g saturated fat; 18 g monounsaturated fat; 3 g polyunsaturated fat; 45 g carb; 10 g fiber; 2 g sugar; 138 mg phosphorus; 43 mg calcium; 2 mg iron; 8 mg sodium; 465 mg potassium; 397 IU vitamin A; 0 mg vitamin E; 55 mg vitamin C; 0 mg cholesterol

Orange Avocado Salad

Fresh and citrusy with a sesame/poppyseed dressing, this salad would dress up any meal. It's particularly good with chicken or fish.

2 tablespoons (40 g) honey

1 tablespoon sesame seeds

1 teaspoon poppyseeds

2 tablespoons (28 ml) vegetable oil

2 tablespoons (28 ml) cider vinegar

¼ teaspoon Worcestershire sauce

¼ teaspoon onion powder

4 cups (220 g) lettuce, torn into bite-size pieces

2 oranges, separated into sections

1 avocado, diced

Combine first 4 ingredients in blender until well blended. With blender running, add oil, vinegar, and Worcestershire sauce in a slow, steady stream. Blend until thickened. Toss lettuce, oranges, and avocado. Drizzle with dressing.

Yield: 4 servings

Each with: 183 g water; 209 calories (51% from fat, 4% from protein, 45% from carb); 2 g protein; 13 g total fat; 2 g saturated fat; 5 g monounsaturated fat; 5 g polyunsaturated fat; 25 g carb; 5 g fiber; 19 g sugar; 54 mg phosphorus; 67 mg calcium; 1 mg iron; 14 mg sodium; 461 mg potassium; 621 IU vitamin A; 0 mg vitamin E; 55 mg vitamin C; 0 mg cholesterol

Spinach and Orange Section Salad

A great salad, this could easily be made a full meal by adding some chicken or shrimp.

1 pound (455 g) spinach, washed, trimmed, and drained

½ pound (35 g) sliced cleaned mushrooms

5 ounces (140 g) water chestnuts, drained and rinsed

4 oranges, peeled and sectioned

2 tablespoons (28 ml) orange juice

1 tablespoon (15 ml) soy sauce

¼ teaspoon dry mustard

⅛ teaspoon black pepper, fresh ground

Tear spinach into bite-size pieces. Toss with mushrooms, water chestnuts, and orange sections. Combine remaining ingredients in a jar with a tight-fitting lid. Shake well. Before serving, pour over spinach mixture; toss lightly.

Yield: 8 servings

Each with: 174 g water; 88 calories (5% from fat, 18% from protein, 78% from carb); 4 g protein; 1 g total fat; 0 g saturated fat; 0 g monounsaturated fat; 0 g polyunsaturated fat; 19 g carb; 5 g fiber; 10 g sugar; 79 mg phosphorus; 127 mg calcium; 1 mg iron; 125 mg sodium; 543 mg potassium; 7049 IU vitamin A; 0 mg vitamin E; 53 mg vitamin C; 0 mg cholesterol

Spinach Salad

This is an easy salad with lots of flavor from an unusual combination of ingredients. And that's not even to mention the fact that it contains almost half your daily target of fiber.

¼ cup (60 ml) lemon juice

1 teaspoon sugar

½ teaspoon minced garlic

¼ teaspoon black pepper

4 cups (120 g) fresh spinach, cleaned and torn

½ cup (50 g) chopped scallions

1 avocado, cubed

14 ounces (397 g) artichoke hearts, drained and halved

Combine first 4 ingredients to make dressing. Toss with remaining ingredients.

Yield: 4 servings

Each with: 305 g water; 175 calories (29% from fat, 22% from protein, 49% from carb); 12 g protein; 7 g total fat; 1 g saturated fat; 3 g monounsaturated fat; 1 g polyunsaturated fat; 25 g carb; 14 g fiber; 4 g sugar; 180 mg phosphorus; 327 mg calcium; 5 mg iron; 242 mg sodium; 1064 mg potassium; 23256 IU vitamin A; 0 mg vitamin E; 22 mg vitamin C; 0 mg cholesterol

Island Slaw

2 cups (140 g) shredded cabbage

½ cup (55 g) shredded carrot

½ cup (36 g) shredded broccoli

¼ cup (50 g) sugar

3 tablespoons (45 ml) white wine vinegar

2 tablespoons (28 ml) olive oil

1 teaspoon vanilla extract

1 teaspoon black pepper

¼ teaspoon ground ginger

⅛ teaspoon cayenne pepper

Mix vegetables in a large bowl. Combine remaining ingredients; stir until well blended. Just before serving, pour over cabbage mixture; toss gently.

Yield: 4 servings

Each with: 79 g water; 137 calories (45% from fat, 4% from protein, 51% from carb); 1 g protein; 7 g total fat; 1 g saturated fat; 5 g monounsaturated fat; 1 g polyunsaturated fat; 18 g carb; 2 g fiber; 14 g sugar; 27 mg phosphorus; 33 mg calcium; 1 mg iron; 21 mg sodium; 189 mg potassium; 3016 IU vitamin A; 0 mg vitamin E; 28 mg vitamin C; 0 mg cholesterol

Mexican Cole Slaw

½ cup (35 g) shredded red cabbage

¼ teaspoon cumin

1 cup (70 g) shredded green cabbage

¼ cup (28 g) pared, grated carrot

¼ teaspoon black pepper, fresh ground

¼ cup (60 g) plain fat-free yogurt

2 tablespoons (28 ml) lime juice

Combine all ingredients in a medium mixing bowl. Serve at once or refrigerate and serve cold.

Yield: 3 servings

Each with: 77 g water; 31 calories (4% from fat, 22% from protein, 73% from carb); 2 g protein; 0 g total fat; 0 g saturated fat; 0 g monounsaturated fat; 0 g polyunsaturated fat; 6 g carb; 2 g fiber; 4 g sugar; 50 mg phosphorus; 66 mg calcium; 0 mg iron; 33 mg sodium; 188 mg potassium; 1997 IU vitamin A; 0 mg vitamin E; 23 mg vitamin C; 0 mg cholesterol

Molded Vegetable Salad

This molded salad is another of those traditional family recipes. This one is seen most often at Easter, along with ham, turkey, and potato salad.

6 ounces (170 g) lemon gelatin

2 cups (475 ml) boiling water

2 ¼ cups (535 ml) cold water, divided

1 tablespoon unflavored gelatin

1 cup (180 g) chopped tomato

½ cup (75 g) chopped green bell pepper

½ cup (80 g) chopped onion

½ cup (60 g) sliced cucumber

½ cup (65 g) sliced carrot

1 cup (70 g) shredded cabbage

¼ cup (60 ml) cider vinegar

Prepare lemon gelatin according to package directions using 2 cups each boiling and cold water. Dissolve 1 tablespoon unflavored gelatin in ¼ cup (60 ml) cold water. Let stand 5 minutes. Add this to the lemon gelatin mixture. Refrigerate until consistency of unbeaten egg whites or soft custard. Combine the remaining ingredients. Stir into chilled gelatin and pour into a 7-cup well-oiled mold or bowl. Chill at least 8 hours in refrigerator until firm.

Yield: 8 servings

Each with: 191 g water; 140 calories (1% from fat, 9% from protein, 91% from carb); 3 g protein; 0 g total fat; 0 g saturated fat; 0 g monounsaturated fat; 0 g polyunsaturated fat; 33 g carb; 1 g fiber; 29 g sugar; 62 mg phosphorus; 18 mg calcium; 0 mg iron; 163 mg sodium; 135 mg potassium; 1513 IU vitamin A; 0 mg vitamin E; 18 mg vitamin C; 0 mg cholesterol

Italian Pasta Salad

Here's a quick and zesty salad with the flavor of Italy. We like this with barbecued chicken.

1 pound (455 g) tricolored pasta

½ cup (50 g) chopped black olives

½ cup (90 g) chopped roasted red pepper

½ cup (150 g) chopped artichoke hearts

1 cup (71 g) broccoli

4 ounces (120 ml) Italian dressing

TIP *For a more flavorful pasta, prepare it 1 day before you plan to eat it so the flavors have time to develop.*

Cook pasta according to package directions. Add other ingredients and salad dressing to cooked pasta while it's still warm. Refrigerate.

Yield: 6 servings

Each with: 63 g water; 359 calories (19% from fat, 12% from protein, 69% from carb); 11 g protein; 8 g total fat; 1 g saturated fat; 2 g monounsaturated fat; 3 g polyunsaturated fat; 62 g carb; 5 g fiber; 2 g sugar; 111 mg phosphorus; 52 mg calcium; 4 mg iron; 615 mg sodium; 327 mg potassium; 351 IU vitamin A; 0 mg vitamin E; 20 mg vitamin C; 0 mg cholesterol

Italian Salad

Try this salad with your next Italian meal. Or add some tuna or salami and make it a meal.

2 cups (110 g) romaine lettuce, torn into bite-size pieces

2 cups (110 g) iceberg lettuce, torn into bite-size pieces

1 cup (160 g) red onion, separated into rings

1 can artichoke hearts, drained and separated

1 cup (71 g) broccoli florets

1 cup (150 g) shredded mozzarella cheese

½ cup (120 ml) Italian dressing

(continued on page 374)

Toss all ingredients together.

Yield: 4 servings

Each with: 191 g water; 227 calories (57% from fat, 16% from protein, 26% from carb); 10 g protein; 15 g total fat; 5 g saturated fat; 4 g monounsaturated fat; 4 g polyunsaturated fat; 16 g carb; 4 g fiber; 6 g sugar; 176 mg phosphorus; 188 mg calcium; 1 mg iron; 706 mg sodium; 419 mg potassium; 2,375 IU vitamin A; 49 mg vitamin E; 29 mg vitamin C; 22 mg cholesterol

Four Bean Salad

If three bean salad is good, why not go it one better?

10 ounces (280 g) green beans

10 ounces (280 g) yellow beans

2 cups (320 g) chickpeas

2 cups (200 g) kidney beans

½ cup (75 g) chopped green bell pepper

½ cup (80 g) chopped onion

1 cup (200 g) sugar

1 cup (235 ml) cider vinegar

¾ cup (180 ml) vegetable oil

½ teaspoon black pepper

TIP *This will keep for up to a week in the refrigerator.*

If beans are frozen, cook until crisp-tender; if canned, drain. Combine with the bell pepper and onion; set aside. Combine remaining ingredients; pour over vegetables, mixing well. Cover and marinate in the refrigerator for 24 hours, stirring occasionally.

Yield: 8 servings

Each with: 145 g water; 351 calories (43% from fat, 8% from protein, 50% from carb); 7 g protein; 17 g total fat; 2 g saturated fat; 5 g monounsaturated fat; 9 g polyunsaturated fat; 44 g carb; 8 g fiber; 21 g sugar; 119 mg phosphorus; 64 mg calcium; 2 mg iron; 150 mg sodium; 392 mg potassium; 271 IU vitamin A; 0 mg vitamin E; 18 mg vitamin C; 0 mg cholesterol

Marinated Cauliflower Salad

Yes, it says cauliflower salad, but this dish also gets a nice fiber boost from tomatoes, carrots, and artichokes.

2 cups (200 g) cauliflower, cut into florets

1 cup (300 g) artichoke hearts, drained and quartered

12 cherry tomatoes, halved

½ cup (65 g) thinly sliced carrot

½ cup (80 g) red onion, peeled, sliced, and separated into rings

1 cup (130 g) frozen peas, thawed and drained

2 tablespoons (16 g) sesame seeds, toasted

½ cup (120 ml) Italian dressing

Combine vegetables and sesame seeds in large container. Stir in dressing. Cover and refrigerate several hours.

Yield: 6 servings

Each with: 116 g water; 143 calories (49% from fat, 11% from protein, 39% from carb); 4 g protein; 8 g total fat; 1 g saturated fat; 2 g monounsaturated fat; 4 g polyunsaturated fat; 15 g carb; 5 g fiber; 5 g sugar; 94 mg phosphorus; 75 mg calcium; 2 mg iron; 440 mg sodium; 338 mg potassium; 2624 IU vitamin A; 0 mg vitamin E; 30 mg vitamin C; 0 mg cholesterol

Marinated Zucchini Salad

This is a nice summer salad that can help to use up those extra zucchini when the garden is producing more than you can eat.

2 cups (220 g) thinly sliced zucchini

½ cup (35 g) thinly sliced mushrooms

1 cup (300 g) artichoke hearts, drained and sliced

1 can bamboo shoots, drained

½ cup (120 ml) Italian dressing

(continued on page 376)

Mix all but dressing together in a large bowl. Pour dressing over ingredients and stir to mix. Marinate several hours or overnight.

Yield: 4 servings

Each with: 181 g water; 129 calories (57% from fat, 10% from protein, 32% from carb); 4 g protein; 9 g total fat; 1 g saturated fat; 2 g monounsaturated fat; 4 g polyunsaturated fat; 11 g carb; 4 g fiber; 5 g sugar; 76 mg phosphorus; 26 mg calcium; 1 mg iron; 520 mg sodium; 368 mg potassium; 212 IU vitamin A; 0 mg vitamin E; 14 mg vitamin C; 0 mg cholesterol

Marinated Vegetable Salad

This is a great salad with just a piece of meat or as the main dish with a little chicken or seafood added.

½ cup (120 ml) olive oil

¼ cup (60 ml) red wine vinegar

1 tablespoon (15 ml) light corn syrup

1 teaspoon dried basil

½ teaspoon black pepper

½ cup (35 g) sliced mushrooms

¾ pound (340 g) fresh asparagus, slightly cooked and cut into 2-inch (5 cm) pieces

1 cup (164 g) cooked chickpeas, drained

¼ cup (25 g) sliced black olives

¼ cup (25 g) sliced green olives

10 ounces (280 g) artichoke hearts, cooked

1 cup (160 g) thinly sliced red onion

Combine first 5 ingredients. Add to all vegetables in nonaluminum bowl. Marinate at least 1 hour or overnight. Drain and serve on lettuce leaves.

Yield: 4 servings

Each with: 255 g water; 419 calories (62% from fat, 7% from protein, 30% from carb); 8 g protein; 30 g total fat; 4 g saturated fat; 21 g monounsaturated fat; 4 g polyunsaturated fat; 33 g carb; 9 g fiber; 5 g sugar; 164 mg phosphorus; 85 mg calcium; 4 mg iron; 372 mg sodium; 565 mg potassium; 859 IU vitamin A; 0 mg vitamin E; 14 mg vitamin C; 0 mg cholesterol

Raspberry-Cranberry Mold

Pineapple and cranberry in a raspberry base ... this recipe has almost all my favorite fruits.

6 ounces (170 g) raspberry gelatin

2 cups (310 g) crushed pineapple with syrup, drained

16 ounces (455 g) whole berry cranberry sauce, undrained

1 cup (120 g) halved walnuts

Dissolve gelatin in 4 cups (950 ml) boiling water; add drained pineapple and the undrained cranberry sauce; mix well. Chill until partially set and then add walnuts and pour into 9 x 13-inch (23 x 33 cm) dish or mold. Chill until set.

Yield: 10 servings

Each with: 71 g water; 237 calories (27% from fat, 7% from protein, 66% from carb); 5 g protein; 8 g total fat; 0 g saturated fat; 2 g monounsaturated fat; 4 g polyunsaturated fat; 41 g carb; 2 g fiber; 38 g sugar; 94 mg phosphorus; 17 mg calcium; 1 mg iron; 93 mg sodium; 131 mg potassium; 43 IU vitamin A; 0 mg vitamin E; 5 mg vitamin C; 0 mg cholesterol

Overnight Layered Fruit Salad

This makes a great presentation if you layer it in a glass trifle bowl. But more importantly, it tastes good.

2 cups (110 g) shredded iceberg lettuce

2 Golden Delicious apples

2 oranges

2 cups (300 g) seedless green grapes

⅓ cup (75 g) mayonnaise

⅓ cup (77 g) sour cream

1 cup (115 g) shredded Cheddar cheese

Spread lettuce on bottom of 2-quart (2 L) serving dish. Core and quarter apples; slice thinly and layer over lettuce. Peel and section oranges; squeeze a teaspoon or so of orange juice onto the apples. Arrange sectioned orange on top of apple slices. Layer grapes. Combine mayonnaise and sour cream in small bowl; spread over grapes. Sprinkle shredded cheese over all. Cover dish tightly with plastic wrap. Refrigerate overnight.

Yield: 6 servings

Each with: 159 g water; 268 calories (61% from fat, 10% from protein, 29% from carb); 7 g protein; 19 g total fat; 7 g saturated fat; 5 g monounsaturated fat; 6 g polyunsaturated fat; 20 g carb; 3 g fiber; 16 g sugar; 150 mg phosphorus; 210 mg calcium; 0 mg iron; 215 mg sodium; 285 mg potassium; 611 IU vitamin A; 80 mg vitamin E; 36 mg vitamin C; 33 mg cholesterol

17

Side Dishes and Salads:
Combinations

Our chapter of combination side dishes contains a wide range of recipes. From stuffed peppers to pasta and veggie dishes to casseroles, salads, and molds, you are sure to find something here when you are looking for something just a little different for your meal.

Rice and Beans

This is an easy stovetop preparation for a tasty rice and bean dish. Use it as a side dish or make it a whole meal.

1 cup (190 g) brown rice

2 cups (475 ml) water

1 cup (160 g) chopped onion

1 tablespoon (15 ml) olive oil

½ teaspoon crushed garlic

1 cup (180 g) diced tomato

1 cup (113 g) chopped zucchini

½ teaspoon oregano

2 cups (200 g) cooked kidney beans, drained (can be pink or red)

1 cup (115 g) shredded Cheddar cheese

In medium saucepan, combine rice and water. Bring to a boil; reduce heat, cover, and simmer 35 minutes. Sauté onion in oil in a large saucepan until tender. Stir in remaining ingredients except cheese. Heat to boiling, reduce heat, and simmer until vegetables are tender. Stir in rice and heat through. Serve with cheese sprinkled over top.

Yield: 4 servings

Each with: 325 g water; 356 calories (37% from fat, 21% from protein, 42% from carb); 19 g protein; 15 g total fat; 8 g saturated fat; 6 g monounsaturated fat; 1 g polyunsaturated fat; 38 g carb; 11 g fiber; 3 g sugar; 364 mg phosphorus; 323 mg calcium; 4 mg iron; 223 mg sodium; 651 mg potassium; 637 IU vitamin A; 85 mg vitamin E; 19 mg vitamin C; 35 mg cholesterol

Moroccan Couscous

This is a delicious side dish with a Middle Eastern flavor. Serve it with grilled chicken for a great meal.

1 cup (160 g) chopped onion

1 cup (130 g) sliced carrot

1 cup (100 g) sliced celery

1 cup (70 g) sliced mushrooms

½ cup (60 g) chopped walnuts

5 tablespoons (75 ml) olive oil, divided

2 cups (328 g) cooked chickpeas, drained

8 ounces (225 g) no-salt-added tomato sauce

½ cup (75 g) raisins

2 teaspoons curry powder

¼ teaspoon cayenne pepper

1 teaspoon paprika

1½ cups (355 ml) water

1 cup (175 g) couscous

To make the vegetable mixture, in a large pan, brown onion, carrot, celery, mushrooms, and walnuts in 3 tablespoons olive oil. Add next 6 ingredients, bring to boil, cover, and simmer for 40 minutes. To make the couscous, boil the water with the remaining olive oil. Pour over couscous, stir, cover, and let stand for 5 minutes or until water is absorbed. Serve vegetables over steaming couscous.

Yield: 4 servings

Each with: 335 g water; 676 calories (37% from fat, 11% from protein, 53% from carb); 18 g protein; 28 g total fat; 3 g saturated fat; 15 g monounsaturated fat; 8 g polyunsaturated fat; 92 g carb; 13 g fiber; 19 g sugar; 351 mg phosphorus; 116 mg calcium; 4 mg iron; 421 mg sodium; 1040 mg potassium; 6085 IU vitamin A; 0 mg vitamin E; 19 mg vitamin C; 0 mg cholesterol

Barley-Stuffed Green Peppers

You can either use these as a side dish with a simple piece of meat or make them a full meal by adding some ground beef or turkey to the mixture.

1 tablespoon (15 ml) olive oil

2 cups (140 g) chopped mushrooms

1 cup (160 g) chopped onion

1½ cups (235 g) cooked pearl barley

2 tablespoons chopped fresh parsley

¼ teaspoon thyme

¼ teaspoon black pepper

1 cup (115 g) shredded Monterey Jack cheese

4 green bell peppers

1 cup (245 g) no-salt-added tomato sauce

TIP *Vary the flavor by adding other spices or using spaghetti sauce.*

Preheat oven to 350°F (180°C, gas mark 4). Heat the oil in a large skillet. Add mushrooms and onion and cook, stirring until the onion is browned. Stir in the barley, parsley, thyme, and pepper. Stir in the cheese; set aside. Cut off the tops of the peppers; remove and discard the seeds. Spoon ¼ of the mixture into each pepper. Stand the peppers upright in a baking dish just large enough to accommodate them. Pour the sauce over the peppers. Bake 30 minutes or until the peppers are tender.

Yield: 4 servings

Each with: 284 g water; 474 calories (28% from fat, 17% from protein, 55% from carb); 20 g protein; 16 g total fat; 7 g saturated fat; 6 g monounsaturated fat; 2 g polyunsaturated fat; 67 g carb; 17 g fiber; 9 g sugar; 421 mg phosphorus; 307 mg calcium; 4 mg iron; 201 mg sodium; 1008 mg potassium; 1193 IU vitamin A; 63 mg vitamin E; 134 mg vitamin C; 29 mg cholesterol

Barley with Mushrooms

Barley by itself can be pretty plain, but mushrooms and other vegetables give this dish a great flavor boost.

1 tablespoon (15 ml) olive oil

½ cup (80 g) chopped onion

½ cup (65 g) finely chopped carrot

½ cup (75 g) chopped red bell pepper

½ teaspoon finely minced garlic

½ pound (225 g) coarsely sliced mushrooms

1 cup (200 g) pearl barley

1¾ cups (410 ml) low-sodium beef broth, divided

2 tablespoons minced fresh parsley

3 tablespoons minced fresh dill

2 tablespoons (30 ml) fresh lemon juice

In a 10-inch (25 cm) sauté pan, heat oil over medium heat. Add onion, carrot, pepper, and garlic. Sauté for 3 minutes. Add mushrooms; sauté and toss for 3 minutes. Add barley and continue cooking until lightly browned, about 5 minutes. Add 1 cup (235 ml) of broth; cover and simmer over medium-low heat for 15 minutes. Add the remaining broth and continue simmering until the liquid is absorbed, about 10 minutes longer, stirring now and then. Stir in the parsley, dill, and lemon juice.

Yield: 4 servings

Each with: 217 g water; 241 calories (18% from fat, 15% from protein, 67% from carb); 10 g protein; 5 g total fat; 1 g saturated fat; 3 g monounsaturated fat; 1 g polyunsaturated fat; 42 g carb; 10 g fiber; 4 g sugar; 215 mg phosphorus; 80 mg calcium; 4 mg iron; 88 mg sodium; 663 mg potassium; 3579 IU vitamin A; 0 mg vitamin E; 35 mg vitamin C; 0 mg cholesterol

Chickpea and Vegetable Casserole

This simple casserole of chickpeas and veggies is good with any meat.

8 ounces (225 g) dried chickpeas

½ cup (65 g) diced carrot

½ cup (50 g) diced scallions

1 cup (180 g) diced tomato

¼ cup (38 g) diced green bell pepper

½ tablespoon vegetable seasoning

½ tablespoon paprika

1 cup (115 g) shredded Cheddar cheese

Soak beans overnight with three times as much water. The next morning rinse the beans, place in a pot with twice as much water, cover, and bring to a boil. Reduce to simmer and simmer for about 35 minutes. Dice carrot into chunks and steam for 15 minutes. Dice other vegetables and mix with chickpeas and seasonings. Place in well-buttered casserole dish, cover, and bake at 325°F (170°C, gas mark 3) for 35 minutes. After 25 minutes, put a layer of cheese on top.

Yield: 6 servings

Each with: 80 g water; 149 calories (47% from fat, 21% from protein, 32% from carb); 8 g protein; 8 g total fat; 5 g saturated fat; 2 g monounsaturated fat; 1 g polyunsaturated fat; 12 g carb; 3 g fiber; 1 g sugar; 163 mg phosphorus; 183 mg calcium; 1 mg iron; 261 mg sodium; 223 mg potassium; 2587 IU vitamin A; 57 mg vitamin E; 15 mg vitamin C; 23 mg cholesterol

Stuffed Oranges

This is a great side dish to have with pork. I can see it for something like Thanksgiving dinner, maybe with a few of the required mini marshmallows on top.

6 yams

4 oranges

½ cup (112 g) unsalted butter, melted

½ cup (115 g) brown sugar

¼ teaspoon nutmeg

¼ teaspoon cinnamon

½ cup (75 g) raisins

1 ounce (28 ml) Grand Marnier

½ cup (55 g) chopped pecans

Bake yams at 350°F (180°C, gas mark 4) until tender. Cut oranges in half, scoop out pulp, and chop half of it. Peel yams, put in mixing bowl with chopped orange pulp, melted butter, sugar, nutmeg, cinnamon, raisins, and Grand Marnier. Mix well and stuff orange halves. Sprinkle top with pecans. Bake in a 350°F (180°C, gas mark 4) oven for 20 minutes.

Yield: 8 servings

Each with: 133 g water; 367 calories (40% from fat, 3% from protein, 57% from carb); 3 g protein; 17 g total fat; 8 g saturated fat; 6 g monounsaturated fat; 2 g polyunsaturated fat; 54 g carb; 6 g fiber; 30 g sugar; 82 mg phosphorus; 72 mg calcium; 1 mg iron; 14 mg sodium; 779 mg potassium; 648 IU vitamin A; 95 mg vitamin E; 58 mg vitamin C; 30 mg cholesterol

Two Bean and Rice Salad

This makes a lot of salad, but it will keep well in the refrigerator for up to a week.

3 cups (495 g) cooked, chilled rice

2 cups (342 g) cooked pinto beans, rinsed and drained

2 cups (344 g) cooked black beans, rinsed and drained

10 ounces (280 g) frozen peas, thawed

1 cup (100 g) sliced celery

1 cup (160 g) chopped red onion

8 ounces (225 g) chopped green chiles, drained

¼ cup chopped fresh cilantro

⅓ cup (78 ml) white wine vinegar

¼ cup (60 ml) olive oil

2 tablespoons (30 ml) water

½ teaspoon garlic powder

½ teaspoon black pepper

In a 2½-quart (2.5 L) covered container, combine cooked rice, pinto beans, black beans, peas, celery, onion, chiles, and cilantro. In screw-top jar, combine remaining ingredients. Cover and shake well to mix. Add dressing to rice mixture; toss gently to mix. Cover and chill several hours.

Yield: 10 servings

Each with: 157 g water; 238 calories (23% from fat, 16% from protein, 61% from carb); 9 g protein; 6 g total fat; 1 g saturated fat; 4 g monounsaturated fat; 1 g polyunsaturated fat; 37 g carb; 9 g fiber; 2 g sugar; 162 mg phosphorus; 59 mg calcium; 3 mg iron; 193 mg sodium; 435 mg potassium; 743 IU vitamin A; 0 mg vitamin E; 13 mg vitamin C; 0 mg cholesterol

Wild Rice and Barley Salad

We like this as a side dish with grilled chicken. Serve it over lettuce.

1¾ cups (410 ml) low-sodium chicken broth

½ cup (85 g) brown and wild rice mix

½ cup (100 g) pearl barley

¾ cup (123 g) cooked chickpeas

⅓ cup (50 g) golden raisins

¼ cup (25 g) sliced scallions

2 tablespoons (28 ml) red wine vinegar

1½ teaspoons (8 ml) olive oil

1 teaspoon Dijon mustard

¼ teaspoon black pepper

2 tablespoons chopped fresh basil

2 tablespoons (18 g) slivered almonds, toasted

Combine first 3 ingredients in a medium saucepan; bring to a boil. Cover, reduce heat, and simmer 40 minutes or until liquid is absorbed. Remove from heat and let stand, covered, 5 minutes. Spoon rice mixture into a medium bowl. Add chickpeas, raisins, and scallions. Combine vinegar and next 3 ingredients in a small bowl; stir with a whisk. Pour over rice mixture; toss well. Cover; chill 2 hours. Stir in basil and almonds before serving.

Yield: 8 servings

Each with: 76 g water; 156 calories (17% from fat, 15% from protein, 69% from carb); 6 g protein; 3 g total fat; 0 g saturated fat; 2 g monounsaturated fat; 1 g polyunsaturated fat; 28 g carb; 4 g fiber; 5 g sugar; 133 mg phosphorus; 39 mg calcium; 2 mg iron; 94 mg sodium; 276 mg potassium; 91 IU vitamin A; 0 mg vitamin E; 2 mg vitamin C; 0 mg cholesterol

Tabbouleh

Tabbouleh is a Middle Eastern salad of bulgur wheat. The chickpeas are not traditional, but they add a nice touch of flavor and up the fiber content.

4 cups (950 ml) water, boiling

1½ cups (210 g) bulgur

¾ cup (123 g) cooked chickpeas

1½ cups (90 g) minced fresh parsley

¾ cup (72 g) fresh mint

¼ cup (25 g) chopped scallions

1 cup (180 g) chopped tomato

½ cup (120 ml) lemon juice

¼ cup (60 ml) olive oil

½ teaspoon black pepper, to taste

Pour boiling water over bulgur. Let stand covered about 2 hours until light and fluffy. Remove excess water by shaking in a strainer and squeezing with hands. Combine cooked, squeezed bulgur, cooked beans, parsley, and mint (if fresh mint is not available, substitute more fresh parsley). Add scallions, tomato, lemon juice, olive oil, and pepper. Chill for at least 1 hour. This may be used as a light meal or as salad.

Yield: 6 servings

Each with: 236 g water; 234 calories (36% from fat, 10% from protein, 55% from carb); 6 g protein; 10 g total fat; 1 g saturated fat; 7 g monounsaturated fat; 1 g polyunsaturated fat; 34 g carb; 9 g fiber; 1 g sugar; 139 mg phosphorus; 70 mg calcium; 4 mg iron; 56 mg sodium; 392 mg potassium; 1932 IU vitamin A; 0 mg vitamin E; 38 mg vitamin C; 0 mg cholesterol

Pasta and Bean Salad

This is another salad that could be a full meal if you want. A simple dressing brings out the flavor of the vegetables.

3 tablespoons (45 ml) vinegar

¼ cup (60 ml) light corn syrup

¼ cup (60 ml) olive oil

10 ounces (280 g) frozen green beans

1 cup (100 g) chopped celery

1 cup (150 g) chopped green bell pepper

1 cup (160 g) thinly sliced red onion

1 cup (182 g) cooked navy beans

2 cups (280 g) cooked whole wheat pasta

In medium saucepan, stir together vinegar and corn syrup. Bring to full boil, remove from heat, and cool. Add oil. Cook frozen beans according to directions. Drain and cool. In large bowl, mix vegetables, navy beans, and pasta. Pour vinegar and oil mixture over vegetables. Refrigerate 24 hours, stirring occasionally.

Yield: 6 servings

Each with: 123 g water; 394 calories (22% from fat, 13% from protein, 65% from carb); 13 g protein; 10 g total fat; 1 g saturated fat; 7 g monounsaturated fat; 2 g polyunsaturated fat; 67 g carb; 11 g fiber; 8 g sugar; 267 mg phosphorus; 100 mg calcium; 4 mg iron; 32 mg sodium; 717 mg potassium; 494 IU vitamin A; 0 mg vitamin E; 31 mg vitamin C; 0 mg cholesterol

Bean and Artichoke Salad

This is a tasty variation on three bean salad. Serve it over lettuce or as a side dish.

½ cup (50 g) green beans, cooked

½ cup (50 g) yellow beans, cooked

½ cup (50 g) cooked kidney beans

1 jar (6 ounces) artichoke hearts

¼ cup (48 g) chopped pimento

¼ cup (60 ml) Italian dressing

Cook and drain beans. Chop artichoke hearts. Save the juice. Combine beans, hearts, and pimento. Add dressing to the juice of the hearts and pour over mixture. Refrigerate at least 2 hours or overnight.

Yield: 4 servings

Each with: 99 g water; 158 calories (25% from fat, 19% from protein, 56% from carb); 8 g protein; 5 g total fat; 1 g saturated fat; 1 g monounsaturated fat; 2 g polyunsaturated fat; 23 g carb; 10 g fiber; 3 g sugar; 144 mg phosphorus; 57 mg calcium; 3 mg iron; 284 mg sodium; 565 mg potassium; 532 IU vitamin A; 0 mg vitamin E; 19 mg vitamin C; 0 mg cholesterol

Black-Eyed Pea Salad

This is a great-tasting salad with Mediterranean flavor. You could make a whole meal of it by increasing the portion and adding a little cooked chicken.

2 cups (344 g) cooked black-eyed peas, drained

¼ cup (40 g) chopped red onion

¼ cup (38 g) chopped green bell pepper

3 ounces (85 g) feta cheese

½ cup (55 g) sun-dried tomatoes, oil packed

¼ cup (60 ml) balsamic vinegar

1 tablespoon (15 ml) Dijon mustard

1 tablespoon (20 g) honey

In a medium bowl, mix the peas, onion, bell pepper, and feta. In a separate bowl, combine the sun-dried tomatoes, vinegar, mustard, and honey. Drizzle over the salad and gently toss to coat. Refrigerate 1 hour before serving.

Yield: 4 servings

Each with: 111 g water; 225 calories (28% from fat, 20% from protein, 52% from carb); 11 g protein; 7 g total fat; 4 g saturated fat; 2 g monounsaturated fat; 1 g polyunsaturated fat; 30 g carb; 7 g fiber; 10 g sugar; 205 mg phosphorus; 138 mg calcium; 2 mg iron; 322 mg sodium; 597 mg potassium; 368 IU vitamin A; 27 mg vitamin E; 25 mg vitamin C; 19 mg cholesterol

Black-Eyed Pea and Rice Salad

This nice side salad of rice and black-eyed peas is the perfect accompaniment to meat grilled with Caribbean spices.

3 cups (660 g) cooked brown rice

1½ cups (258 g) cooked black-eyed peas

1 tablespoon (15 ml) Dijon mustard

½ teaspoon black pepper, fresh ground

¼ cup (60 ml) red wine vinegar

¼ cup (60 ml) olive oil

½ cup (80 g) sliced red onion

½ teaspoon minced garlic

½ cup (55 g) grated carrot

¼ cup chopped fresh parsley

TIP *This can be prepared a day ahead and stored in the refrigerator. Allow it to come to room temperature before serving.*

Cook the rice and the peas in advance. Whisk the mustard, pepper, and vinegar until dissolved. Drizzle in the oil while whisking. Toss the black-eyed peas and the rice with the vinaigrette. Mix in the onion, garlic, carrot, and parsley. Serve over romaine or Boston lettuce.

Yield: 8 servings

Each with: 56 g water; 371 calories (22% from fat, 9% from protein, 69% from carb); 9 g protein; 9 g total fat; 1 g saturated fat; 6 g monounsaturated fat; 2 g polyunsaturated fat; 64 g carb; 5 g fiber; 3 g sugar; 280 mg phosphorus; 32 mg calcium; 2 mg iron; 37 mg sodium; 335 mg potassium; 2043 IU vitamin A; 0 mg vitamin E; 2 mg vitamin C; 0 mg cholesterol

Chickpea Salad

This is a nice combination of salad ingredients that is set off by a fresh homemade dressing. Serve it over lettuce leaves.

2 cups (328 g) cooked chickpeas

1 cup (150 g) green bell pepper, cut in strips

¼ cup (40 g) chopped onion

1 cup (180 g) tomato, cut in thin wedges or 12 cherry tomatoes

2 tablespoons chopped fresh parsley

Dressing

1 tablespoon (15 ml) lemon juice

2 tablespoons (28 ml) olive oil

3 tablespoons (45 ml) water

⅛ teaspoon cayenne pepper

¼ cup (60 ml) rice vinegar

2 teaspoons fresh basil

½ teaspoon dry mustard

Place chickpeas in a nonmetal bowl. Combine dressing ingredients, pour over chickpeas, and marinate in the refrigerator for an hour or two. Add rest of ingredients, toss well, and serve.

Yield: 4 servings

Each with: 158 g water; 220 calories (36% from fat, 14% from protein, 49% from carb); 8 g protein; 9 g total fat; 1 g saturated fat; 5 g monounsaturated fat; 2 g polyunsaturated fat; 28 g carb; 8 g fiber; 5 g sugar; 161 mg phosphorus; 60 mg calcium; 3 mg iron; 13 mg sodium; 442 mg potassium; 607 IU vitamin A; 0 mg vitamin E; 46 mg vitamin C; 0 mg cholesterol

Broccoli, Navy Bean, and Cashew Salad

Either as a main dish or side salad, this will fill you up as well as satisfy your taste buds.

1 cup (71 g) broccoli

½ cup (91 g) cooked navy beans

½ cup (120 ml) Italian dressing

4 cups (220 g) iceberg lettuce

¼ cup (35 g) cashews

¼ cup (60 g) plain fat-free yogurt

Steam broccoli until tender but still crunchy and combine with navy beans. Marinade in Italian dressing; chill overnight. Wash and dry lettuce and tear into bite-size pieces. Drain beans and broccoli; add them to lettuce. Add cashews and yogurt just before serving.

Yield: 4 servings

Each with: 123 g water; 249 calories (45% from fat, 13% from protein, 42% from carb); 9 g protein; 13 g total fat; 2 g saturated fat; 4 g monounsaturated fat; 5 g polyunsaturated fat; 27 g carb; 6 g fiber; 7 g sugar; 204 mg phosphorus; 98 mg calcium; 3 mg iron; 515 mg sodium; 584 mg potassium; 517 IU vitamin A; 0 mg vitamin E; 23 mg vitamin C; 0 mg cholesterol

Confetti Salad

Colorful, tasty, and good for you—what more could you ask? This makes a lot of salad, so you might want to cut the amount in half, which is easier if you use frozen vegetables.

1 cup (150 g) peas

1 cup (164 g) white corn

2 cups (328 g) chickpeas

4 ounces (115 g) pimento, cut in strips

1 cup (150 g) green bell pepper, cut in strips

1 cup (100 g) green beans

1 cup (130 g) sliced carrot

1 cup (100 g) sliced celery

¼ cup (25 g) sliced scallions

½ teaspoon black pepper, fresh ground

1 teaspoon celery seed

Dressing
¾ cup (180 ml) vinegar

1 cup (200 g) sugar

½ cup (120 ml) olive oil

Drain liquid from any canned vegetables. Layer vegetables in bowl. Sprinkle with pepper and celery seed. To make the dressing, heat vinegar and sugar until sugar dissolves. Add oil. Cool slightly, pour over vegetables. Stir gently. Cover tightly. Marinate at least a day before serving.

Yield: 15 servings

Each with: 89 g water; 185 calories (37% from fat, 6% from protein, 57% from carb); 3 g protein; 8 g total fat; 1 g saturated fat; 5 g monounsaturated fat; 1 g polyunsaturated fat; 27 g carb; 3 g fiber; 15 g sugar; 58 mg phosphorus; 28 mg calcium; 1 mg iron; 171 mg sodium; 195 mg potassium; 2002 IU vitamin A; 0 mg vitamin E; 19 mg vitamin C; 0 mg cholesterol

Marinated Bean and Corn Salad

This Mexican-flavored salad recipe makes a big batch, but it keeps well in the refrigerator. I like it just as is for a quick lunch to take to work.

1 cup (100 g) cooked kidney beans

1 cup (171 g) cooked pinto beans

1 cup (164 g) cooked chickpeas

1 cup (172 g) cooked black beans

10 ounces (280 g) frozen corn, thawed

½ cup (80 g) chopped onion

¼ cup chopped fresh parsley

½ cup (50 g) thinly sliced celery

(continued on page 396)

1/3 cup (80 ml) olive oil

1/4 cup (60 ml) red wine vinegar

1/2 teaspoon minced garlic

1/4 teaspoon chili powder

1/4 teaspoon cumin

1/4 teaspoon red pepper flakes

Drain beans; put into large bowl. Add corn, onion, and parsley; toss to mix. Mix remaining ingredients in small bowl. Pour over bean and corn mixture; toss to coat. Refrigerate covered overnight. Taste and adjust seasonings. Serve at room temperature.

Yield: 8 servings

Each with: 104 g water; 291 calories (30% from fat, 16% from protein, 54% from carb); 12 g protein; 10 g total fat; 1 g saturated fat; 7 g monounsaturated fat; 1 g polyunsaturated fat; 40 g carb; 10 g fiber; 2 g sugar; 214 mg phosphorus; 68 mg calcium; 3 mg iron; 104 mg sodium; 658 mg potassium; 244 IU vitamin A; 0 mg vitamin E; 8 mg vitamin C; 0 mg cholesterol

Marinated Vegetable Salad

I really like marinated vegetables, especially in the summer when you can just add them to some lettuce to make a refreshing and filling salad.

1/2 cup (56 g) sliced zucchini

1/2 cup (56 g) sliced yellow squash

1/2 cup (36 g) broccoli florets

1/2 cup (50 g) cauliflower florets

1/4 cup (33 g) sliced carrot

1/4 cup (40 g) thinly sliced red onion

15 cherry tomatoes, halved

4 ounces (115 g) mushrooms, sliced

Marinade

1 cup (235 ml) olive oil

1/2 cup (120 ml) red wine vinegar

1/4 cup (60 ml) lemon juice

1 teaspoon oregano

1 teaspoon dry mustard

1 teaspoon minced onion

1/2 teaspoon pressed garlic

Mix vegetables in a bowl. Combine marinade ingredients and pour over vegetables. Refrigerate for several hours or overnight.

Yield: 8 servings

Each with: 71 g water; 265 calories (91% from fat, 2% from protein, 7% from carb); 1 g protein; 27 g total fat; 4 g saturated fat; 20 g monounsaturated fat; 3 g polyunsaturated fat; 5 g carb; 2 g fiber; 1 g sugar; 29 mg phosphorus; 16 mg calcium; 1 mg iron; 10 mg sodium; 228 mg potassium; 1046 IU vitamin A; 0 mg vitamin E; 21 mg vitamin C; 0 mg cholesterol

Mexican Bean and Corn Salad

Although a fairly simple salad, it's full of flavor and loaded with fiber, providing 13 grams.

1 cup (164 g) cooked corn

1½ cups (150 g) cooked kidney beans

2 cups (110 g) shredded lettuce

¼ cup (25 g) sliced black olives

2 tablespoons (18 g) chopped green chiles

½ cup (60 g) shredded Monterey Jack cheese

½ tablespoon tomato paste

2 tablespoons (28 ml) cider vinegar

6 tablespoons (90 ml) olive oil

½ teaspoon chili powder

Combine first 6 ingredients. Mix remaining ingredients thoroughly; add to salad and toss.

Yield: 6 servings

Each with: 67 g water; 349 calories (45% from fat, 16% from protein, 39% from carb); 15 g protein; 18 g total fat; 4 g saturated fat; 11 g monounsaturated fat; 2 g polyunsaturated fat; 35 g carb; 13 g fiber; 3 g sugar; 259 mg phosphorus; 161 mg calcium; 4 mg iron; 148 mg sodium; 755 mg potassium; 315 IU vitamin A; 21 mg vitamin E; 5 mg vitamin C; 10 mg cholesterol

Pasta, White Bean, and Tuna Salad

This tasty main dish salad has two-thirds of your daily fiber requirements in one helping.

Vegetables

1 can artichoke hearts

6 ounces (170 g) green beans, blanched and drained

½ pound (225 g) beets, cooked or canned, drained, and sliced

1½ cups (270 g) tomato, sliced in wedges

Pasta Mixture

½ pound (225 g) whole wheat pasta, cooked, rinsed, and drained

2 cups (200 g) cooked white beans, drained

1 can tuna, drained

Vinaigrette

¼ cup (60 ml) olive oil

½ cup (120 ml) fresh lemon juice

½ teaspoon garlic, peeled and minced

1 teaspoon dried basil

½ teaspoon black pepper

Whisk all vinaigrette ingredients together. Using half the vinaigrette mixture, marinate the vegetables for at least 1 hour before serving. Stir together drained pasta, beans, and tuna and mix. Immediately before serving, toss vegetables and pasta mixture with the remaining vinaigrette.

Yield: 5 servings

Each with: 216 g water; 629 calories (19% from fat, 22% from protein, 59% from carb); 37 g protein; 14 g total fat; 2 g saturated fat; 8 g monounsaturated fat; 2 g polyunsaturated fat; 97 g carb; 21 g fiber; 6 g sugar; 498 mg phosphorus; 255 mg calcium; 12 mg iron; 154 mg sodium; 2033 mg potassium; 628 IU vitamin A; 2 mg vitamin E; 33 mg vitamin C; 14 mg cholesterol

Pinto Bean and Wild Rice Salad

This salad offers a variety of options on the basic recipe. Feel free to substitute other greens like endive or radicchio, brown rice for the wild, and other beans for the pintos. It will still be healthy and delicious.

¾ cup (145 g) dried pinto beans

1½ cups (83 g) lettuce

1½ cups (247 g) cooked wild rice

½ cup (120 ml) olive oil

3 tablespoons (45 ml) red wine vinegar

2 tablespoons chopped fresh chives

½ teaspoon minced garlic

¼ teaspoon black pepper

TIP *You may use canned beans that have been rinsed and drained in place of the cooked dried beans.*

Soak the beans overnight in water to cover. Drain the beans, rinse them under cold running water, and place them in a saucepan with fresh water to cover. Bring to a boil over high heat and then reduce the heat and simmer several hours until the beans are soft and the skins begin to split. Add water when necessary to keep the beans from drying and stir occasionally to prevent them from burning and sticking. Remove from the heat, drain, and allow to cool. In a bowl, toss together the lettuce, beans, and rice. Cover and chill in the refrigerator at least 30 minutes. In a blender, combine the oil, vinegar, chives, garlic, and pepper. Blend until the chives and garlic are finely pureed. Pour the dressing over the salad just before serving.

Yield: 6 servings

Each with: 42 g water; 337 calories (49% from fat, 9% from protein, 42% from carb); 8 g protein; 19 g total fat; 3 g saturated fat; 13 g monounsaturated fat; 2 g polyunsaturated fat; 36 g carb; 5 g fiber; 1 g sugar; 210 mg phosphorus; 24 mg calcium; 1 mg iron; 6 mg sodium; 298 mg potassium; 142 IU vitamin A; 0 mg vitamin E; 1 mg vitamin C; 0 mg cholesterol

Spinach and Black-Eyed Pea Salad

This is a tasty salad of marinated black-eyed peas over spinach.

½ pound (225 g) black-eyed peas

1 cup (160 g) chopped onion

½ teaspoon minced garlic

4 cups (950 ml) water

14 ounces (400 g) artichoke hearts

1 tablespoon (15 ml) Dijon mustard

1 tablespoon (15 ml) Worcestershire sauce

½ pound (225 g) spinach leaves

4 slices bacon, cooked and crumbled

Sort and wash peas; place in a Dutch oven with next 3 ingredients. Bring to a boil; reduce heat and simmer 40 minutes or until peas are tender. Drain. Keep peas warm. Drain artichoke hearts, reserving marinade. Chop artichoke hearts and add to black-eyed peas. Combine reserved marinade, mustard, and Worcestershire; pour over peas and toss gently. Arrange spinach leaves on individual salad plates; spoon salad onto spinach. Sprinkle with crumbled bacon and serve warm.

Yield: 6 servings

Each with: 302 g water; 132 calories (20% from fat, 25% from protein, 56% from carb); 9 g protein; 3 g total fat; 1 g saturated fat; 1 g monounsaturated fat; 1 g polyunsaturated fat; 20 g carb; 7 g fiber; 4 g sugar; 147 mg phosphorus; 73 mg calcium; 3 mg iron; 249 mg sodium; 622 mg potassium; 3688 IU vitamin A; 1 mg vitamin E; 21 mg vitamin C; 6 mg cholesterol

Spinach and Toasted Walnut Salad

This is a simple two-ingredient salad. Raspberry-walnut vinaigrette dressing (such as Wish-Bone) goes perfectly with this.

¼ cup (30 g) chopped walnuts

1 pound (455 g) fresh spinach, deveined and torn into bite-size pieces

Place walnuts in preheated 350°F (180°C, gas mark 4) oven for 8 to 10 minutes. Watch carefully, as they do burn easily. Set aside. Place 1 cup spinach on each of 4 chilled plates and spoon 1 tablespoon raspberry-walnut vinaigrette dressing (such as Wish-Bone) over the top. Top each with 1 tablespoon toasted walnuts.

Yield: 4 servings

Each with: 101 g water; 85 calories (47% from fat, 26% from protein, 27% from carb); 6 g protein; 5 g total fat; 0 g saturated fat; 1 g monounsaturated fat; 3 g polyunsaturated fat; 7 g carb; 5 g fiber; 1 g sugar; 97 mg phosphorus; 178 mg calcium; 2 mg iron; 110 mg sodium; 383 mg potassium; 13680 IU vitamin A; 0 mg vitamin E; 3 mg vitamin C; 0 mg cholesterol

Cranberry Walnut Mold

This mold always reminds me of fall, with its cranberries and apples.

1 cup ground (110 g) cranberries

1 cup (245 g) ground apples

1 cup (200 g) sugar

3 ounces (85 g) lemon gelatin

1 cup (235 ml) hot water

1 cup (235 ml) pineapple juice

½ cup (75 g) seedless green grapes, cut up

¼ cup (30 g) chopped walnuts

Combine cranberries, apples, and sugar. Dissolve gelatin in hot water. Add juice, chill. Add cranberry mixture, grapes, and nuts. Put in mold and chill in the refrigerator until set.

Yield: 6 servings

Each with: 101 g water; 314 calories (9% from fat, 3% from protein, 87% from carb); 3 g protein; 3 g total fat; 0 g saturated fat; 1 g monounsaturated fat; 2 g polyunsaturated fat; 73 g carb; 2 g fiber; 66 g sugar; 54 mg phosphorus; 15 mg calcium; 0 mg iron; 69 mg sodium; 123 mg potassium; 19 IU vitamin A; 0 mg vitamin E; 5 mg vitamin C; 0 mg cholesterol

18

Breads

Whole grain breads and rolls are a great way to add extra fiber to your diet. We have a number of yeast bread recipes here that will help you do just that. But don't stop there; we also have recipes for whole grain biscuits and cornbread and for making your own higher-fiber tortillas, flatbread, pizza crust, and bagels.

100% Whole Wheat Bread

This recipe is a variation of one that came with my bread machine. It makes a reasonably light, very tasty bread, good for sandwiches.

1¼ cups (295 ml) water

2 tablespoons (28 g) unsalted butter

3 cups (360 g) whole wheat flour

¼ cup (60 g) brown sugar

1¾ teaspoons yeast

1 tablespoon vital wheat gluten

Place ingredients in bread machine in order specified by manufacturer. Process on whole wheat cycle.

Yield: 12 servings

Each with: 28 g water; 140 calories (15% from fat, 13% from protein, 72% from carb); 5 g protein; 2 g total fat; 0 g saturated fat; 1 g monounsaturated fat; 1 g polyunsaturated fat; 27 g carb; 4 g fiber; 5 g sugar; 113 mg phosphorus; 16 mg calcium; 1 mg iron; 4 mg sodium; 150 mg potassium; 87 IU vitamin A; 18 mg vitamin E; 0 mg vitamin C; 0 mg cholesterol

Sunflower Honey Wheat Bread

This makes a nice bread with soup or for sandwiches. It has a lot of flavor, and the seeds add texture.

1¼ cups (295 ml) water

3 tablespoons (60 g) honey

2 tablespoons (28 g) unsalted butter

2 cups (240 g) whole wheat flour

1½ cups (187 g) bread flour

1 tablespoon vital wheat gluten

½ cup (72 g) shelled sunflower seeds, toasted

1¼ teaspoons yeast

(continued on page 404)

Place ingredients in bread machine in order specified by manufacturer. Process on whole wheat cycle.

Yield: 12 servings

Each with: 30 g water; 197 calories (23% from fat, 13% from protein, 64% from carb); 7 g protein; 5 g total fat; 2 g saturated fat; 1 g monounsaturated fat; 2 g polyunsaturated fat; 33 g carb; 4 g fiber; 5 g sugar; 154 mg phosphorus; 15 mg calcium; 2 mg iron; 3 mg sodium; 155 mg potassium; 62 IU vitamin A; 16 mg vitamin E; 0 mg vitamin C; 5 mg cholesterol

Whole Wheat Beer Bread

This bread is good with soups and chili, and it makes excellent toast. The flavor of the bread will change, depending on type of beer used.

1½ cups (187 g) all-purpose flour

1½ cups (180 g) whole wheat flour

4½ teaspoons (20 g) baking powder

1 tablespoon baking soda

⅓ cup (75 g) brown sugar

12 ounces (355 ml) beer

Preheat oven to 350°F (180°C, gas mark 4). Coat a 9 × 5-inch (23 × 13 cm) loaf pan with nonstick vegetable oil spray. In a large mixing bowl, combine all-purpose flour, whole wheat flour, baking powder, baking soda, and brown sugar. Pour in beer; stir until a stiff batter is formed. It may be necessary to mix dough with your hands. Scrape dough into prepared loaf pan. Bake in preheated oven for 50 to 60 minutes until a toothpick inserted into center of the loaf comes out clean.

Yield: 12 servings

Each with: 30 g water; 140 calories (3% from fat, 11% from protein, 86% from carb); 4 g protein; 0 g total fat; 0 g saturated fat; 0 g monounsaturated fat; 0 g polyunsaturated fat; 30 g carb; 2 g fiber; 6 g sugar; 111 mg phosphorus; 115 mg calcium; 2 mg iron; 187 mg sodium; 105 mg potassium; 1 IU vitamin A; 0 mg vitamin E; 0 mg vitamin C; 0 mg cholesterol

Oatmeal Bread

The wonderful, slightly sweet flavor of this bread is great toasted for breakfast or for sandwiches.

1 cup (80 g) quick-cooking oats

⅔ cup (157 ml) skim milk

⅓ cup (78 ml) water

1 tablespoon unsalted butter

½ cup (60 g) whole wheat flour

2 cups (274 g) bread flour

3 tablespoons (45 g) brown sugar

1 teaspoon yeast

Spread the oats in a baking pan and toast in a 350°F (180°C, gas mark 4) oven until lightly browned, about 15 minutes, stirring occasionally. Place ingredients in bread machine in order specified by manufacturer. Process on whole wheat cycle.

Yield: 12 servings

Each with: 24 g water; 178 calories (12% from fat, 14% from protein, 74% from carb); 6 g protein; 2 g total fat; 1 g saturated fat; 1 g monounsaturated fat; 1 g polyunsaturated fat; 33 g carb; 3 g fiber; 3 g sugar; 128 mg phosphorus; 35 mg calcium; 2 mg iron; 11 mg sodium; 143 mg potassium; 58 IU vitamin A; 16 mg vitamin E; 0 mg vitamin C; 3 mg cholesterol

Oatmeal Bread to Live For

This is a sturdy loaf—very nourishing. It is great with salads, soups, as sandwiches, or toasted with jam.

1¼ cups (295 ml) water

2 teaspoons (10 ml) canola oil

1 tablespoon (15 g) brown sugar

1 cup (80 g) quick-cooking oats

2¼ cups (270 g) whole wheat flour, divided

(continued on page 406)

1 tablespoon vital wheat gluten

1¼ teaspoons yeast

1 tablespoon shelled sunflower seeds

Put water, oil, and sugar in the bread machine. Add the oats and let it sit for 5 minutes. Add 2 cups (240 g) of flour and the gluten. Make a well in the middle of the flour for the yeast. Turn on the bread machine. (Use a setting for 1½-pound [680 g] loaf, dark if you have it.) If the dough seems too sticky, add additional flour as required. Add the sunflower seeds at the beep.

Yield: 12 servings

Each with: 28 g water; 146 calories (14% from fat, 16% from protein, 70% from carb); 6 g protein; 2 g total fat; 0 g saturated fat; 1 g monounsaturated fat; 1 g polyunsaturated fat; 27 g carb; 4 g fiber; 1 g sugar; 159 mg phosphorus; 17 mg calcium; 2 mg iron; 3 mg sodium; 165 mg potassium; 2 IU vitamin A; 0 mg vitamin E; 0 mg vitamin C; 0 mg cholesterol

Oatmeal Sunflower Bread

This has a lovely crunchy texture.

1 cup (235 ml) water

¼ cup (85 g) honey

2 tablespoons (28 g) unsalted butter

3 cups (411 g) bread flour

½ cup (40 g) quick-cooking oats

2 tablespoons nonfat dry milk powder

2 teaspoons yeast

1 tablespoon vital wheat gluten

½ cup (72 g) unsalted shelled sunflower seeds

Place all ingredients except the sunflower seeds in bread machine in order specified by manufacturer. Process on large white loaf cycle. Add the sunflower seeds at the beep or 5 minutes before the end of kneading.

Yield: 12 servings

Each with: 27 g water; 225 calories (22% from fat, 13% from protein, 65% from carb); 7 g protein; 6 g total fat; 2 g saturated fat; 1 g monounsaturated fat; 2 g polyunsaturated fat; 37 g carb; 2 g fiber; 6 g sugar; 145 mg phosphorus; 23 mg calcium; 2 mg iron; 6 mg sodium; 137 mg potassium; 77 IU vitamin A; 21 mg vitamin E; 0 mg vitamin C; 5 mg cholesterol

Maple Oatmeal Bread

Being a slightly sweet bread with maple flavor, this one is just made for breakfast. It seems to me it would be perfect for French toast.

1¾ teaspoons yeast

⅔ cup (157 ml) warm water

2½ cups (342 g) bread flour

½ cup (60 g) whole wheat flour

⅓ cup (27 g) rolled oats

⅓ cup (80 ml) maple syrup

¼ cup (17 g) nonfat dry milk

2 tablespoons (28 g) unsalted butter, room temperature

Add ingredients to the bread machine in the order specified by manufacturer. Process on sweet bread or whole wheat cycle.

Yield: 12 servings

Each with: 21 g water; 178 calories (14% from fat, 12% from protein, 74% from carb); 6 g protein; 3 g total fat; 1 g saturated fat; 1 g monounsaturated fat; 0 g polyunsaturated fat; 33 g carb; 2 g fiber; 6 g sugar; 89 mg phosphorus; 32 mg calcium; 2 mg iron; 11 mg sodium; 129 mg potassium; 94 IU vitamin A; 26 mg vitamin E; 0 mg vitamin C; 5 mg cholesterol

German Dark Bread

To me this is almost purely a sandwich bread. Other than maybe a pork-chops-and-cabbage meal, I can't picture it for anything else. But it's perfect with mild-flavored fillings like chicken, turkey, or egg salad.

1 cup (235 ml) water

¼ cup (85 g) molasses

1 tablespoon unsalted butter

2 cups (274 g) bread flour

1¼ cups (160 g) rye flour

2 tablespoons cocoa powder

1½ teaspoons yeast

1 tablespoon vital wheat gluten

Place ingredients in bread machine in order specified by the manufacturer. Process on whole wheat cycle.

Yield: 12 servings

Each with: 25 g water; 156 calories (9% from fat, 11% from protein, 79% from carb); 5 g protein; 2 g total fat; 1 g saturated fat; 0 g monounsaturated fat; 0 g polyunsaturated fat; 31 g carb; 3 g fiber; 4 g sugar; 58 mg phosphorus; 22 mg calcium; 2 mg iron; 4 mg sodium; 175 mg potassium; 30 IU vitamin A; 8 mg vitamin E; 0 mg vitamin C; 3 mg cholesterol

Onion and Garlic Wheat Bread

Looking for a bread with a little more flavor to stand up to some of your spicier meals? This may be just the one.

½ cup (80 g) finely chopped onion

½ teaspoon finely chopped garlic

1 tablespoon sugar

½ cup (60 g) whole wheat flour

2½ cups (342 g) bread flour

1½ tablespoons nonfat dry milk

1½ teaspoons yeast

¾ cup (175 ml) water

1½ tablespoons (21 g) unsalted butter

Place ingredients in bread machine in order specified by manufacturer. Process on white bread cycle.

Yield: 12 servings

Each with: 25 g water; 143 calories (13% from fat, 13% from protein, 74% from carb); 5 g protein; 2 g total fat; 1 g saturated fat; 0 g monounsaturated fat; 0 g polyunsaturated fat; 27 g carb; 2 g fiber; 2 g sugar; 59 mg phosphorus; 15 mg calcium; 2 mg iron; 5 mg sodium; 79 mg potassium; 58 IU vitamin A; 16 mg vitamin E; 1 mg vitamin C; 4 mg cholesterol

Rich Granola Bread

This makes a wonderful breakfast bread, either plain or with a little cream cheese.

½ cup (112 g) unsalted butter, softened

¼ cup (85 g) molasses

1 egg

1¾ cups (210 g) whole wheat pastry flour

1 teaspoon baking powder

1 teaspoon baking soda

1 cup (230 g) plain fat-free yogurt

¼ cup (60 g) brown sugar

1¼ cups (105 g) granola

(continued on page 410)

Coat 1 loaf pan generously with nonstick vegetable oil spray. Preheat oven to 350°F (180°C, gas mark 4). In a large bowl, beat together butter, molasses, and egg. Sift together the flour, baking powder, and baking soda. Add the dry mixture to butter mixture in batches alternately with the yogurt and brown sugar, blending well. Mix in granola and turn batter into the prepared loaf pan. Bake for 1 hour or until done.

Yield: 12 servings

Each with: 24 g water; 226 calories (35% from fat, 8% from protein, 57% from carb); 5 g protein; 9 g total fat; 5 g saturated fat; 3 g monounsaturated fat; 1 g polyunsaturated fat; 33 g carb; 3 g fiber; 15 g sugar; 128 mg phosphorus; 83 mg calcium; 1 mg iron; 98 mg sodium; 258 mg potassium; 274 IU vitamin A; 73 mg vitamin E; 0 mg vitamin C; 39 mg cholesterol

Raisin Bread

This bread is great for breakfast; it's sweet enough that it doesn't need anything added.

1¼ cups (295 ml) water

2 tablespoons (28 g) unsalted butter, softened

2½ cups (342 g) bread flour

¾ cup (90 g) whole wheat flour

¼ cup (50 g) sugar

1½ teaspoons yeast

2 teaspoons cinnamon

¾ cup (110 g) raisins

Place all ingredients except raisins in bread machine in order specified by manufacturer. Bake on sweet bread or white bread cycle. Add raisins at the beep or after first kneading.

Yield: 12 servings

Each with: 31 g water; 195 calories (12% from fat, 10% from protein, 78% from carb); 5 g protein; 3 g total fat; 1 g saturated fat; 1 g monounsaturated fat; 0 g polyunsaturated fat; 39 g carb; 2 g fiber; 10 g sugar; 71 mg phosphorus; 18 mg calcium; 2 mg iron; 3 mg sodium; 149 mg potassium; 61 IU vitamin A; 16 mg vitamin E; 0 mg vitamin C; 5 mg cholesterol

Banana Raisin Bread

This makes a great breakfast bread. I like it with toasted with a little peanut butter and a drizzle of honey, but I'll leave it up to you how (and if) to make it more tasty and less healthy.

¾ (175 ml) cup + 2 tablespoons (28 ml) water

½ cup (112 g) mashed banana

3 cups (411 g) bread flour

2 tablespoons (30 g) brown sugar

1 teaspoon cinnamon

2 teaspoons yeast

½ cup (75 g) raisins

Place all ingredients except raisins in bread machine in order specified by manufacturer. Process on white bread cycle. Add raisins at the beep or 5 minutes before the end of the kneading cycle.

Yield: 12 servings

Each with: 30 g water; 164 calories (4% from fat, 11% from protein, 85% from carb); 5 g protein; 1 g total fat; 0 g saturated fat; 0 g monounsaturated fat; 0 g polyunsaturated fat; 35 g carb; 2 g fiber; 8 g sugar; 51 mg phosphorus; 14 mg calcium; 2 mg iron; 3 mg sodium; 142 mg potassium; 7 IU vitamin A; 0 mg vitamin E; 1 mg vitamin C; 0 mg cholesterol

Banana Chip Bread

This is a sweet bread that's good for breakfast. I don't know about you, but we always seem to have a couple of bananas at that stage where you'd prefer they not be quite as ripe, so I'm always on the lookout for ways to use them. This particular recipe was a big hit.

½ cup (120 ml) orange juice

1¼ cups (281 g) mashed banana

2 tablespoons (28 ml) oil

¼ cup (85 g) honey

1 teaspoon orange peel

(continued on page 412)

3½ cups (479 g) bread flour

1 cup (80 g) coconut

1½ teaspoons yeast

¾ cup (75 g) crushed banana chips

Place all ingredients except banana chips in bread machine in order specified by manufacturer. Process on sweet bread cycle. Add the banana chips at the beep or 5 minutes before the end of kneading.

Yield: 12 servings

Each with: 35 g water; 266 calories (22% from fat, 8% from protein, 69% from carb); 6 g protein; 7 g total fat; 4 g saturated fat; 1 g monounsaturated fat; 2 g polyunsaturated fat; 47 g carb; 2 g fiber; 10 g sugar; 61 mg phosphorus; 11 mg calcium; 2 mg iron; 3 mg sodium; 204 mg potassium; 29 IU vitamin A; 0 mg vitamin E; 6 mg vitamin C; 0 mg cholesterol

Diet Soda Bread

A newsletter subscriber sent me this bread recipe, which uses diet soda instead of beer. She says she's also tried it with tangerine soda, and it came out great that way too.

12 ounces (355 ml) diet cola

1 cup (80 g) quick-cooking oats

3 cups (411 g) bread flour

2¾ teaspoons yeast

Place all ingredients in bread machine in order directed by manufacturer and set for 1½-pound (710 g) loaf, light or regular setting, white bread.

Yield: 12 servings

Each with: 34 g water; 177 calories (8% from fat, 15% from protein, 77% from carb); 7 g protein; 2 g total fat; 0 g saturated fat; 0 g monounsaturated fat; 1 g polyunsaturated fat; 34 g carb; 2 g fiber; 0 g sugar; 116 mg phosphorus; 14 mg calcium; 2 mg iron; 4 mg sodium; 111 mg potassium; 1 IU vitamin A; 0 mg vitamin E; 0 mg vitamin C; 0 mg cholesterol

Nut Bread

Another good use for ripe bananas, this provides grab-and-go breakfast for most of the week when I make it.

1¾ cups (210 g) whole wheat pastry flour

1¼ teaspoons baking powder

1 teaspoon baking soda

⅔ cup (133 g) sugar

½ cup (112 g) unsalted butter

2 eggs

2 tablespoons (28 ml) skim milk

1 cup (225 g) mashed banana

¼ cup (28 g) chopped pecans

Stir together flour, baking powder, and baking soda. In a mixing bowl, cream sugar and butter with electric mixer until light. Add eggs and milk, beating until smooth. Add dry ingredients and banana alternately, beating until smooth after each addition. Stir in pecans. Pour batter into 9 × 4 × 2-inch (23 × 10 × 5 cm) loaf pan coated with nonstick vegetable oil spray. Bake at 350°F (180°C, gas mark 4) for 60 to 65 minutes until knife inserted near center comes out clean. Cool 10 minutes before removing from pan.

Yield: 12 servings

Each with: 27 g water; 218 calories (42% from fat, 7% from protein, 51% from carb); 4 g protein; 11 g total fat; 5 g saturated fat; 3 g monounsaturated fat; 1 g polyunsaturated fat; 29 g carb; 3 g fiber; 14 g sugar; 104 mg phosphorus; 48 mg calcium; 1 mg iron; 67 mg sodium; 167 mg potassium; 302 IU vitamin A; 78 mg vitamin E; 2 mg vitamin C; 60 mg cholesterol

Fruited Focaccia

This has been popular as a Christmas morning breakfast. It's a great idea, combining traditional bread with the holiday fruits.

1 cup (235 ml) water

2 tablespoons (28 ml) canola oil

3¼ cups (445 g) bread flour

3 tablespoons (39 g) sugar

1 teaspoon grated lemon peel

½ teaspoon cardamom

2½ teaspoons yeast

½ cup candied fruit

¼ cup (35 g) raisins

⅓ cup (37 g) chopped almonds

1 tablespoon unsalted butter

2 tablespoons (26 g) sugar

Place first 7 ingredients in bread machine in order specified by manufacturer. Process on dough cycle. Add the fruit and almonds at the beep or 5 minutes before the end of kneading. Remove dough from machine and form into ball. Spread to a 12-inch (30 cm) circle on a baking sheet coated with nonstick vegetable oil spray. Melt butter and brush over bread. Prick several times with fork. Cover and let rise in a warm place until doubled, 40 to 50 minutes. Uncover dough. Sprinkle with sugar. Bake at 400°F (200°C, gas mark 6) for 15 to 20 minutes or until golden brown. Remove from baking sheet and cut into wedges.

Yield: 12 servings

Each with: 219 calories (24% from fat, 10% from protein, 65% from carb); 6 g protein; 6 g total fat; 1 g saturated fat; 2 g monounsaturated fat; 36 g carb; 2 g fiber; 0 g sugar; 18 mg calcium; 2 mg iron; 3 mg sodium; 109 mg potassium; 43 IU vitamin A; 0 mg vitamin C; 0 mg cholesterol

Holiday Scones

I created this recipe one year when I was looking for a use for leftover candied fruit from the Christmas baking season. I'd only had scones a few times and they'd struck me as kind of dry and not very exciting, but this version turned out really well.

2 cups (240 g) whole wheat pastry flour

⅓ cup (67 g) sugar

1 tablespoon baking powder

6 tablespoons (85 g) unsalted butter

¾ cup candied fruit

1 egg

½ cup (120 ml) skim milk

½ teaspoon lemon peel

¾ cup (75 g) confectioners' sugar

2 tablespoons (30 ml) lemon juice

In a medium bowl, stir together dry ingredients. With a pastry blender, cut in butter until mixture resembles coarse crumbs. Stir in fruit. Stir together egg, milk, and lemon peel. Add to dry ingredients, stir until just moistened. On a floured surface, knead dough 5 or 6 times until it forms a ball. Place dough on baking sheet coated with nonstick vegetable oil spray and spread to 8-inch (20 cm) circle, about 1 inch (2.5 cm) thick. Cut into 8 wedges. Separate wedges slightly. Bake at 400°F (200°C, gas mark 6) for 15 to 20 minutes or until light golden brown and center is set. Combine confectioners' sugar and lemon juice. Mix well. Drizzle over warm scones.

Yield: 8 servings

Each with: 33 g water; 325 calories (27% from fat, 7% from protein, 66% from carb); 6 g protein; 10 g total fat; 6 g saturated fat; 3 g monounsaturated fat; 1 g polyunsaturated fat; 57 g carb; 5 g fiber; 20 g sugar; 190 mg phosphorus; 148 mg calcium; 2 mg iron; 210 mg sodium; 335 mg potassium; 862 IU vitamin A; 92 mg vitamin E; 3 mg vitamin C; 49 mg cholesterol

Wheat Dinner Rolls

Sometimes you want fresh hot rolls with a special dinner like Thanksgiving. This recipe is the same as the one I use for hamburger buns. The only difference is in the shaping.

1 cup (235 ml) water

2 tablespoons (28 g) unsalted butter

1 egg

2 cups (274 g) bread flour

1¼ cups (150 g) whole wheat flour

¼ cup (50 g) sugar

1 tablespoon yeast

Place all ingredients in bread machine in order specified by manufacturer. Process on dough cycle. At end of cycle, remove to a floured board. Pull into 16 pieces. Shape each into a rounded roll and place in 9 × 13-inch (23 × 33 cm) pan coated with nonstick vegetable oil spray or in individual muffin cups. Cover and let rise until double, about 30 minutes. Bake in preheated 375°F (190°C, gas mark 5) oven 12 to 15 minutes or until golden brown.

Yield: 16 servings

Each with: 20 g water; 126 calories (17% from fat, 13% from protein, 71% from carb); 4 g protein; 2 g total fat; 1 g saturated fat; 1 g monounsaturated fat; 0 g polyunsaturated fat; 23 g carb; 2 g fiber; 3 g sugar; 65 mg phosphorus; 9 mg calcium; 1 mg iron; 8 mg sodium; 75 mg potassium; 66 IU vitamin A; 17 mg vitamin E; 0 mg vitamin C; 17 mg cholesterol

Multigrain Rolls

This makes a nice crunchy, chewy sort of roll, perfect for mild-flavored fillings like turkey or egg salad.

1¼ (295 ml) cups water

3 tablespoons nonfat dry milk powder

1½ tablespoons (25 ml) oil

3 tablespoons (60 g) molasses

2½ cups (342 g) bread flour

1 cup 7-grain cereal

2 teaspoons yeast

3 tablespoons (24 g) sesame seeds

Place all ingredients in bread machine in order specified by manufacturer. Process on dough cycle. Remove from bread machine at the end of cycle, form into rolls, cover, and let rise until doubled. Bake at 375°F (190°C, gas mark 5) until golden brown, about 15 minutes.

Yield: 10 servings

Each with: 37 g water; 212 calories (18% from fat, 12% from protein, 70% from carb); 7 g protein; 4 g total fat; 1 g saturated fat; 1 g monounsaturated fat; 2 g polyunsaturated fat; 38 g carb; 3 g fiber; 4 g sugar; 119 mg phosphorus; 68 mg calcium; 3 mg iron; 12 mg sodium; 239 mg potassium; 31 IU vitamin A; 9 mg vitamin E; 0 mg vitamin C; 0 mg cholesterol

Rye Rolls

This is another good sandwich roll. I like my roast beef on rye, personally.

1 cup (235 ml) skim milk

1½ tablespoons (21 g) unsalted butter

1 egg

1½ cups (205 g) bread flour

2 cups (256 g) rye flour

¼ cup (50 g) sugar

1 tablespoon caraway seed

2 tablespoons (24 g) yeast

Place all ingredients in bread machine in order specified by manufacturer. Process on dough cycle. At end of cycle, remove to a floured board. Pull into 10 pieces. Shape each into a rounded, flattened roll and place on baking sheet coated with nonstick vegetable oil spray. Cover and let rise until double, about 30 minutes. Bake in preheated 375°F (190°C, gas mark 5) oven 12 to 15 minutes or until golden brown.

Yield: 10 servings

(continued on page 418)

Each with: 30 g water; 212 calories (14% from fat, 13% from protein, 73% from carb); 7 g protein; 3 g total fat; 1 g saturated fat; 1 g monounsaturated fat; 0 g polyunsaturated fat; 39 g carb; 4 g fiber; 5 g sugar; 132 mg phosphorus; 52 mg calcium; 2 mg iron; 26 mg sodium; 177 mg potassium; 139 IU vitamin A; 38 mg vitamin E; 0 mg vitamin C; 26 mg cholesterol

Focaccia Rolls

These rolls makes marvelous sandwiches. I particularly like them with egg and Swiss cheese for breakfast.

¾ cup (180 ml) water

2 tablespoons (28 ml) olive oil

2 cups (274 g) bread flour

1 tablespoon sugar

1½ tablespoons (16 g) yeast

1 tablespoon basil

1 teaspoon rosemary

2 tablespoons grated Parmesan cheese

Place first 5 ingredients in bread machine in order specified by manufacturer. Process on dough cycle. Remove the dough from machine when cycle ends. Pat into 8 × 12-inch (20 × 30 cm) rectangle on a floured board. Cut into six 4-inch (10 cm) squares. Place on baking sheet sprayed with nonstick vegetable oil spray. Cover and let rise until doubled, about 30 minutes. Make depressions in top at 1-inch (2.5 cm) intervals with finger. Sprinkle herbs and cheese over top. Bake at 400°F (200°C, gas mark 6) until done, 15 to 18 minutes.

Yield: 6 servings

Each with: 36 g water; 230 calories (23% from fat, 13% from protein, 64% from carb); 7 g protein; 6 g total fat; 1 g saturated fat; 4 g monounsaturated fat; 1 g polyunsaturated fat; 37 g carb; 2 g fiber; 2 g sugar; 97 mg phosphorus; 38 mg calcium; 3 mg iron; 32 mg sodium; 120 mg potassium; 47 IU vitamin A; 2 mg vitamin E; 0 mg vitamin C; 1 mg cholesterol

Whole Grain Veggie Focaccia Bread

I just happened to see a loaf of foccacia bread in the bakery section of a local supermarket that was topped this way. It looks great and tastes pretty good too.

¾ cup (180 ml) water

2 tablespoons (28 ml) olive oil

1½ cups (205 g) bread flour

½ cup (60 g) whole wheat flour

1 tablespoon vital wheat gluten

1 tablespoon sugar

1½ tablespoons (16 g) yeast

½ cup (80 g) sliced onion

½ cup (75 g) sliced green bell pepper

½ cup (75 g) sliced red bell pepper

2 tablespoons grated Parmesan cheese

Place first 7 ingredients in bread machine in order specified by manufacturer. Process on dough cycle. Remove the dough from machine when cycle ends. Pat into 8 × 12-inch (20 × 30 cm) rectangle on baking sheet sprayed with nonstick vegetable oil spray. Cover and let rise until doubled, about 30 minutes. Thinly slice onion and separate into rings. Thinly slice bell peppers into rings. Place onion and pepper on top of dough. Sprinkle Parmesan cheese over top. Bake at 400°F (200°C, gas mark 6) until done, 15 to 18 minutes.

Yield: 6 servings

Each with: 71 g water; 239 calories (22% from fat, 14% from protein, 63% from carb); 9 g protein; 6 g total fat; 1 g saturated fat; 4 g monounsaturated fat; 1 g polyunsaturated fat; 38 g carb; 3 g fiber; 4 g sugar; 131 mg phosphorus; 40 mg calcium; 3 mg iron; 37 mg sodium; 205 mg potassium; 446 IU vitamin A; 2 mg vitamin E; 27 mg vitamin C; 2 mg cholesterol

Whole Wheat Flatbread

Make your own flatbread for roll-ups or other filled sandwiches.

1½ teaspoons yeast

¾ cup (180 ml) water, warm (100–110°F or 38–43°C)

1½ cups (205 g) bread flour

1½ cups (180 g) whole wheat flour

2 tablespoons (28 g) unsalted butter, melted

In small bowl dissolve yeast in warm water. Let stand 5 minutes. Place flours in bowl of food processor. Turn on machine and slowly add yeast-water mixture. Keep machine running until dough just forms a ball. Place ball in bowl coated with nonstick vegetable oil spray. Cover with towel and let rise 1 hour in warm place. Punch down dough and turn out on lightly floured surface. Roll dough into a log about 1½ inches (4 cm) thick. Cut log vertically into 12 equal pieces. Roll each piece into a 6-inch (15 cm) circle. In large cast-iron or heavy skillet over high heat, cook breads one at a time, 1 to 2 minutes, until they begin to form bubbles. With tongs, turn and cook other side 1 to 2 minutes, until golden brown. Brush with melted butter. Store tightly wrapped in the refrigerator for 1 week. To reheat, cook in microwave on high 1 minute on microwave-safe dish lightly covered with plastic wrap.

Yield: 12 servings

Each with: 19 g water; 131 calories (17% from fat, 13% from protein, 70% from carb); 4 g protein; 3 g total fat; 1 g saturated fat; 1 g monounsaturated fat; 0 g polyunsaturated fat; 23 g carb; 2 g fiber; 0 g sugar; 76 mg phosphorus; 9 mg calcium; 1 mg iron; 2 mg sodium; 89 mg potassium; 61 IU vitamin A; 16 mg vitamin E; 0 mg vitamin C; 5 mg cholesterol

Whole Wheat Tortillas

It's easier than you think to make your own tortillas. For a long while I was afraid that I wouldn't be able to roll them thin enough. Then I realized it doesn't matter. The ones the real Mexican restaurants make on site are a lot thicker than the ones you get from the grocer's refrigerator.

1 cup (120 g) whole wheat flour

¼ teaspoon baking powder

¼ teaspoon salt

1½ teaspoons (8 ml) oil

¼ cup (60 ml) cold water

In bowl of food processor, combine flour, baking powder, and salt. Turn food processor on high and add oil. Add water gradually until mixture cleans sides of bowl and forms ball in center of bowl. Let the machine knead the dough for 2 minutes. Remove dough and divide into 4 parts. Let rest 10 minutes. Roll very thin on flour-covered board. Bake on lightly oiled or sprayed griddle. Turn when little bubbles appear and bake other side.

Yield: 4 servings

Each with: 18 g water; 117 calories (16% from fat, 13% from protein, 70% from carb); 4 g protein; 2 g total fat; 0 g saturated fat; 1 g monounsaturated fat; 1 g polyunsaturated fat; 22 g carb; 4 g fiber; 0 g sugar; 110 mg phosphorus; 28 mg calcium; 1 mg iron; 180 mg sodium; 122 mg potassium; 3 IU vitamin A; 0 mg vitamin E; 0 mg vitamin C; 0 mg cholesterol

Whole Wheat Pizza Dough

We used this dough to make a pizza full of fresh veggies from the garden, but you could use it with any toppings you desire.

2 teaspoons active dry yeast

2 cups (274 g) bread flour

1½ cups (180 g) whole wheat flour

1 tablespoon sugar

2 tablespoons (28 ml) olive oil

1½ cups (355 ml) water

Place ingredients in bread machine in order specified by manufacturer and process on dough cycle. Turn out the dough onto a floured board. At this point, you may form the pizzas or refrigerate the dough for several hours, well wrapped in plastic so it won't dry out. This recipe makes enough dough for two 12-inch (30 cm) pizzas or two 10-inch (25 cm) thick-crust pizzas. Bake at 400°F (200°C, gas mark 6) until lightly browned around the edges. Top as desired and return to oven until cheese is melted and crust is browned, about 15 minutes total.

Yield: 16 servings

Each with: 26 g water; 119 calories (16% from fat, 12% from protein, 71% from carb); 4 g protein; 2 g total fat; 0 g saturated fat; 1 g monounsaturated fat; 0 g polyunsaturated fat; 22 g carb; 2 g fiber; 1 g sugar; 62 mg phosphorus; 7 mg calcium; 1 mg iron; 2 mg sodium; 73 mg potassium; 1 IU vitamin A; 0 mg vitamin E; 0 mg vitamin C; 0 mg cholesterol

Whole Wheat Biscuits

This is a small variation on a standard biscuit recipe, but it's one that I prefer with some meals. You could also add a little cheese or other herbs and spices. If you don't have a biscuit cutter, you can use a glass or just cut it into squares with a knife.

1½ cups (187 g) flour

½ cup (60 g) whole wheat flour

2 teaspoons sugar

3 tablespoons (27 g) baking powder

½ cup (112 g) unsalted butter

²/₃ cup (160 ml) skim milk

Stir together dry ingredients. Cut in butter until mixture resembles coarse crumbs. Add milk. Stir until just mixed. Knead gently on floured surface a few times. Press to ½-inch (1 cm) thickness. Cut out with 2½-inch (6 cm) biscuit cutter. Transfer to ungreased baking sheet. Bake at 450°F (230°C, gas mark 8) for 10 to 12 minutes or until golden brown.

Yield: 10 servings

Each with: 20 g water; 182 calories (46% from fat, 8% from protein, 46% from carb); 4 g protein; 10 g total fat; 6 g saturated fat; 2 g monounsaturated fat; 0 g polyunsaturated fat; 22 g carb; 1 g fiber; 1 g sugar; 153 mg phosphorus; 274 mg calcium; 2 mg iron; 450 mg sodium; 78 mg potassium; 317 IU vitamin A; 86 mg vitamin E; 0 mg vitamin C; 25 mg cholesterol

Corn Fritters

This recipe is for a fried bread typical of the New Orleans area. They are similar to hush puppies and can also be served as a side dish with fish or other traditional southern foods like black-eyed peas.

2 cups (240 g) whole wheat pastry flour

1 tablespoon baking powder

¼ cup (50 g) sugar

2 eggs

1 cup (235 ml) skim milk

¼ cup (55 g) unsalted butter, melted

1½ cups (246 g) frozen corn, thawed

Stir together flour, baking powder, and sugar. Combine eggs, milk, and butter. Fold in dry ingredients; add corn last. Drop by tablespoons into hot vegetable oil and deep-fry about 5 minutes or until golden brown. Sprinkle with confectioners' sugar or serve with syrup.

Yield: 6 servings

(continued on page 424)

Each with: 86 g water; 321 calories (28% from fat, 13% from protein, 59% from carb); 11 g protein; 11 g total fat; 6 g saturated fat; 3 g monounsaturated fat; 1 g polyunsaturated fat; 50 g carb; 6 g fiber; 10 g sugar; 308 mg phosphorus; 221 mg calcium; 2 mg iron; 299 mg sodium; 385 mg potassium; 514 IU vitamin A; 114 mg vitamin E; 3 mg vitamin C; 100 mg cholesterol

Whole Wheat Bagels

Bagels really aren't as difficult to make as they sound. This recipe produces big, soft bagels . . . crispy on the outside and just a little chewy on the inside. They are good cold for sandwiches, toasted, or warm right out of the oven.

1½ cups (355 ml) warm water

2 tablespoons (40 g) honey

1 tablespoon (15 ml) vinegar

2 cups (240 g) whole wheat flour

1¼ cups (171 g) bread flour

1½ tablespoons (25 ml) olive oil

2 teaspoons yeast

Place ingredients in bread machine in the order specified by the manufacturer. Process on dough cycle. At end of cycle, separate into 8 pieces. Shape each into a flattened ball. Using your thumbs, pull a hole in the center of each and stretch to a doughnut shape. Place on baking sheet coated with nonstick vegetable oil spray, cover, and let rise until doubled, about 30 minutes. While dough is rising, bring about 2 inches (5 cm) of water to boil in a large pan. Drop bagels a few at a time into boiling water and boil 1 minute, turning once. Remove with slotted spoon or spatula and return to baking sheet. When all bagels have been boiled, bake at 350°F (180°C, gas mark 4) until golden brown, 20 to 25 minutes.

Yield: 8 servings

Each with: 53 g water; 221 calories (14% from fat, 12% from protein, 74% from carb); 7 g protein; 3 g total fat; 1 g saturated fat; 2 g monounsaturated fat; 1 g polyunsaturated fat; 42 g carb; 4 g fiber; 5 g sugar; 138 mg phosphorus; 16 mg calcium; 2 mg iron; 4 mg sodium; 167 mg potassium; 3 IU vitamin A; 0 mg vitamin E; 0 mg vitamin C; 0 mg cholesterol

Mexican-Style Cornbread

This cornbread goes well with any chili.

1 cup (140 g) cornmeal

1 cup (120 g) whole wheat pastry flour

3 tablespoons (41 g) baking powder

¼ cup (55 g) unsalted butter

1 cup (235 ml) skim milk

1 egg

1 cup (164 g) frozen corn

1 can chopped jalapeño peppers

½ cup (58 g) shredded Cheddar cheese

Stir dry ingredients together. Cut in butter until mixture resembles coarse crumbs. Stir together milk and egg. Add to dry ingredients and stir until just mixed. Stir in remaining ingredients. Place in 8 × 8-inch (20 × 20 cm) baking dish coated with nonstick vegetable oil spray and bake at 425°F (220°C, gas mark 7) until done, about 20 minutes.

Yield: 9 servings

Each with: 37 g water; 209 calories (37% from fat, 13% from protein, 50% from carb); 7 g protein; 9 g total fat; 5 g saturated fat; 2 g monounsaturated fat; 1 g polyunsaturated fat; 27 g carb; 2 g fiber; 0 g sugar; 242 mg phosphorus; 369 mg calcium; 2 mg iron; 561 mg sodium; 153 mg potassium; 375 IU vitamin A; 88 mg vitamin E; 1 mg vitamin C; 44 mg cholesterol

Whole Wheat Baking Mix

This can be used in any recipe that calls for Bisquick or a similar baking mix. I usually use butter-flavored Crisco, but any shortening that doesn't require refrigeration will do. If you use regular butter or margarine, it will need to be refrigerated. The nutritional information is based on a half cup of the mix, which may be more than a serving would contain.

4 cups (500 g) all-purpose flour

2 cups (240 g) whole wheat flour

2 tablespoons (27 g) sodium-free baking powder

1¼ cups (281 g) shortening

Stir flours and baking powder together. Cut in shortening with pastry blender or 2 knives until mixture resembles coarse crumbs. Store in a container with a tight-fitting lid.

Yield: 14 servings

Each with: 6 g water; 352 calories (48% from fat, 7% from protein, 45% from carb); 6 g protein; 19 g total fat; 5 g saturated fat; 8 g monounsaturated fat; 5 g polyunsaturated fat; 41 g carb; 3 g fiber; 0 g sugar; 245 mg phosphorus; 104 mg calcium; 2 mg iron; 4 mg sodium; 324 mg potassium; 2 IU vitamin A; 0 mg vitamin E; 0 mg vitamin C; 0 mg cholesterol

19

Desserts and Other Sweets:
Legumes

Yes, there actually are recipes for desserts made with legumes. Admittedly there aren't a lot, and a lot of them tend to be kind of similar, but I was so impressed with the whole idea that I decided to go ahead and make it a separate chapter, even if it does only contain two recipes. You really should try the bean pie—it will not be what you expect.

Bean Pie

Bean pies were something I'd never heard of until I started looking for ways to add fiber to my diet. It turns out a bean pie is a sweet custard pie whose filling consists of mashed beans, usually navy beans, sugar, butter, milk, and spices. It is similar to a pumpkin pie. Bean pies are commonly associated with soul food or southern cuisine. They are also associated with the Nation of Islam movement: Its leader, Elijah Muhammad, encouraged their consumption in lieu of richer foods associated with African American cuisine, and the followers of his community commonly sell bean pies as part of their fund-raising efforts.

3 cups (531 g) cooked great northern beans, drained

3 eggs

1¼ cups (250 g) sugar

¼ cup (55 g) unsalted butter, melted

1 teaspoon vanilla extract

1 teaspoon ground cinnamon

1 teaspoon ground nutmeg

¼ teaspoon ground allspice

1 teaspoon baking powder

⅓ cup (80 ml) fat-free evaporated milk

1 piecrust, 9 inch (23 cm), baked and cooled

In mixing bowl with electric mixer, beat the drained beans until smooth. Beat in eggs, sugar, butter, vanilla, cinnamon, nutmeg, and allspice. In a separate bowl, combine baking powder and milk. Add to bean mixture. Beat mixture well to blend; pour into the cooled pie shell. Bake the pie in preheated 350°F (180°C, gas mark 4) oven for 50 minutes or until set. Let pie cool before slicing.

Yield: 8 servings

Each with: 99 g water; 441 calories (32% from fat, 11% from protein, 57% from carb); 12 g protein; 16 g total fat; 6 g saturated fat; 6 g monounsaturated fat; 3 g polyunsaturated fat; 64 g carb; 6 g fiber; 33 g sugar; 224 mg phosphorus; 137 mg calcium; 3 mg iron; 224 mg sodium; 429 mg potassium; 323 IU vitamin A; 89 mg vitamin E; 2 mg vitamin C; 105 mg cholesterol

Pinto Bean Pecan Pie

Like a pecan pie, but with the added fiber boost of a secret ingredient, pinto beans. You won't believe it unless you try it.

⅓ cup (75 g) unsalted butter

1 cup (200 g) sugar

⅔ cup (150 g) packed brown sugar

3 eggs, slightly beaten

1 cup (171 g) pinto beans, cooked and mashed

⅓ cup (37 g) chopped pecans

1 piecrust, unbaked

Preheat oven to 350°F (180°C, gas mark 4). Cream together butter, sugars, and eggs. Add beans and nuts, mix well, and pour into unbaked pie shell. Bake for 35 to 40 minutes.

Yield: 8 servings

Each with: 25 g water; 493 calories (37% from fat, 8% from protein, 55% from carb); 10 g protein; 21 g total fat; 8 g saturated fat; 8 g monounsaturated fat; 4 g polyunsaturated fat; 69 g carb; 5 g fiber; 44 g sugar; 173 mg phosphorus; 62 mg calcium; 3 mg iron; 211 mg sodium; 463 mg potassium; 341 IU vitamin A; 93 mg vitamin E; 2 mg vitamin C; 109 mg cholesterol

20

Desserts and Other Sweets:
Grains

Grains are a primary ingredient in many desserts and sweets. We have recipes here for cookies, brownies, and cakes, as well as piecrusts and a couple of rice desserts. The key concept here is the use of whole wheat pastry flour to replace the regular white flour in these recipes. I tried many of these cookie recipes made this way for the first time last Christmas, and I have to say I like the extra flavor the whole grain flour gives them.

Chocolate Peanut Cookies

This a quick and easy treat. It only makes 6 cookies, but the nonbake method makes it possible to stir up a batch whenever you want them. (I've found you can cheat on the 30 minutes and take them out of the freezer a little early too.)

1⅝ ounces (45 g) chocolate candy bar

4 tablespoons (64 g) crunchy peanut butter

1 cup (60 g) lightly sweetened bran cereal, such as Fiber One

Melt the chocolate bar and peanut butter in microwave until smooth, checking at 30-second intervals. Be careful not to burn. Stir to mix melted chocolate and peanut butter. Add cereal and gently toss until coated. Drop on waxed paper or foil, making 6 cookies. Freeze for 30 minutes. Put in resealable plastic bags and refrigerate.

Yield: 6 servings

Each with: 1 g water; 124 calories (49% from fat, 10% from protein, 41% from carb); 4 g protein; 8 g total fat; 2 g saturated fat; 4 g monounsaturated fat; 2 g polyunsaturated fat; 15 g carb; 6 g fiber; 5 g sugar; 100 mg phosphorus; 53 mg calcium; 2 mg iron; 93 mg sodium; 169 mg potassium; 17 IU vitamin A; 4 mg vitamin E; 2 mg vitamin C; 2 mg cholesterol

Whole Wheat–Chocolate Chip Cookies

What's not to like about chocolate chip cookies?

1 cup (225 g) unsalted butter

¼ cup (64 g) peanut butter

1 cup (340 g) honey

2 eggs

1½ cups (180 g) whole wheat pastry flour

1 teaspoon baking soda

2 cups (160 g) rolled oats

(continued on page 432)

2 cups (350 g) chocolate chips

1 cup (110 g) chopped pecans

Cream together first 4 ingredients. Add next 5 ingredients and mix well. Add enough flour for stiff dough. Drop by teaspoon on baking sheet. Bake at 375°F (190°C, gas mark 5) for 10 minutes.

Yield: 48 servings

Each with: 6 g water; 194 calories (52% from fat, 7% from protein, 41% from carb); 3 g protein; 12 g total fat; 5 g saturated fat; 4 g monounsaturated fat; 1 g polyunsaturated fat; 21 g carb; 2 g fiber; 13 g sugar; 80 mg phosphorus; 28 mg calcium; 1 mg iron; 22 mg sodium; 107 mg potassium; 191 IU vitamin A; 51 mg vitamin E; 0 mg vitamin C; 29 mg cholesterol

Good-for-You Chocolate Chip Cookies

These are oatmeal chocolate chip cookies that you'll never suspect have been made more healthy.

¼ cup (55 g) unsalted butter

⅔ cup (150 g) packed brown sugar

¼ cup (85 g) honey

1 egg

1 teaspoon vanilla extract

¼ cup (60 ml) skim milk

1 teaspoon baking soda

½ teaspoon baking powder

1 cup (82 g) granola

¾ cup (60 g) quick-cooking oats

2 cups (240 g) whole wheat pastry flour

1 cup (175 g) chocolate chips

Cream together butter and brown sugar. Mix in honey, egg, vanilla, and milk, then baking soda and baking powder. Add granola, oats, and flour. Mix all ingredients. Stir in chocolate chips. Place on nonstick baking sheet by teaspoons. Bake at 325°F (170°C, gas mark 3) for 10 minutes.

Yield: 36 servings

Each with: 4 g water; 100 calories (28% from fat, 8% from protein, 64% from carb); 2 g protein; 3 g total fat; 2 g saturated fat; 1 g monounsaturated fat; 0 g polyunsaturated fat; 17 g carb; 1 g fiber; 9 g sugar; 54 mg phosphorus; 24 mg calcium; 1 mg iron; 25 mg sodium; 78 mg potassium; 61 IU vitamin A; 16 mg vitamin E; 0 mg vitamin C; 10 mg cholesterol

Oat and Wheat Cookies

This is a simple and easy-to-make cookie. But don't let the simplicity fool you, I find them to be just the little bit of sweetness I want after dinner.

¾ cup (165 g) unsalted butter

½ cup (130 g) peanut butter

²/₃ cup (150 g) brown sugar

1¼ cups (150 g) whole wheat pastry flour

1 teaspoon baking soda

1¼ cups (100 g) rolled oats

Mix all ingredients. Drop by rounded teaspoons onto ungreased baking sheet. Bake at 375°F (190°C, gas mark 5) for 10 to 12 minutes or until golden brown. Cool on baking sheet 1 minute and then cool on racks.

Yield: 36 servings

Each with: 2 g water; 95 calories (53% from fat, 8% from protein, 39% from carb); 2 g protein; 6 g total fat; 3 g saturated fat; 2 g monounsaturated fat; 1 g polyunsaturated fat; 10 g carb; 1 g fiber; 4 g sugar; 41 mg phosphorus; 9 mg calcium; 0 mg iron; 20 mg sodium; 69 mg potassium; 119 IU vitamin A; 32 mg vitamin E; 0 mg vitamin C; 10 mg cholesterol

Oatmeal Spice Cookies

A subscriber contributed this excellent recipe for oatmeal cookies. They have become family favorites.

1 cup (145 g) raisins

1 cup (235 ml) water

½ cup (112 g) unsalted butter, softened

¼ cup (60 ml) vegetable oil

1½ cups (300 g) sugar

2 eggs

1 teaspoon vanilla extract

2½ cups (300 g) whole wheat pastry flour

½ teaspoon baking powder

1 teaspoon baking soda

2 teaspoons cinnamon

¼ teaspoon nutmeg

2 cups (160 g) quick-cooking oats

½ cup (60 g) chopped walnuts

Preheat oven to 350°F (180°C, gas mark 4). Simmer raisins and water in saucepan on low until plump, approximately 20 minutes. Drain liquid into measuring cup and add water to make ½ cup liquid. Cream butter, oil, and sugar. Add eggs and vanilla. Stir in raisin liquid. Sift flour and spices; add to sugar mixture. Add oats, nuts, and raisins. Drop by rounded teaspoons onto ungreased baking sheet. Flatten slightly and then bake 8 to 10 minutes or until slightly brown.

Yield: 48 servings

Each with: 9 g water; 120 calories (33% from fat, 9% from protein, 58% from carb); 3 g protein; 5 g total fat; 2 g saturated fat; 1 g monounsaturated fat; 1 g polyunsaturated fat; 18 g carb; 2 g fiber; 8 g sugar; 72 mg phosphorus; 14 mg calcium; 1 mg iron; 10 mg sodium; 90 mg potassium; 72 IU vitamin A; 19 mg vitamin E; 0 mg vitamin C; 15 mg cholesterol

Trail Mix Cookies

This was an experiment that went right. The nutritional information will vary somewhat depending on the ingredients of the trail mix you find.

¾ cup (165 g) unsalted butter

¾ cup (150 g) sugar

1 egg

1 teaspoon vanilla extract

2 cups (240 g) whole wheat pastry flour

1 teaspoon baking soda

1 teaspoon cinnamon

¼ teaspoon nutmeg

¾ cup (175 ml) skim milk

1¾ cups (140 g) quick-cooking oats

1½ cups (200 g) trail mix

Cream together butter and sugar. Add egg and vanilla and beat well. Stir together dry ingredients. Add dry ingredients to mixture alternately with milk, mixing well. Stir in oats and trail mix. Drop by tablespoons on a baking sheet covered with nonstick vegetable oil spray. Bake at 400°F (200°C, gas mark 6) until lightly browned, 8 to 10 minutes.

Yield: 60 servings

Each with: 5 g water; 82 calories (42% from fat, 10% from protein, 49% from carb); 2 g protein; 4 g total fat; 2 g saturated fat; 1 g monounsaturated fat; 1 g polyunsaturated fat; 10 g carb; 1 g fiber; 3 g sugar; 56 mg phosphorus; 13 mg calcium; 1 mg iron; 4 mg sodium; 69 mg potassium; 84 IU vitamin A; 22 mg vitamin E; 0 mg vitamin C; 10 mg cholesterol

White Chocolate–Cranberry Cookies

These were inspired by cookies that were served as a snack at a training session I had at work. I was looking for a soft cookie with white chips and dried cranberries.

½ cup (112 g) shortening

1 cup (225 g) brown sugar

1 egg

1 teaspoon vanilla extract

1¾ cups (210 g) whole wheat pastry flour

1 teaspoon baking soda

¼ cup (60 ml) buttermilk

½ cup (87 g) white chocolate chips

½ cup (60 g) dried cranberries

TIP *If you like softer cookies, replace the butter with shortening like butter-flavored Crisco and the white sugar with brown.*

Beat shortening until light. Add sugar and beat until fluffy. Beat in egg and vanilla. Stir together dry ingredients. Add dry ingredients to mixture alternately with buttermilk. Beat until smooth. Stir in chips and cranberries. Drop about 2 inches (5 cm) apart on baking sheet coated with nonstick vegetable oil spray. Bake at 375°F (190°C, gas mark 5) 8 to 10 minutes, until lightly browned.

Yield: 36 servings

Each with: 4 g water; 91 calories (37% from fat, 5% from protein, 57% from carb); 1 g protein; 4 g total fat; 1 g saturated fat; 2 g monounsaturated fat; 1 g polyunsaturated fat; 13 g carb; 1 g fiber; 9 g sugar; 33 mg phosphorus; 15 mg calcium; 0 mg iron; 9 mg sodium; 75 mg potassium; 14 IU vitamin A; 4 mg vitamin E; 0 mg vitamin C; 6 mg cholesterol

Poppyseed Cookies

If you like poppyseeds, you'll love these. If you don't like poppyseeds, you still may ...

½ cup (112 g) unsalted butter, softened

¾ cup (170 g) packed brown sugar

2 eggs, beaten

½ teaspoon vanilla extract

½ teaspoon lemon peel

⅓ cup poppyseeds

2 cups (240 g) whole wheat pastry flour

2 teaspoons baking powder

Cream together butter and sugar. Beat until light. Add eggs and vanilla. Beat until creamy. Combine dry ingredients. Add and stir until well mixed. Drop by teaspoons on baking sheet. Bake at 350°F (180°C, gas mark 4) until lightly browned, about 10 minutes.

Yield: 30 servings

Each with: 5 g water; 89 calories (42% from fat, 8% from protein, 50% from carb); 2 g protein; 4 g total fat; 2 g saturated fat; 1 g monounsaturated fat; 1 g polyunsaturated fat; 12 g carb; 1 g fiber; 6 g sugar; 57 mg phosphorus; 51 mg calcium; 1 mg iron; 41 mg sodium; 69 mg potassium; 113 IU vitamin A; 31 mg vitamin E; 0 mg vitamin C; 24 mg cholesterol

Whole Wheat Sunflower Seed Cookies

These are crunchy sweet nuggets of goodness.

4 tablespoons (55 g) unsalted butter

½ cup (170 g) honey

1½ cups (180 g) whole wheat pastry flour

1 cup (68 g) nonfat dry milk

½ teaspoon baking soda

(continued on page 438)

2 tablespoons (28 ml) water

2 eggs

½ teaspoon vanilla extract

1 cup (175 g) chocolate chips

½ cup (72 g) sunflower seeds

¼ cup (37 g) chopped peanuts

Combine all ingredients. Drop by teaspoon onto baking sheet coated with nonstick vegetable oil spray. Bake in 350°F (180°C, gas mark 4) oven for 12 minutes.

Yield: 48 servings

Each with: 4 g water; 68 calories (39% from fat, 11% from protein, 50% from carb); 2 g protein; 3 g total fat; 1 g saturated fat; 1 g monounsaturated fat; 1 g polyunsaturated fat; 9 g carb; 1 g fiber; 6 g sugar; 55 mg phosphorus; 28 mg calcium; 0 mg iron; 17 mg sodium; 70 mg potassium; 81 IU vitamin A; 23 mg vitamin E; 0 mg vitamin C; 13 mg cholesterol

High-Fiber Cookies

These tasty cookies get extra bran and flavor from two kinds of cereal.

1 cup (100 g) oat bran

1 cup (80 g) rolled oats

1 cup (60 g) lightly sweetened bran cereal, such as Fiber One

1 cup (40 g) bran flakes cereal

1 cup (145 g) raisins

1 cup (120 g) chopped walnuts

¾ cup (150 g) sugar

¾ cup (170 g) brown sugar

1 cup (225 g) unsalted butter

1 egg

2 teaspoons vanilla extract

2 cups (240 g) whole wheat pastry flour

1 teaspoon baking powder

1 teaspoon baking soda

½ cup (120 ml) water, room temperature

Place oat bran, rolled oats, bran cereal, bran flakes, raisins, and walnuts in a bowl. Mix lightly and set aside. Place sugars and butter in mixing bowl and mix at medium speed until light and fluffy. Add egg and vanilla and mix lightly, scraping the bowl before and after adding the egg. In a separate bowl, combine the flour, baking powder, and baking soda and mix at low speed about 30 seconds to blend well. Add flour mixture and water to sugar mixture and mix at medium speed only until flour is moistened. Add bran mixture and mix at medium speed until well blended. Drop by heaping tablespoons onto a baking sheet that has been sprayed with nonstick vegetable oil spray or lined with aluminum foil. Bake at 375°F (190°C, gas mark 5) for 12 to 14 minutes or until lightly browned. Remove from oven and let sit for 1 minute. Remove cookies to wire rack and cool to room temperature.

Yield: 48 servings

Each with: 6 g water; 120 calories (41% from fat, 7% from protein, 52% from carb); 2 g protein; 6 g total fat; 3 g saturated fat; 2 g monounsaturated fat; 1 g polyunsaturated fat; 17 g carb; 2 g fiber; 9 g sugar; 64 mg phosphorus; 23 mg calcium; 1 mg iron; 28 mg sodium; 97 mg potassium; 171 IU vitamin A; 47 mg vitamin E; 2 mg vitamin C; 15 mg cholesterol

Molasses Cookies

This is the perfect cookie dough for making gingerbread men.

1 cup (225 g) unsalted butter, softened

1 cup (200 g) sugar

1 cup (340 g) molasses

⅓ cup (78 ml) water, boiling

1 tablespoon (15 ml) vinegar

5 cups (600 g) whole wheat pastry flour

2 teaspoons baking soda

1 teaspoon ginger

1 teaspoon cinnamon

(continued on page 440)

Cream butter and sugar. Add molasses, water, and vinegar. Combine dry ingredients. Beat into creamed mixture. Cover and chill for at least 3 hours. On a lightly floured surface, roll dough to ¼-inch (0.5 cm) thickness. Cut out cookies with cookie cutter or glass dipped in flour. Place on baking sheets coated with nonstick vegetable oil spray. Bake at 375°F (190°C, gas mark 5) for 8 minutes or until edges are lightly browned.

Yield: 72 servings

Each with: 4 g water; 75 calories (31% from fat, 6% from protein, 63% from carb); 1 g protein; 3 g total fat; 2 g saturated fat; 1 g monounsaturated fat; 0 g polyunsaturated fat; 12 g carb; 1 g fiber; 5 g sugar; 31 mg phosphorus; 14 mg calcium; 1 mg iron; 3 mg sodium; 104 mg potassium; 80 IU vitamin A; 21 mg vitamin E; 0 mg vitamin C; 7 mg cholesterol

Fudgy Brownies

This quick brownie recipe gets a fiber boost not just from the whole wheat flour but also from the cocoa.

1 cup (225 g) unsalted butter

½ cup (45 g) cocoa powder

2 cups (400 g) sugar

4 eggs

2 teaspoons vanilla extract

1 cup (120 g) whole wheat pastry flour

Heat oven to 350°F (180°C, gas mark 4). In microwave, melt butter and cocoa together, stirring once or twice. When melted, add sugar, eggs, and vanilla. Stir to mix well and then add flour. Pour into 13 × 9-inch (33 × 23 cm) pan coated with nonstick vegetable oil spray. Bake 25 minutes.

Yield: 18 servings

Each with: 13 g water; 224 calories (46% from fat, 5% from protein, 49% from carb); 3 g protein; 12 g total fat; 7 g saturated fat; 3 g monounsaturated fat; 1 g polyunsaturated fat; 29 g carb; 2 g fiber; 23 g sugar; 67 mg phosphorus; 15 mg calcium; 1 mg iron; 20 mg sodium; 84 mg potassium; 376 IU vitamin A; 102 mg vitamin E; 0 mg vitamin C; 80 mg cholesterol

Granola Bars

You can add unsalted nuts to this if you want or substitute chocolate chips or other dried fruit for the raisins to vary the flavor.

3 cups (240 g) quick-cooking oats

½ cup (115 g) brown sugar

¼ cup (28 g) wheat germ

½ cup (112 g) unsalted butter

¼ cup (60 ml) corn syrup

¼ cup (85 g) honey

½ cup (75 g) raisins

½ cup (40 g) sweetened coconut

Combine the oats, sugar, and wheat germ. Cut in the butter until the mixture is crumbly. Stir in the corn syrup and honey. Add the raisins and coconut. Press into a 9-inch (23 cm) square pan coated with nonstick vegetable oil spray. Bake in a 350°F (180°C, gas mark 4) oven for 20 to 25 minutes. Let cool 10 minutes and then cut into bars.

Yield: 27 servings

Each with: 4 g water; 153 calories (30% from fat, 8% from protein, 61% from carb); 3 g protein; 5 g total fat; 3 g saturated fat; 1 g monounsaturated fat; 1 g polyunsaturated fat; 24 g carb; 2 g fiber; 10 g sugar; 107 mg phosphorus; 17 mg calcium; 1 mg iron; 9 mg sodium; 129 mg potassium; 105 IU vitamin A; 28 mg vitamin E; 0 mg vitamin C; 9 mg cholesterol

Honey Oatmeal Cake

This makes a great breakfast or snack cake. Of course, I happen to be very fond of the flavor of honey.

1¼ cups (295 ml) water, boiling

1 cup (80 g) rolled oats

½ cup (112 g) unsalted butter, softened

1½ cups (510 g) honey

2 eggs

1 teaspoon vanilla extract

1¾ cups (210 g) whole wheat pastry flour

1 teaspoon baking soda

1 teaspoon ground cinnamon

¼ teaspoon ground nutmeg

Combine first 3 ingredients in a large bowl; stir well. Set aside for 20 minutes. Add honey, eggs, and vanilla; stir well. Combine whole wheat flour and remaining ingredients; gradually add to honey mixture. Pour into a greased and floured 13 × 9 × 2-inch (33 × 23 × 5 cm) baking pan. Bake at 350°F (180°C, gas mark 4) for 30 to 40 minutes or until toothpick comes out clean. Cool in pan. Frost if desired or sprinkle with confectioners' sugar.

Yield: 15 servings

Each with: 35 g water; 238 calories (27% from fat, 6% from protein, 67% from carb); 4 g protein; 8 g total fat; 4 g saturated fat; 2 g monounsaturated fat; 1 g polyunsaturated fat; 42 g carb; 2 g fiber; 28 g sugar; 92 mg phosphorus; 18 mg calcium; 1 mg iron; 14 mg sodium; 107 mg potassium; 227 IU vitamin A; 61 mg vitamin E; 0 mg vitamin C; 48 mg cholesterol

Red Velvet Cake

This is one of those old-time traditional cakes, updated to provide a little extra fiber by using whole wheat flour.

2½ cups (300 g) whole wheat pastry flour

1½ cups (300 g) sugar

2 teaspoons cocoa powder

1 teaspoon baking soda

2 eggs

½ cup (120 ml) canola oil

½ cup (120 ml) buttermilk

2 tablespoons (28 ml) red food coloring

1 teaspoon vanilla extract

Icing

¼ cup (55 g) unsalted butter

4 cups (400 g) confectioners' sugar

½ teaspoon vanilla extract

8 ounces (225 g) cream cheese

1 cup (110 g) chopped pecans

Mix together all dry ingredients in a large bowl. Blend eggs with a fork, add oil, and blend again. Add the dry ingredients and mix with whisk till smooth. Add and blend in buttermilk, food coloring, and vanilla. Pour into 3 greased and floured 8-inch (20 cm) cake pans. Bake at 350°F (180°C, gas mark 4) for 30 minutes. Cool for 10 minutes and gently remove from pan. To make icing, mix ingredients until light and fluffy. Frost cake when cool.

Yield: 16 servings

Each with: 23 g water; 457 calories (39% from fat, 6% from protein, 55% from carb); 7 g protein; 20 g total fat; 6 g saturated fat; 9 g monounsaturated fat; 4 g polyunsaturated fat; 65 g carb; 3 g fiber; 49 g sugar; 137 mg phosphorus; 40 mg calcium; 1 mg iron; 63 mg sodium; 184 mg potassium; 317 IU vitamin A; 85 mg vitamin E; 0 mg vitamin C; 53 mg cholesterol

Brown Rice Pudding

This quick rice pudding recipe uses leftover rice. (I tend to make a lot of rice when I cook it so I can use it in all these recipes calling for leftovers.)

2 cups (440 g) cooked brown rice

1½ cups (355 ml) skim milk

½ cup (170 g) honey

1 cup (145 g) golden raisins

1 tablespoon unsalted butter

1 teaspoon cinnamon

In medium saucepan, combine rice, milk, honey, and raisins and bring to boil. Reduce heat and simmer 20 minutes, stirring frequently. Remove from heat and stir in butter and cinnamon.

Yield: 4 servings

Each with: 168 g water; 426 calories (8% from fat, 7% from protein, 85% from carb); 8 g protein; 4 g total fat; 2 g saturated fat; 1 g monounsaturated fat; 0 g polyunsaturated fat; 96 g carb; 4 g fiber; 60 g sugar; 235 mg phosphorus; 174 mg calcium; 2 mg iron; 66 mg sodium; 543 mg potassium; 277 IU vitamin A; 80 mg vitamin E; 3 mg vitamin C; 9 mg cholesterol

Cool Rice

This is a kind of instant rice pudding and similar to the dish served at many family get-togethers during my childhood.

½ pound (225 g) brown rice

6 ounces (170 g) nondairy whipped topping, such as Cool Whip

¼ cup (50 g) sugar

1 teaspoon vanilla extract

10 ounces (284 g) crushed pineapple

5 maraschino cherries, halved

Cook rice according to package directions and cool. Combine all ingredients in large bowl. Refrigerate until ready to serve.

Yield: 5 servings

Each with: 106 g water; 217 calories (33% from fat, 4% from protein, 63% from carb); 2 g protein; 8 g total fat; 5 g saturated fat; 2 g monounsaturated fat; 0 g polyunsaturated fat; 35 g carb; 1 g fiber; 22 g sugar; 72 mg phosphorus; 50 mg calcium; 0 mg iron; 47 mg sodium; 132 mg potassium; 257 IU vitamin A; 63 mg vitamin E; 4 mg vitamin C; 26 mg cholesterol

Whole Wheat Piecrust

I find this oil-based piecrust easier to work with than with solid shortening. And it seems to stay flaky through more handling.

⅓ cup (80 ml) canola oil

1⅓ cups (160 g) whole wheat pastry flour

2 tablespoons (28 ml) water, cold

Add oil to flour and mix well with fork. Sprinkle water over and mix well. With hands press into ball and flatten. Roll between 2 pieces of waxed paper. Remove top waxed paper, invert over pan, and remove other paper. Press into place. For pies that do not require a baked filling, bake at 400°F (200°C, gas mark 6) until lighted browned, about 12 to 15 minutes.

Yield: 8 servings

Each with: 6 g water; 150 calories (56% from fat, 7% from protein, 37% from carb); 3 g protein; 10 g total fat; 1 g saturated fat; 6 g monounsaturated fat; 3 g polyunsaturated fat; 15 g carb; 2 g fiber; 0 g sugar; 69 mg phosphorus; 7 mg calcium; 1 mg iron; 1 mg sodium; 81 mg potassium; 2 IU vitamin A; 0 mg vitamin E; 0 mg vitamin C; 0 mg cholesterol

High-Fiber Piecrust

This is a really simple piecrust with 4 grams of fiber. You can add sugar or other sweeteners or spices like cinnamon depending on the final flavor you want.

1 cup (60 g) lightly sweetetened bran cereal, such as Fiber One
½ cup (120 ml) water, approximately

Crush cereal to a powder in a resealable plastic bag. Add any sweetener or spice desired to taste here and shake together. Pour evenly into a 9-inch (23 cm) springform or pie plate. Drizzle a little water at a time just to moisten the crumbs. Spread and press crust evenly. Use as stated in recipe, either baking before or simply pouring filling in and then baking or refrigerating.

Yield: 8 servings

Each with: 15 g water; 15 calories (8% from fat, 7% from protein, 85% from carb); 1 g protein; 0 g total fat; 0 g saturated fat; 0 g monounsaturated fat; 0 g polyunsaturated fat; 6 g carb; 4 g fiber; 0 g sugar; 38 mg phosphorus; 25 mg calcium; 1 mg iron; 27 mg sodium; 45 mg potassium; 3 IU vitamin A; 0 mg vitamin E; 2 mg vitamin C; 0 mg cholesterol

21

Desserts and Other Sweets:
Vegetables and Fruits

Fruit makes a great dessert choice. It has all kinds of great nutritional benefits and tends to be lower in calories than many other desserts. We have recipes here ranging from good old-fashioned ambrosia to pie fillings, fruit salads, and molds.

Ambrosia

This is one of the lighter desserts, the sort of refreshing end you might want with a heavy meal or something like a spicy curry. But it still contains 5 grams of fiber per serving.

4 cups orange slices

2 cups (300 g) sliced banana

1 cup (110 g) coarsely chopped pecans

2 ounces (57 g) coconut

In a large glass bowl, arrange alternate layers of orange slices, banana, pecans, and coconut. Drizzle a small amount of orange juice between layers if desired. Repeat layers. Chill several hours.

Yield: 8 servings

Each with: 122 g water; 218 calories (47% from fat, 5% from protein, 48% from carb); 3 g protein; 12 g total fat; 3 g saturated fat; 6 g monounsaturated fat; 3 g polyunsaturated fat; 28 g carb; 5 g fiber; 16 g sugar; 70 mg phosphorus; 49 mg calcium; 1 mg iron; 2 mg sodium; 443 mg potassium; 246 IU vitamin A; 0 mg vitamin E; 53 mg vitamin C; 0 mg cholesterol

Fresh Fruit Compote

This makes a refreshing ending to just about any meal, especially in the spring when berries are in season.

2 peaches, sliced

2 cups (290 g) blueberries

2 cups (300 g) sliced banana

2 cups (290 g) strawberries, hulled and halved

¼ cup (50 g) sugar

2 cups (460 g) plain fat-free yogurt

Combine fruit with sugar in a large bowl. Toss and transfer to a serving bowl. Serve with yogurt.

Yield: 4 servings

Each with: 378 g water; 309 calories (3% from fat, 12% from protein, 85% from carb); 10 g protein; 1 g total fat; 0 g saturated fat; 0 g monounsaturated fat; 0 g polyunsaturated fat; 70 g carb; 7 g fiber; 52 g sugar; 257 mg phosphorus; 270 mg calcium; 1 mg iron; 97 mg sodium; 1012 mg potassium; 341 IU vitamin A; 2 mg vitamin E; 67 mg vitamin C; 2 mg cholesterol

Fruit Soup

This is a cool, refreshing soup. This is another of those recipes where you can pick and choose the ingredients to get your favorites.

24 ounces (709 ml) grapefruit juice

16 ounces (455 g) plums

16 ounces (455 g) canned apricots, drained

20 ounces (567 g) frozen raspberries

¼ cup (38 g) quick-cooking tapioca

2 cinnamon sticks

6 whole cloves

3 cups (450 g) sliced banana

In a large pan, combine all ingredients except banana. Cook slowly 30 minutes or until heated through. It can be served hot or cold. Remove cinnamon sticks and whole cloves before serving. Ladle soup into bowls. Top with sliced banana or strawberries.

Yield: 16 servings

Each with: 87 g water; 70 calories (4% from fat, 6% from protein, 90% from carb); 1 g protein; 0 g total fat; 0 g saturated fat; 0 g monounsaturated fat; 0 g polyunsaturated fat; 17 g carb; 4 g fiber; 10 g sugar; 25 mg phosphorus; 14 mg calcium; 0 mg iron; 2 mg sodium; 251 mg potassium; 518 IU vitamin A; 0 mg vitamin E; 14 mg vitamin C; 0 mg cholesterol

Hawaiian Fruit Salad

The little extras in the dressing for this salad, like lime juice and crystallized ginger, are what really make it special.

2 cups (310 g) diced pineapple

1 cup (170 g) diced honeydew melon

1 cup (175 g) diced mango

2 tablespoons (28 ml) lime juice

2 tablespoons (40 g) honey

1 tablespoon chopped fresh cilantro

1 tablespoon minced crystallized ginger

½ cup (75 g) minced red bell pepper

1 tablespoon sesame seeds

Mix all ingredients except sesame seeds in large bowl. Let stand 10 minutes for flavors to blend. Divide fruit mixture among wineglasses and sprinkle with sesame seeds.

Yield: 6 servings

Each with: 139 g water; 110 calories (8% from fat, 4% from protein, 88% from carb); 1 g protein; 1 g total fat; 0 g saturated fat; 0 g monounsaturated fat; 0 g polyunsaturated fat; 27 g carb; 2 g fiber; 24 g sugar; 27 mg phosphorus; 34 mg calcium; 1 mg iron; 8 mg sodium; 256 mg potassium; 679 IU vitamin A; 0 mg vitamin E; 37 mg vitamin C; 0 mg cholesterol

Tropical Twist

This is a light, yet still satisfying, dessert full of fruit and other good things.

2 oranges

2 cups (300 g) sliced banana

2 kiwifruits, peeled and sliced

10 ounces (280 g) miniature marshmallows

1½ cups (345 g) sour cream

¼ cup (85 g) honey

½ teaspoon vanilla extract

⅓ cup (27 g) coconut, toasted

¼ cup (27 g) slivered almonds

From 1 orange, grate peel to equal ½ teaspoon (1 g) peel and section oranges. Place in large bowl with banana and kiwifruit. Stir in next 4 ingredients; toss to coat well. Spoon into 4 dessert bowls. Top with coconut and almonds.

Yield: 8 servings

Each with: 146 g water; 332 calories (23% from fat, 5% from protein, 72% from carb); 4 g protein; 9 g total fat; 5 g saturated fat; 3 g monounsaturated fat; 1 g polyunsaturated fat; 63 g carb; 4 g fiber; 43 g sugar; 97 mg phosphorus; 90 mg calcium; 1 mg iron; 49 mg sodium; 464 mg potassium; 328 IU vitamin A; 45 mg vitamin E; 51 mg vitamin C; 18 mg cholesterol

Winter Fruit Bowl

This is a great blending of fruit flavors, with the tartness of the grapefruit and cranberries offset by the sweetness of the banana and marmalade.

2 grapefruits

½ cup (100 g) sugar

¼ cup (75 g) orange marmalade

1 cup (100 g) cranberries, fresh or frozen

1½ cups (225 g) sliced banana

Section grapefruit. Reserve juice and add water to make 1 cup (235 ml). Combine juice with sugar and marmalade. Heat to boiling. Stir to dissolve sugar. Add cranberries; cook and stir until skins pop, 5 to 8 minutes. Cool. Add grapefruit, cover, and chill. Add sliced banana just before serving.

Yield: 5 servings

Each with: 180 g water; 295 calories (2% from fat, 2% from protein, 96% from carb); 2 g protein; 1 g total fat; 0 g saturated fat; 0 g monounsaturated fat; 0 g polyunsaturated fat; 77 g carb; 5 g fiber; 63 g sugar; 28 mg phosphorus; 28 mg calcium; 0 mg iron; 10 mg sodium; 442 mg potassium; 1284 IU vitamin A; 0 mg vitamin E; 52 mg vitamin C; 0 mg cholesterol

Ribbon Fruit Mold

This makes a mold that is not only tasty but also very pretty with its different-colored layers.

Raspberry Layer

1 cup (235 ml) boiling water

3 ounces (85 g) raspberry gelatin

10 ounces (284 g) frozen raspberries

Orange Layer

1 cup (235 ml) boiling water

3 ounces (85 g) orange gelatin

8 ounces (225 g) cream cheese, softened

11 ounces (310 g) mandarin oranges

Lime Layer

1 cup (235 ml) boiling water

3 ounces (85 g) lime gelatin

1 cup (155 g) crushed pineapple with syrup

Make raspberry layer: Pour boiling water on raspberry gelatin in large bowl. Stir until gelatin is dissolved. Stir in frozen raspberries. Chill until thickened. Pour into 9 × 13 × 2-inch (23 × 33 × 5 cm) baking pan. Chill until almost firm. Make orange layer: Pour boiling water on orange gelatin in large bowl. Stir until gelatin is dissolved. Stir gradually into cream cheese. Chill until thickened slightly. Mix in orange segments (with syrup). Pour evenly on raspberry layer. Chill. Make lime layer: Pour boiling water on lime gelatin in a large bowl. Stir until gelatin is dissolved. Stir in pineapple (with syrup). Chill slightly. Pour over orange layer. Chill until firm.

Yield: 8 servings

Each with: 196 g water; 270 calories (33% from fat, 8% from protein, 60% from carb); 5 g protein; 10 g total fat; 6 g saturated fat; 3 g monounsaturated fat; 1 g polyunsaturated fat; 42 g carb; 3 g fiber; 37 g sugar; 91 mg phosphorus; 44 mg calcium; 1 mg iron; 238 mg sodium; 175 mg potassium; 737 IU vitamin A; 102 mg vitamin E; 25 mg vitamin C; 31 mg cholesterol

Brandied Fruit

The flavor of this develops more and more over time. Use over ice cream, pound cake, or just as a little special snack.

15 ounces (425 g) pineapple chunks, drained

16 ounces (455 g) canned sliced peaches, drained

16 ounces (455 g) canned apricot halves, drained

10 ounces (280 g) maraschino cherries, drained

1¼ cups (250 g) sugar

1¼ cups (295 ml) brandy

Combine all ingredients in a clean, nonmetal bowl; stir gently. Cover and let stand at room temperature for 3 weeks, stirring fruit twice a week. Serve fruit over ice cream or pound cake, reserving at least 1 cup starter at all times. To replenish starter, add 1 cup sugar and 1 of the first 4 ingredients every 1 to 3 weeks, alternating fruits each time; stir gently. Cover and let stand at room temperature 3 days before using.

Yield: 12 servings

Each with: 126 g water; 224 calories (1% from fat, 2% from protein, 98% from carb); 1 g protein; 0 g total fat; 0 g saturated fat; 0 g monounsaturated fat; 0 g polyunsaturated fat; 43 g carb; 2 g fiber; 41 g sugar; 17 mg phosphorus; 25 mg calcium; 0 mg iron; 4 mg sodium; 161 mg potassium; 807 IU vitamin A; 0 mg vitamin E; 6 mg vitamin C; 0 mg cholesterol

Apple Topping

You can use this on pancakes or as a topping for ice cream or even a side dish with pork.

3 apples, peeled, cored, and chopped

¼ cup (85 g) honey

1 teaspoon cinnamon

(continued on page 454)

Combine ingredients in a microwave-safe bowl. Microwave on high until apples are soft, about 5 minutes

Yield: 4 servings

Each with: 87 g water; 112 calories (1% from fat, 1% from protein, 98% from carb); 0 g protein; 0 g total fat; 0 g saturated fat; 0 g monounsaturated fat; 0 g polyunsaturated fat; 30 g carb; 2 g fiber; 27 g sugar; 12 mg phosphorus; 13 mg calcium; 0 mg iron; 1 mg sodium; 100 mg potassium; 38 IU vitamin A; 0 mg vitamin E; 4 mg vitamin C; 0 mg cholesterol

Pear Pie Filling

Try this with the whole wheat piecrust on page 445.

½ cup (100 g) sugar

3 tablespoons (24 g) flour

1 teaspoon cinnamon

1 teaspoon lemon peel

5 cups pears, peeled and sliced

1 tablespoon unsalted butter

1 tablespoon (15 ml) lemon juice

Combine sugar, flour, cinnamon, and lemon peel in mixing bowl. Arrange pears in layers in a 9-inch (23 cm) pastry-lined pan, sprinkling sugar mixture over each layer. Dot with butter. Sprinkle with lemon juice. Roll out remaining dough; cut slits for escape of steam. Moisten rim of bottom crust. Place top crust over filling. Fold edge under bottom crust, pressing to seal. Flute edge. Bake at 450°F (230°C, gas mark 8) for 10 minutes. Reduce temperature to 350°F (180°C, gas mark 4) and bake for an additional 35 to 40 minutes.

Yield: 8 servings

Each with: 80 g water; 127 calories (11% from fat, 2% from protein, 87% from carb); 1 g protein; 2 g total fat; 1 g saturated fat; 0 g monounsaturated fat; 0 g polyunsaturated fat; 30 g carb; 3 g fiber; 22 g sugar; 14 mg phosphorus; 13 mg calcium; 0 mg iron; 1 mg sodium; 118 mg potassium; 67 IU vitamin A; 12 mg vitamin E; 5 mg vitamin C; 4 mg cholesterol

Strawberry Rhubarb Pie Filling

This makes a great pie filling or topping for ice cream or pudding. (Or use it on pancakes, if it's time for breakfast.)

2 cups chopped rhubarb

2 cups (340 g) slightly chopped strawberries

½ cup (100 g) sugar

3 tablespoons (24 g) cornstarch

Place fruit and sugar in bowl and let stand 15 minutes, stirring occasionally. Stir in cornstarch. Cook and stir until mixture is thickened and bubbly.

Yield: 8 servings

Each with: 79 g water; 86 calories (1% from fat, 2% from protein, 96% from carb); 1 g protein; 0 g total fat; 0 g saturated fat; 0 g monounsaturated fat; 0 g polyunsaturated fat; 22 g carb; 2 g fiber; 15 g sugar; 12 mg phosphorus; 35 mg calcium; 0 mg iron; 3 mg sodium; 170 mg potassium; 56 IU vitamin A; 0 mg vitamin E; 25 mg vitamin C; 0 mg cholesterol

Raspberry Cobbler

Raspberries are one of the higher-fiber fruits available, so this is a good choice when they are in season.

2 tablespoons (16 g) cornstarch

¼ cup (60 ml) cold water

1½ cups (300 g) sugar, divided

1 tablespoon (15 ml) lemon juice

4 cups (500 g) raspberries

1 cup (120 g) whole wheat pastry flour

1 teaspoon baking powder

6 tablespoons (85 g) unsalted butter

¼ cup (60 ml) boiling water

(continued on page 456)

In a saucepan, stir together the cornstarch and cold water until cornstarch is completely dissolved. Add 1 cup (200 g) sugar, lemon juice, and raspberries; combine gently. In a bowl, combine the flour, remaining sugar, and baking powder. Blend in the butter until the mixture resembles coarse meal. Add the boiling water and stir the mixture until it just forms a dough. Bring the raspberry mixture to a boil, stirring constantly. Transfer to a 1½-quart (1.5 L) baking dish. Drop spoonfuls of the dough carefully onto the mixture. Bake the cobbler on a baking sheet in the middle of a preheated 400°F (200°C, gas mark 6) oven for 20 to 25 minutes or until the topping is golden. Serve warm with vanilla ice cream or whipped cream.

Yield: 8 servings

Each with: 73 g water; 314 calories (26% from fat, 4% from protein, 71% from carb); 3 g protein; 9 g total fat; 6 g saturated fat; 2 g monounsaturated fat; 1 g polyunsaturated fat; 58 g carb; 6 g fiber; 41 g sugar; 85 mg phosphorus; 58 mg calcium; 1 mg iron; 64 mg sodium; 160 mg potassium; 288 IU vitamin A; 71 mg vitamin E; 17 mg vitamin C; 23 mg cholesterol

Cranberry Apple Crisp

Cranberry apple is a popular flavor combination. Here a can of cranberry sauce adds kick to an apple crisp.

2½ pounds (1 kg) apple, peeled, cored, and cut into ½-inch (1-cm) chunks

16 ounces (455 g) whole berry cranberry sauce

2 tablespoons (30 ml) lemon juice

1 cup (80 g) rolled oats

½ cup (60 g) whole wheat pastry flour

⅓ cup (40 g) chopped walnuts

¼ cup (60 g) packed brown sugar

¼ cup (65 g) apple juice concentrate, thawed

1 tablespoon (15 ml) canola oil

Preheat oven to 350°F (180°C, gas mark 4). Combine apple, cranberry sauce, and lemon juice in a large bowl. Transfer to a 9½-inch (24-cm) deep-dish pie pan. Whisk oats, flour, walnuts, and brown sugar in a medium bowl. Whisk apple juice concentrate and oil in a small bowl until blended; drizzle over dry ingredients and mix until moistened. Sprinkle over apples. Bake until apples are tender and top is golden, 40 to 45 minutes.

Yield: 8 servings

Each with: 167 g water; 304 calories (16% from fat, 6% from protein, 78% from carb); 4 g protein; 6 g total fat; 0 g saturated fat; 2 g monounsaturated fat; 3 g polyunsaturated fat; 63 g carb; 5 g fiber; 45 g sugar; 123 mg phosphorus; 28 mg calcium; 1 mg iron; 22 mg sodium; 296 mg potassium; 81 IU vitamin A; 0 mg vitamin E; 15 mg vitamin C; 0 mg cholesterol

Pumpkin Custard

This is basically a pumpkin pie without the crust. This recipe is also a little less sweet than most pies.

2 eggs

1 tablespoon sugar

1 cup (235 ml) skim milk

2 cups (490 g) pumpkin, cooked or canned

1 teaspoon cinnamon

1 teaspoon ginger

Beat the eggs and combine with the sugar. Add the milk and pumpkin and mix well. Add the spices and pour into an 8-inch (20 cm) pie pan. Bake in a 350°F (180°C, gas mark 4) for 50 to 60 minutes. Test by inserting a knife near the edge. When it comes out clean, the custard is finished. Cut into 6 equal portions when chilled. This custard will keep the pie-wedge shape without a crust.

Yield: 6 servings

Each with: 125 g water; 81 calories (23% from fat, 23% from protein, 54% from carb); 5 g protein; 2 g total fat; 1 g saturated fat; 1 g monounsaturated fat; 0 g polyunsaturated fat; 11 g carb; 3 g fiber; 5 g sugar; 111 mg phosphorus; 94 mg calcium; 2 mg iron; 55 mg sodium; 271 mg potassium; 12885 IU vitamin A; 51 mg vitamin E; 4 mg vitamin C; 80 mg cholesterol

Cranberry Rice

Use this as an alternative to cranberry sauce ... or just a nice sweet dish for your holiday. This can be either a side dish or a dessert.

2 cups (475 ml) water, divided

1⅓ cups (267 g) sugar, divided

2 cups (200 g) cranberries

1⅓ cups (292 g) cooked, cooled brown rice

¼ teaspoon cinnamon

1 apple, peeled and sliced

In a saucepan, combine ½ cup (120 ml) of the water and 1 cup (200 g) of the sugar. Bring to boil. Add cranberries, return to boil, reduce heat, and simmer 10 minutes or until most of the berries have popped. Add rice, cinnamon, and the remaining water and sugar. Bring to boil. Reduce heat, cover, and simmer 5 minutes. Remove from heat and stir in apple. Cover and let stand for 10 minutes.

Yield: 6 servings

Each with: 161 g water; 249 calories (2% from fat, 2% from protein, 96% from carb); 1 g protein; 0 g total fat; 0 g saturated fat; 0 g monounsaturated fat; 0 g polyunsaturated fat; 62 g carb; 3 g fiber; 49 g sugar; 43 mg phosphorus; 12 mg calcium; 0 mg iron; 5 mg sodium; 71 mg potassium; 30 IU vitamin A; 0 mg vitamin E; 6 mg vitamin C; 0 mg cholesterol

Cranberry Orange Ring

This molded dessert or salad goes well with chicken, turkey, or ham.

2 oranges

6 ounces (170 g) strawberry-flavored gelatin, such as Jell-O

1½ cups (355 ml) boiling water

1½ cups (415 g) jellied cranberry sauce

1 tablespoon orange peel

⅔ cup (74 g) chopped pecans

Section oranges. Finely dice and drain sections. Dissolve gelatin in boiling water. Stir cranberry sauce until smooth; blend into gelatin with orange peel. Chill until slightly thick and then fold in diced oranges and pecans. Pour into 5-cup ring mold. Chill until firm. Unmold to serve.

Yield: 8 servings

Each with: 117 g water; 245 calories (23% from fat, 5% from protein, 72% from carb); 3 g protein; 7 g total fat; 1 g saturated fat; 4 g monounsaturated fat; 2 g polyunsaturated fat; 46 g carb; 3 g fiber; 43 g sugar; 65 mg phosphorus; 30 mg calcium; 0 mg iron; 115 mg sodium; 138 mg potassium; 134 IU vitamin A; 0 mg vitamin E; 27 mg vitamin C; 0 mg cholesterol

Fruit Pizza

This is a great dessert for a kids' party, but it's also popular with older people.

20 ounces (570 g) sugar cookie dough

8 ounces (225 g) cream cheese

⅓ cup (67 g) sugar

½ teaspoon vanilla extract

2 cups (300 g) sliced banana

3 kiwifruits, sliced

1 pound (455 g) strawberries, sliced

1 cup (145 g) blueberries

½ cup (160 g) peach preserves

2 tablespoons (28 ml) water

Freeze dough for 1 hour. Line a 14-inch (36 cm) pizza pan with foil. Slice dough ⅛ inch (0.3 cm) thick and line pan; overlap slices but don't flatten into pan. Bake at 375°F (190°C, gas mark 5) for 12 minutes or until browned. Cool completely. Invert crust onto another pan, remove foil, and put on serving plate. Combine cream cheese, sugar, and vanilla until blended. Spread on crust; arrange fruit. Put preserves and water in bowl and stir to glaze-like consistency. Pour over fruit; chill. To serve, cut into wedges.

Yield: 14 servings

(continued on page 460)

Each with: 99 g water; 341 calories (37% from fat, 4% from protein, 59% from carb); 4 g protein; 14 g total fat; 6 g saturated fat; 6 g monounsaturated fat; 1 g polyunsaturated fat; 51 g carb; 3 g fiber; 27 g sugar; 110 mg phosphorus; 62 mg calcium; 1 mg iron; 224 mg sodium; 322 mg potassium; 280 IU vitamin A; 63 mg vitamin E; 42 mg vitamin C; 30 mg cholesterol

Chocolate Caramel Apples

This is decadence defined. Yes, coating an apple with both caramel and chocolate is overdoing it a bit, but it sure tastes good.

5 apples

5 wooden craft sticks

14 ounces (400 g) caramels, individual candies unwrapped

2 tablespoons (28 ml) water

7 ounces (200 g) chocolate candy bar, broken into pieces

1 tablespoon shortening

Bring a large pot of water to a boil. Dip apples into boiling water briefly, using a slotted spoon, to remove any wax that may be present. Wipe dry and set aside to cool. Insert sticks into the apples through the cores. Line a baking sheet with waxed paper and coat with nonstick vegetable oil spray. Place the unwrapped caramels into a microwave-safe medium bowl along with 2 tablespoons (28 ml) of water. Cook on high for 2 minutes and then stir and continue cooking and stirring at 1-minute intervals until caramel is melted and smooth. Hold apples by the stick and dip into the caramel to coat. Set on waxed paper; refrigerate for about 15 minutes to set. Heat the chocolate with the shortening in a microwave-safe bowl until melted and smooth. Dip apples into the chocolate to cover the layer of caramel. Return to the waxed paper to set.

Yield: 5 servings

Each with: 124 g water; 600 calories (30% from fat, 5% from protein, 65% from carb); 7 g protein; 21 g total fat; 8 g saturated fat; 8 g monounsaturated fat; 4 g polyunsaturated fat; 101 g carb; 3 g fiber; 85 g sugar; 187 mg phosphorus; 191 mg calcium; 1 mg iron; 226 mg sodium; 433 mg potassium; 151 IU vitamin A; 28 mg vitamin E; 5 mg vitamin C; 15 mg cholesterol

Easy Pumpkin Cupcakes

Use a cake mix and canned pumpkin pie filling to make these tasty cupcakes quick and easy to prepare.

1 package yellow cake mix

2 cups (490 g) pumpkin pie filling

2 eggs

6 ounces (170 g) butterscotch chips

Mix all ingredients together and place in greased or lined cupcake pan. Bake at 350°F (180°C, gas mark 4) for 15 to 20 minutes.

Yield: 24 servings

Each with: 20 g water; 65 calories (12% from fat, 5% from protein, 83% from carb); 1 g protein; 1 g total fat; 0 g saturated fat; 0 g monounsaturated fat; 0 g polyunsaturated fat; 14 g carb; 2 g fiber; 7 g sugar; 19 mg phosphorus; 14 mg calcium; 0 mg iron; 93 mg sodium; 38 mg potassium; 1897 IU vitamin A; 8 mg vitamin E; 1 mg vitamin C; 20 mg cholesterol

22

Desserts and Other Sweets:
Combinations

There are a couple of main themes in the combination dessert chapter. We start off with some good cookie recipes containing whole grain flour and nuts, but then we move quickly into fruit and grain dishes like cobblers, apple dumplings, and fruit breads. You should be able to find a number of things here that your family will love.

Almond Crunch Cookies

I love the almond and butter brickle taste of these cookies. The inch-and-a-half balls make pretty big cookies. You could make them smaller if you like.

1 cup (200 g) sugar

1 cup (100 g) confectioners' sugar, sifted

1 cup (225 g) unsalted butter, softened

1 cup (235 ml) canola oil

2 eggs

2 teaspoons almond extract

4½ cups (540 g) whole wheat pastry flour

1 teaspoon baking soda

1 teaspoon cream of tartar

2 cups (220 g) chopped almonds

6 ounces (170 g) Heath Bar chips

Combine sugar, confectioners' sugar, butter, and oil in a large mixing bowl; beat at medium speed with electric mixer until blended. Add eggs and almond extract, beating well. Combine flour, soda, and cream of tartar; gradually add to creamed mixture, beating just until blended after each addition. Stir in almonds and chips. Chill dough 3 to 4 hours. Shape dough into 1½-inch (4 cm) balls and place at least 3 inches (7.5 cm) apart on ungreased baking sheets. Flatten cookies with a fork dipped in sugar, making a crisscross pattern. Bake at 350°F (180°C, gas mark 4) for 14 to 15 minutes or until lightly browned. Transfer to racks to cool. Store in an airtight container.

Yield: 48 servings

Each with: 4 g water; 197 calories (58% from fat, 7% from protein, 36% from carb); 3 g protein; 13 g total fat; 4 g saturated fat; 6 g monounsaturated fat; 2 g polyunsaturated fat; 18 g carb; 2 g fiber; 9 g sugar; 76 mg phosphorus; 22 mg calcium; 1 mg iron; 15 mg sodium; 109 mg potassium; 139 IU vitamin A; 35 mg vitamin E; 0 mg vitamin C; 21 mg cholesterol

Apple Cookies

This is a nice, soft, chewy cookie … and it includes things that are good for you.

2 cups (240 g) whole wheat pastry flour

1 teaspoon baking soda

1 teaspoon cinnamon

½ teaspoon cloves

½ teaspoon nutmeg

½ cup (112 g) unsalted butter

1¼ cups (210 g) firmly packed brown sugar

1 egg

1 cup (110 g) chopped pecans

1 cup (125 g) finely chopped apple

1 cup (145 g) raisins

¼ cup (60 ml) skim milk

Sift flour with baking soda, cinnamon, cloves, and nutmeg. In a large mixing bowl, cream butter and brown sugar; beat in egg until well-blended. Stir in half of flour and spice mixture and then stir in pecans, apple, and raisins. Blend in milk, then remaining flour mixture. Drop by rounded tablespoons of dough, about 2 inches (5 cm) apart, onto baking sheets coated with nonstick vegetable oil spray. Bake at 375°F (190°C, gas mark 5) for 12 to 15 minutes or until done. Transfer to racks to cool. Store in an airtight container.

Yield: 36 servings

Each with: 8 g water; 114 calories (38% from fat, 5% from protein, 56% from carb); 2 g protein; 5 g total fat; 2 g saturated fat; 2 g monounsaturated fat; 1 g polyunsaturated fat; 17 g carb; 1 g fiber; 11 g sugar; 44 mg phosphorus; 18 mg calcium; 1 mg iron; 7 mg sodium; 110 mg potassium; 94 IU vitamin A; 24 mg vitamin E; 0 mg vitamin C; 13 mg cholesterol

Crunchy Orange Cookies

This is a different kind of oatmeal cookie, with a nice, unexpected orange flavor.

1 cup (225 g) unsalted butter

1 cup (200 g) sugar

2 eggs

¼ cup (60 ml) orange juice

1 teaspoon vanilla extract

2 teaspoons grated orange peel

2 cups (240 g) whole wheat pastry flour

1 teaspoon baking soda

2 cups (160 g) quick-cooking oats

1 cup (145 g) raisins

½ cup (55 g) chopped pecans

Cream butter and sugar until light. Beat in eggs, juice, vanilla, and orange peel. Add dry ingredients and mix well. Stir in oats, raisins, and pecans by hand. Drop by rounded teaspoons on baking sheet coated with nonstick vegetable oil spray. Bake at 375°F (190°C, gas mark 5) for 10 to 15 minutes. Transfer to racks to cool. Store in an airtight container.

Yield: 42 servings

Each with: 6 g water; 117 calories (44% from fat, 7% from protein, 49% from carb); 2 g protein; 6 g total fat; 3 g saturated fat; 2 g monounsaturated fat; 1 g polyunsaturated fat; 15 g carb; 1 g fiber; 7 g sugar; 52 mg phosphorus; 10 mg calcium; 1 mg iron; 5 mg sodium; 80 mg potassium; 151 IU vitamin A; 40 mg vitamin E; 1 mg vitamin C; 23 mg cholesterol

Fruit Cookies

Pick your favorite fruit or fruits to make these cookies your own. My personal favorites are cranberries, cherries, and pineapple.

1½ cups (337 g) mashed banana

⅓ cup (80 ml) canola oil

1 teaspoon vanilla extract

1½ cups (120 g) rolled oats

½ cup (50 g) oat bran

1½ cups (240 g) mixed dried fruits, coarsely chopped

½ cup (60 g) chopped walnuts

Preheat oven to 350°F (180°C, gas mark 4). Coat 2 baking sheets with nonstick vegetable oil spray. Mash bananas in a large bowl until smooth. Stir in oil and vanilla. Add oats, oat bran, mixed fruits, and walnuts. Stir well to combine. Drop by rounded teaspoons on baking sheets about 1 inch (2.5 cm) apart. Flatten slightly with back of a spoon. Bake 20 to 25 minutes or until bottom and edges are lightly brown. Cool completely; refrigerate.

Yield: 24 servings

Each with: 23 g water; 115 calories (38% from fat, 6% from protein, 56% from carb); 2 g protein; 5 g total fat; 0 g saturated fat; 2 g monounsaturated fat; 2 g polyunsaturated fat; 17 g carb; 2 g fiber; 9 g sugar; 49 mg phosphorus; 8 mg calcium; 1 mg iron; 4 mg sodium; 139 mg potassium; 28 IU vitamin A; 3 mg vitamin E; 3 mg vitamin C; 0 mg cholesterol

Graham Cracker Praline Cookies

These are an easy sort of toffee cookie.

24 graham crackers

1 cup (225 g) unsalted butter

1 cup (225 g) packed dark brown sugar

1 cup (110 g) chopped pecans

Place crackers on ungreased baking sheet with an edge. Melt butter and sugar. Bring to a boil. Add pecans and boil 2 minutes, no longer. Pour over graham crackers and bake in 275°F (140°C, gas mark 1) oven for 10 minutes. Remove, let cool slightly, and cut into fingers while still warm.

Yield: 48 servings

Each with: 1 g water; 86 calories (61% from fat, 3% from protein, 37% from carb); 1 g protein; 6 g total fat; 3 g saturated fat; 2 g monounsaturated fat; 1 g polyunsaturated fat; 8 g carb; 1 g fiber; 6 g sugar; 12 mg phosphorus; 4 mg calcium; 0 mg iron; 29 mg sodium; 17 mg potassium; 120 IU vitamin A; 32 mg vitamin E; 0 mg vitamin C; 10 mg cholesterol

Granola Cookies

These make tasty treats for breakfast or a snack, and they are healthy besides.

1 cup (145 g) firmly packed dates

1 cup (260 g) apple juice concentrate

3 tablespoons (48 g) peanut butter

3 tablespoons (60 g) honey

1 teaspoon vanilla extract

1 tablespoon (20 g) molasses

1 tablespoon chopped walnuts

½ cup (40 g) coconut

½ cup (75 g) raisins

2⅓ cups (280 g) whole wheat flour

2 cups (160 g) quick-cooking oats

Blend dates and apple juice until smooth. Add peanut butter, honey, vanilla, and molasses. Blend well and place in mixing bowl. Add nuts, coconut, raisins, and flour and mix well. Add oats and blend. Spoon onto nonstick baking sheet; press with wet fork until ¼ inch (0.5 cm) thick. Bake at 300°F (150°C, gas mark 2) about 20 minutes. Cool completely on racks and store in airtight container.

Yield: 36 servings

(continued on page 468)

Each with: 5 g water; 91 calories (15% from fat, 10% from protein, 75% from carb); 2 g protein; 2 g total fat; 0 g saturated fat; 0 g monounsaturated fat; 0 g polyunsaturated fat; 18 g carb; 2 g fiber; 8 g sugar; 61 mg phosphorus; 11 mg calcium; 1 mg iron; 9 mg sodium; 135 mg potassium; 1 IU vitamin A; 0 mg vitamin E; 3 mg vitamin C; 0 mg cholesterol

Raisin-Granola Cookies

These are good-tasting snacks that you can feel good about.

1¾ (145 g) cups granola

1½ cups (180 g) whole wheat pastry flour

1 cup (225 g) unsalted butter, softened

¾ cup (150 g) sugar

¾ cup (170 g) packed dark brown sugar

1 teaspoon baking soda

1 teaspoon vanilla extract

1 egg

1½ cups (220 g) raisins

Preheat oven to 375°F (190°C, gas mark 5). Coat baking sheets with nonstick vegetable oil spray. Into large bowl measure all ingredients except raisins. With mixer at low speed, beat ingredients just until mixed. Increase speed to medium and beat 2 minutes, occasionally scraping bowl with rubber spatula. Stir in raisins until mixture is well blended. Drop dough by heaping teaspoons about 2 inches (5 cm) apart on baking sheets. Bake 12 to 15 minutes until cookies are lightly browned around edges. Remove to wire racks and allow to cool. Store cookies in a tightly covered container up to 1 week.

Yield: 48 servings

Each with: 3 g water; 97 calories (39% from fat, 4% from protein, 57% from carb); 1 g protein; 4 g total fat; 3 g saturated fat; 1 g monounsaturated fat; 0 g polyunsaturated fat; 14 g carb; 1 g fiber; 9 g sugar; 29 mg phosphorus; 6 mg calcium; 0 mg iron; 19 mg sodium; 53 mg potassium; 126 IU vitamin A; 34 mg vitamin E; 0 mg vitamin C; 15 mg cholesterol

Pecan Cookies

Full of pecans and other good things, these are another cookie that you can eat with a little less guilt than usual.

1 cup (110 g) chopped pecans

½ cup (40 g) coconut

¼ cup (36 g) sesame seeds

½ cup (112 g) unsalted butter

½ cup (100 g) sugar

1 egg

1 teaspoon vanilla extract

¼ cup (60 ml) skim milk

1 cup (120 g) whole wheat pastry flour

½ teaspoon baking soda

1 cup (82 g) granola

½ cup (75 g) raisins

Combine pecans, coconut, and sesame seeds on baking sheet, and heat at 350°F (180°C, gas mark 4) until lightly toasted. Cream butter and sugar. Beat in egg, vanilla, and milk. Sift together flour and baking soda. Stir into egg mixture until blended. Stir in granola, pecan mixture, and raisins. Drop by spoonfuls onto baking sheets coated with nonstick vegetable oil spray.
Bake at 375°F (190°C, gas mark 5) for 15 to 20 minutes until lightly browned.

Yield: 36 servings

Each with: 4 g water; 95 calories (54% from fat, 6% from protein, 40% from carb); 1 g protein; 6 g total fat; 2 g saturated fat; 2 g monounsaturated fat; 1 g polyunsaturated fat; 10 g carb; 1 g fiber; 5 g sugar; 41 mg phosphorus; 19 mg calcium; 0 mg iron; 13 mg sodium; 64 mg potassium; 94 IU vitamin A; 25 mg vitamin E; 0 mg vitamin C; 13 mg cholesterol

Peanut-Granola Cookies

These make a nice, soft, chewy cookie with a great granola flavor.

1¾ cups (145 g) granola

1½ cups (180 g) whole wheat pastry flour

1 cup (225 g) unsalted butter, softened

¾ cup (150 g) sugar

¾ cup (170 g) packed dark brown sugar

1 teaspoon baking soda

1 teaspoon vanilla extract

1 egg

1 cup (145 g) peanuts, unsalted and coarsely chopped

Preheat oven to 375°F (190°C, gas mark 5). Coat baking sheets with nonstick vegetable oil spray. Measure all ingredients into a large bowl except peanuts. With mixer at low speed, beat ingredients just until mixed. Increase speed to medium and beat 2 minutes. Stir in peanuts until well blended. Drop dough by heaping teaspoons, about 2 inches (5 cm) apart. Bake 12 to 15 minutes until lightly browned around edges. Remove to rack and cool completely. Store in container with tight lid.

Yield: 48 servings

Each with: 3 g water; 97 calories (39% from fat, 4% from protein, 57% from carb); 1 g protein; 4 g total fat; 3 g saturated fat; 1 g monounsaturated fat; 0 g polyunsaturated fat; 14 g carb; 1 g fiber; 9 g sugar; 29 mg phosphorus; 6 mg calcium; 0 mg iron; 19 mg sodium; 53 mg potassium; 126 IU vitamin A; 34 mg vitamin E; 0 mg vitamin C; 15 mg cholesterol

Zucchini Cookies

No one will ever guess the secret ingredient in these supermoist cookies.

½ cup (112 g) unsalted butter, softened

¾ cup (150 g) sugar

1 egg

½ teaspoon vanilla extract

1½ cups (187 g) flour

1 teaspoon cinnamon

½ teaspoon baking soda

1 cup (80 g) quick-cooking oats

1½ cups (169 g) shredded zucchini

1 cup (82 g) granola

12 ounces (340 g) chocolate chips

Mix all ingredients in a large bowl. Drop by heaping teaspoons onto baking sheet. Bake in 350°F (180°C, gas mark 4) oven for 10 to 12 minutes. Cool completely before storing in an airtight container.

Yield: 48 servings

Each with: 6 g water; 97 calories (40% from fat, 6% from protein, 53% from carb); 2 g protein; 4 g total fat; 2 g saturated fat; 2 g monounsaturated fat; 0 g polyunsaturated fat; 13 g carb; 1 g fiber; 7 g sugar; 36 mg phosphorus; 18 mg calcium; 1 mg iron; 15 mg sodium; 54 mg potassium; 86 IU vitamin A; 21 mg vitamin E; 1 mg vitamin C; 11 mg cholesterol

Zucchini Bars

Sweet and moist, these are almost perfect, in my humble opinion.

3 eggs

2 cups (400 g) sugar

1 cup (225 g) unsalted butter, melted

2 cups (226 g) grated zucchini

1 tablespoon vanilla extract

3 cups (360 g) whole wheat pastry flour

1 teaspoon baking soda

½ teaspoon baking powder

1 tablespoon cinnamon

1 cup (120 g) chopped walnuts

Topping

½ cup (56 g) wheat germ

½ cup (115 g) brown sugar

1 teaspoon cinnamon

Beat eggs until light and foamy. Add sugar, butter, zucchini, and vanilla. Combine flour, baking soda, baking powder, and cinnamon. Add to egg-zucchini mixture. Stir until well blended; add walnuts. Pour into a 13 × 9 × 2-inch (33 × 23 × 5 cm) baking pan coated with nonstick vegetable oil spray. Make the topping: Mix wheat germ, brown sugar, and cinnamon together and sprinkle over batter. Bake in a 350°F (180°C, gas mark 4) oven for 15 to 20 minutes. Cool on rack. Cut into bars, and store in an airtight container.

Yield: 18 servings

Each with: 25 g water; 342 calories (40% from fat, 8% from protein, 52% from carb); 7 g protein; 16 g total fat; 7 g saturated fat; 4 g monounsaturated fat; 3 g polyunsaturated fat; 46 g carb; 4 g fiber; 29 g sugar; 171 mg phosphorus; 42 mg calcium; 2 mg iron; 33 mg sodium; 224 mg potassium; 397 IU vitamin A; 98 mg vitamin E; 3 mg vitamin C; 67 mg cholesterol

Trail Bars

These no-bake bars make a great grab-and-go breakfast or snack.

1 cup (235 ml) light corn syrup

½ cup (115 g) packed brown sugar

1½ cups (390 g) crunchy peanut butter

1 teaspoon vanilla extract

1 cup (68 g) nonfat dry milk

1 cup (82 g) granola

1 cup (40 g) bran flakes cereal

1 cup (145 g) raisins

1 cup (175 g) chocolate chips

Line 9 × 13-inch (23 × 33 cm) pan with waxed paper. In heavy saucepan (or large bowl in microwave) combine syrup and sugar; bring to boil. Remove from heat; stir in peanut butter and vanilla. Add remaining ingredients except chocolate; cool slightly. Add chocolate pieces; press into prepared pan. Refrigerate 30 minutes; cut into bars. Store in refrigerator.

Yield: 24 servings

Each with: 5 g water; 241 calories (37% from fat, 10% from protein, 54% from carb); 6 g protein; 10 g total fat; 2 g saturated fat; 5 g monounsaturated fat; 2 g polyunsaturated fat; 34 g carb; 2 g fiber; 20 g sugar; 123 mg phosphorus; 67 mg calcium; 1 mg iron; 143 mg sodium; 284 mg potassium; 169 IU vitamin A; 23 mg vitamin E; 1 mg vitamin C; 2 mg cholesterol

Johnny Appleseed Squares

These apple snack bars have lots of flavor and nutrition too.

1½ cups (180 g) whole wheat pastry flour

½ teaspoon baking soda

1½ cups (120 g) rolled oats

1 cup (225 g) brown sugar

(continued on page 474)

2 eggs

½ cup (112 g) unsalted butter, melted

2 cups (250 g) chopped apples

1 tablespoon (15 ml) lemon juice

⅓ cup (50 g) raisins

⅓ cup (37 g) chopped pecans

2 tablespoons (16 g) confectioners' sugar

Mix together flour and baking soda. Stir in oats and brown sugar. Gradually add eggs and butter, stirring with fork until crumbly. Firmly press half of mixture into bottom of 9-inch (23 cm) square pan coated with nonstick vegetable oil spray. Mix apples and lemon juice; stir in raisins and pecans. Place apple mixture in even layer over crumb base. Roll remaining oats mixture between 2 sheets of waxed paper to form a 9-inch (23 cm) square. Remove top of waxed paper and invert dough over filling, pressing dough down lightly. Remove paper. Bake in 375°F (190°C, gas mark 5) oven for 30 minutes. Sprinkle confectioners' sugar over top, if desired.

Yield: 12 servings

Each with: 29 g water; 284 calories (36% from fat, 7% from protein, 57% from carb); 5 g protein; 12 g total fat; 6 g saturated fat; 4 g monounsaturated fat; 1 g polyunsaturated fat; 42 g carb; 4 g fiber; 23 g sugar; 139 mg phosphorus; 39 mg calcium; 2 mg iron; 23 mg sodium; 239 mg potassium; 292 IU vitamin A; 76 mg vitamin E; 1 mg vitamin C; 60 mg cholesterol

Peanut Bars

These bar cookies are super-easy to make and very good to eat.

½ cup (112 g) unsalted butter

½ cup (115 g) brown sugar

½ cup (100 g) sugar

1 egg

½ teaspoon vanilla extract

1½ cups (120 g) quick-cooking oats

¾ cup (90 g) whole wheat pastry flour

½ teaspoon baking soda

1 cup (260 g) crunchy peanut butter

½ cup (75 g) raisins

Combine all ingredients and mix well. Pat mixture evenly into a 9-inch (23-cm) square baking dish coated with nonstick vegetable oil spray. Bake at 350°F (180°C, gas mark 4) for 30 minutes. Cool in pan. Cut into bars, and store in an airtight container.

Yield: 18 servings

Each with: 5 g water; 236 calories (48% from fat, 9% from protein, 43% from carb); 6 g protein; 13 g total fat; 5 g saturated fat; 5 g monounsaturated fat; 3 g polyunsaturated fat; 26 g carb; 3 g fiber; 16 g sugar; 108 mg phosphorus; 22 mg calcium; 1 mg iron; 79 mg sodium; 212 mg potassium; 177 IU vitamin A; 47 mg vitamin E; 0 mg vitamin C; 25 mg cholesterol

Apricot Pecan Balls

Here are some no-bake cookies with great apricot flavor.

1½ cups crushed vanilla wafers

1 cup (110 g) chopped pecans

½ cup (50 g) confectioners' sugar

½ cup (65 g) chopped dried apricots

¼ cup (60 ml) light corn syrup

2 tablespoons (28 ml) apricot brandy

½ cup (50 g) confectioners' sugar, sifted

In a bowl, stir together vanilla wafers, pecans, confectioners' sugar, and the apricots. Stir in corn syrup and brandy. Using 1 level tablespoon for each cookie, shape mixture into balls. Roll each ball in sifted confectioners' sugar. Store in a covered container.

Yield: 36 servings

Each with: 4 g water; 60 calories (41% from fat, 3% from protein, 56% from carb); 0 g protein; 3 g total fat; 0 g saturated fat; 1 g monounsaturated fat; 1 g polyunsaturated fat; 9 g carb; 1 g fiber; 6 g sugar; 13 mg phosphorus; 5 mg calcium; 0 mg iron; 13 mg sodium; 22 mg potassium; 65 IU vitamin A; 2 mg vitamin E; 0 mg vitamin C; 2 mg cholesterol

Apple Cobbler

A newsletter subscriber sent me this recipe originally. And as she pointed out, for those of us who don't like to peel apples, it doesn't take as many as a "real" apple pie. (I'm still hoping for an apple peeler for Christmas some year.)

4 apples, peeled and sliced

1 teaspoon cinnamon

1 tablespoon sugar

1 egg

¾ cup (165 g) unsalted butter, melted

½ cup (100 g) sugar

½ teaspoon baking powder

1 cup (120 g) whole wheat pastry flour

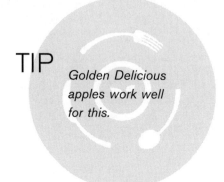

TIP *Golden Delicious apples work well for this.*

Slice the apples and place in a bowl. Add cinnamon and 1 tablespoon sugar and mix well. Pour into a 10-inch (25 cm) glass pie pan that has been sprayed with nonstick vegetable oil spray. In the same bowl, beat the egg. Add melted butter, ½ cup (100 g) sugar, baking powder, and flour. Pour over apples. (It'll be thick, so I actually put little spoonfuls all over to make sure it all gets covered.) Bake at 350°F (180°C, gas mark 4) for 40 to 45 minutes until golden brown and a toothpick inserted comes out clean.

Yield: 8 servings

Each with: 65 g water; 301 calories (53% from fat, 4% from protein, 43% from carb); 3 g protein; 19 g total fat; 11 g saturated fat; 5 g monounsaturated fat; 1 g polyunsaturated fat; 34 g carb; 3 g fiber; 21 g sugar; 82 mg phosphorus; 37 mg calcium; 1 mg iron; 45 mg sodium; 134 mg potassium; 600 IU vitamin A; 154 mg vitamin E; 3 mg vitamin C; 72 mg cholesterol

Apple Crunch

This is a tasty apple dessert with a crunchy topping.

½ cup (100 g) sugar

5 tablespoons (40 g) flour, divided

½ teaspoon cinnamon

¼ teaspoon nutmeg

5 cups (550 g) sliced apples

1 tablespoon unsalted butter

2 cups (164 g) granola

½ cup (115 g) brown sugar, packed

⅓ cup (75 g) unsalted butter, softened

TIP

Serve warm with milk poured over.

Coat a 9-inch-square (23 cm) pan with nonstick vegetable oil spray. Mix sugar, 3 tablespoons (24 g) flour, cinnamon, and nutmeg. Stir in apples and pour into pan. Dot with butter. Mix remaining ingredients; sprinkle over apples. Bake at 350°F (180°C, gas mark 4) for 25 to 30 minutes.

Yield: 12 servings

Each with: 43 g water; 208 calories (29% from fat, 3% from protein, 68% from carb); 2 g protein; 7 g total fat; 4 g saturated fat; 2 g monounsaturated fat; 0 g polyunsaturated fat; 37 g carb; 1 g fiber; 26 g sugar; 50 mg phosphorus; 19 mg calcium; 1 mg iron; 56 mg sodium; 117 mg potassium; 205 IU vitamin A; 50 mg vitamin E; 2 mg vitamin C; 16 mg cholesterol

Apple Dumplings

I remember having apple dumplings for dinner occasionally when I was young. But when I went looking for recipes, most were nothing like what I remember, which was a whole apple wrapped in pastry. Many seem to call for chopping the apples and most include a sugar syrup that my mother never made. This one is a compromise, downsized to half an apple to make it more appropriate for dessert. If it were me, I'd serve them warm with milk.

3 cups (360 g) whole wheat pastry flour

2 teaspoons baking powder

¼ cup (56 g) shortening

¾ cup (175 ml) milk

3 apples (Winesap, York, or other baking apples)

2 tablespoons (28 g) unsalted butter, divided

1 tablespoon sugar

1½ teaspoons cinnamon

Combine first 2 ingredients. Cut in shortening with pastry blender until mixture resembles coarse meal; gradually add milk, stirring to make a soft dough. Roll dough on lightly floured surface to make ¼-inch (0.5 cm) thickness, shaping into a 21 × 14-inch (53 × 36 cm) rectangle. Cut dough with a pastry cutter into six 7-inch (18 cm) squares. Peel and core apples, cut in half, place 1 apple half on each pastry square; dot each with 1 teaspoon butter. Sprinkle each with ½ teaspoon sugar and ¼ teaspoon cinnamon. Moisten edges of each dumpling with water, bringing corners to middle and pinching edges to seal. Place the dumplings in a 12 × 8 × 2-inch (30 × 20 × 5 cm) baking dish coated with nonstick vegetable oil spray and bake in a 375°F (190°C, gas mark 5) oven for 35 minutes.

Yield: 6 servings

Each with: 90 g water; 364 calories (32% from fat, 10% from protein, 58% from carb); 9 g protein; 14 g total fat; 5 g saturated fat; 5 g monounsaturated fat; 3 g polyunsaturated fat; 56 g carb; 8 g fiber; 10 g sugar; 281 mg phosphorus; 160 mg calcium; 3 mg iron; 179 mg sodium; 353 mg potassium; 212 IU vitamin A; 50 mg vitamin E; 3 mg vitamin C; 11 mg cholesterol

Crunchy Baked Apples

Granola adds crunch to these apples, while honey and apple and orange juices provide sweetness.

4 Granny Smith apples

½ cup (41 g) granola

2 cinnamon sticks, broken in half

½ cup (170 g) honey

1 cup (235 ml) apple juice

1 cup (235 ml) orange juice

Slice tops off apples. Seed and core. Do not cut off bottom of apple. Place apples in a baking dish. Fill opening with granola. Place cinnamon sticks in top of apples. Dribble honey over apples. Pour apple and orange juice in dish to cook the apples. Bake uncovered for 2 hours at 300°F (150°C, gas mark 2). Remove cinnamon sticks before serving.

Yield: 4 servings

Each with: 226 g water; 286 calories (3% from fat, 2% from protein, 95% from carb); 2 g protein; 1 g total fat; 0 g saturated fat; 0 g monounsaturated fat; 0 g polyunsaturated fat; 73 g carb; 2 g fiber; 58 g sugar; 55 mg phosphorus; 22 mg calcium; 1 mg iron; 45 mg sodium; 360 mg potassium; 97 IU vitamin A; 0 mg vitamin E; 26 mg vitamin C; 0 mg cholesterol

Date Nut Loaf

This is a sweet bread that's great for either breakfast or dessert. I like it with a little bit of apple butter.

1 cup (235 ml) water, boiling

1 cup (145 g) chopped dates

¼ cup (55 g) unsalted butter

½ cup (115 g) packed brown sugar

¼ cup (50 g) sugar

1 egg

1¾ cups (210 g) whole wheat pastry flour

½ teaspoon baking soda

½ teaspoon baking powder

¾ cup (84 g) coarsely chopped pecans

TIP *This will keep for at least a week refrigerated. For longer storage, freeze.*

Preheat oven to 350°F (180°C, gas mark 4). Spray 8 × 4-inch (20 × 10 cm) loaf pan with nonstick vegetable oil spray. Pour boiling water over dates and let soften. Beat butter until creamy in large bowl. Gradually beat in the sugars and cream well; beat in the egg. Beat in the dates and their liquid (at lowest speed). Sift together flour, baking soda, and baking powder. Add gradually, on lowest speed, to the creamed mixture; stir in the pecans. Pour into loaf pan coated with nonstick vegetable oil spray. Bake 45 minutes or until knife inserted in middle of loaf comes out clean. Cool loaf in pan on rack for 10 minutes and turn out on rack to cool.

Yield: 8 servings

Each with: 43 g water; 361 calories (34% from fat, 6% from protein, 60% from carb); 6 g protein; 15 g total fat; 5 g saturated fat; 6 g monounsaturated fat; 3 g polyunsaturated fat; 57 g carb; 6 g fiber; 34 g sugar; 156 mg phosphorus; 59 mg calcium; 2 mg iron; 51 mg sodium; 353 mg potassium; 230 IU vitamin A; 59 mg vitamin E; 0 mg vitamin C; 42 mg cholesterol

Double Apricot Bread

This is a great bread for those mornings when you want a little something sweet. It doesn't require anything on it, but you could add a little apricot jam and make it a triple.

16 ounces (455 g) canned apricots, drained

2½ cups (300 g) whole wheat pastry flour

1¼ cups (250 g) sugar

3½ teaspoons (16 g) baking powder

½ teaspoon pumpkin pie spice

2 eggs, beaten

½ cup (120 ml) skim milk

3 tablespoons (45 ml) canola oil

1 cup (130 g) chopped dried apricots

In a blender container or food processor bowl, blend or process canned apricot halves until smooth. Set aside. In a large bowl combine flour, sugar, baking powder, and pumpkin pie spice. In another bowl combine eggs, the apricot puree, milk, and oil. Add to flour mixture, stirring just until combined. Stir in dried apricots. Pour into two 8 × 4 × 2-inch (20 × 10 × 5 cm) loaf pans coated with nonstick vegetable oil spray. Bake in a 350°F (180°C, gas mark 4) oven 45 to 50 minutes or until a toothpick inserted near center comes out clean. Cool in pans 10 minutes. Remove from pans. Cool completely. Slice and serve.

Yield: 16 servings

Each with: 41 g water; 195 calories (16% from fat, 8% from protein, 75% from carb); 4 g protein; 4 g total fat; 0 g saturated fat; 2 g monounsaturated fat; 1 g polyunsaturated fat; 39 g carb; 3 g fiber; 23 g sugar; 120 mg phosphorus; 89 mg calcium; 1 mg iron; 124 mg sodium; 241 mg potassium; 824 IU vitamin A; 14 mg vitamin E; 2 mg vitamin C; 30 mg cholesterol

Apple Cake

Everyone wants something sweet every once in a while. But that doesn't mean that it can't still be good for you. Whole wheat flour and apples bump up the nutrition and fiber levels of this cake, but the taste just says "good."

2¼ cups (270 g) whole wheat pastry flour

1 cup (200 g) sugar

¾ cup (170 g) packed brown sugar

1 tablespoon cinnamon

2 teaspoons baking powder

½ teaspoon baking soda

¾ cup (175 ml) canola oil

1 teaspoon vanilla extract

3 eggs

2 cups (250 g) finely chopped apple

1 cup (120 g) chopped walnuts

¼ cup (25 g) confectioners' sugar, sifted

Generously grease and flour a 10-inch (25 cm) fluted tube pan; set aside. In a large mixing bowl, combine the flour, sugars, cinnamon, baking powder, and baking soda. Add oil, vanilla, and the eggs; beat until well mixed. Stir in the chopped apples and walnuts. Spoon batter evenly into prepared pan. Bake in a 350°F (180°C, gas mark 4) oven for 45 to 50 minutes or until cake tests done. Cool in pan 12 minutes; invert cake onto a wire rack. Cool thoroughly. Sprinkle with confectioners' sugar.

Yield: 16 servings

Each with: 22 g water; 317 calories (45% from fat, 7% from protein, 48% from carb); 6 g protein; 17 g total fat; 1 g saturated fat; 8 g monounsaturated fat; 6 g polyunsaturated fat; 40 g carb; 3 g fiber; 26 g sugar; 135 mg phosphorus; 65 mg calcium; 2 mg iron; 81 mg sodium; 174 mg potassium; 62 IU vitamin A; 15 mg vitamin E; 1 mg vitamin C; 44 mg cholesterol

Applesauce Date Cake

This is further proof that something sweet and delicious can still have significant nutritional value. This cake keeps well and is great for snacks or with lunches.

2 cups (240 g) whole wheat pastry flour

2 teaspoons baking soda

1 teaspoon cinnamon

½ teaspoon allspice

½ teaspoon nutmeg

¼ teaspoon ground cloves

2 eggs

1 cup (225 g) packed brown sugar

½ cup (112 g) unsalted butter, softened

2 cups applesauce, divided

1 cup (145 g) chopped dates

¾ cup (84 g) coarsely chopped pecans

Preheat oven to 350°F (180°C, gas mark 4). Spray a 9 × 9 × 2-inch (23 × 23 × 5 cm) pan with nonstick vegetable oil spray. Stir together flour, baking soda, and spices. Add eggs, brown sugar, butter, and 1 cup applesauce. Beat at low speed just until the ingredients are combined. At medium speed, beat 2 minutes longer, occasionally scraping the side of the bowl. Add remaining applesauce, dates, and pecans; beat 1 minute. Pour batter into pan. Bake 50 minutes or until knife inserted in center comes out clean. Cool 10 minutes in pan.

Yield: 12 servings

Each with: 48 g water; 341 calories (35% from fat, 6% from protein, 59% from carb); 5 g protein; 14 g total fat; 6 g saturated fat; 5 g monounsaturated fat; 2 g polyunsaturated fat; 53 g carb; 5 g fiber; 35 g sugar; 125 mg phosphorus; 45 mg calcium; 2 mg iron; 24 mg sodium; 313 mg potassium; 295 IU vitamin A; 76 mg vitamin E; 1 mg vitamin C; 60 mg cholesterol

Chocolate Cherry Cake

This is a great special occasion cake (Valentine's Day comes immediately to mind).

2 cups (240 g) whole wheat pastry flour

1½ cups (300 g) sugar

1¼ teaspoons baking soda

1 teaspoon baking powder

3 tablespoons nonfat dry milk powder

⅔ cup (135 g) shortening

⅓ cup (30 g) cocoa powder

1 can cherry pie filling

2 eggs

1 teaspoon almond extract

Combine all ingredients. Pour into greased and floured 13 × 9-inch (33 × 23 cm) pan. Bake at 350°F (180°C, gas mark 4) until done, about 30 minutes.

Yield: 16 servings

Each with: 34 g water; 260 calories (33% from fat, 5% from protein, 62% from carb); 4 g protein; 10 g total fat; 3 g saturated fat; 4 g monounsaturated fat; 2 g polyunsaturated fat; 42 g carb; 3 g fiber; 19 g sugar; 98 mg phosphorus; 42 mg calcium; 1 mg iron; 52 mg sodium; 151 mg potassium; 131 IU vitamin A; 15 mg vitamin E; 1 mg vitamin C; 30 mg cholesterol

Irish Apple Cake

I was searching for Irish dessert recipes last St. Patrick's Day and came across one similar to this one. It's like a half cake/half pie and absolutely delicious.

¼ pound (113 g) unsalted butter

1¾ cups (210 g) whole wheat pastry flour

¼ teaspoon baking powder

½ cup (100 g) sugar

1 egg, beaten

½ cup (120 ml) skim milk

2 apples

1 tablespoon sugar

½ teaspoon ground cloves

Cut butter into flour and baking powder to make dry crumbs. Add sugar, beaten egg, and enough milk to make a soft dough. Divide dough in two. Roll one half into a circle to fit an ovenproof pie pan coated with nonstick vegetable oil spray. Peel and core apples. Slice them onto the dough and add sugar and cloves. Roll out the remaining pastry and fit on top. Press the sides together; cut a slit through the lid. Bake at 350°F (180°C, gas mark 4) about 40 minutes or until apples are cooked through and the pastry is nicely browned.

Yield: 6 servings

Each with: 69 g water; 370 calories (40% from fat, 7% from protein, 53% from carb); 7 g protein; 17 g total fat; 10 g saturated fat; 4 g monounsaturated fat; 1 g polyunsaturated fat; 51 g carb; 5 g fiber; 23 g sugar; 176 mg phosphorus; 65 mg calcium; 2 mg iron; 50 mg sodium; 237 mg potassium; 580 IU vitamin A; 152 mg vitamin E; 2 mg vitamin C; 81 mg cholesterol

Orange Zucchini Cake

So moist and sweet, this makes a great snack cake.

1 cup (120 g) whole wheat pastry flour

1 teaspoon baking powder

½ teaspoon baking soda

1 teaspoon ground cinnamon

½ teaspoon ground nutmeg

¾ cup (150 g) sugar

½ cup (120 ml) canola oil

2 eggs

½ cup (30 g) all-bran cereal

(continued on page 486)

1½ teaspoons grated orange peel

1 teaspoon vanilla extract

1 cup (113 g) grated zucchini

½ cup (55 g) chopped pecans

¾ cup (110 g) raisins

Combine flour, baking powder, baking soda, cinnamon, and nutmeg. Set aside. In large bowl, beat sugar, oil, and eggs until well combined. Stir in cereal, orange peel, and vanilla. Add flour mixture, zucchini, pecans, and raisins. Mix well. Spread evenly in 10 × 6-inch (25 × 15-cm) baking dish coated with nonstick vegetable oil spray. Bake at 325°F (170°C, gas mark 3) for 35 minutes or until wooden pick inserted near center comes out clean. Cool completely.

Yield: 12 servings

Each with: 20 g water; 252 calories (47% from fat, 6% from protein, 47% from carb); 4 g protein; 14 g total fat; 1 g saturated fat; 8 g monounsaturated fat; 4 g polyunsaturated fat; 31 g carb; 3 g fiber; 20 g sugar; 118 mg phosphorus; 54 mg calcium; 1 mg iron; 63 mg sodium; 205 mg potassium; 116 IU vitamin A; 27 mg vitamin E; 3 mg vitamin C; 39 mg cholesterol

Pineapple Upside-Down Cake

I hadn't had one of these in many years when I recently made this. Having had the first warm slice, I wondered why.

6 tablespoons (85 g) unsalted butter, divided

½ cup (115 g) dark brown sugar

5 slices pineapple

5 maraschino cherries

½ cup (120 ml) skim milk

1 egg

1 teaspoon vanilla extract

1¼ cups (150 g) whole wheat pastry flour

½ cup (100 g) sugar

2 teaspoons baking powder

Preheat the oven to 375°F (190°C, gas mark 5). Melt half of the butter in a heavy cast-iron skillet or ovenproof pan. Add the brown sugar and stir well. Whisk in 2 teaspoons (10 ml) of water. Remove from the heat and add a single layer of pineapple slices. Place a cherry in the middle of each. Set aside. Melt the rest of the butter. Whisk in the milk, egg, and vanilla. Combine the flour, sugar, and baking powder in a separate mixing bowl. Beat the milk mixture into the flour mixture until a smooth batter forms. Pour over the pineapple in the skillet. Bake for 30 to 35 minutes or until the center is firm. Allow to cool for 10 minutes. Invert the pan onto a serving plate. Serve warm or at room temperature.

Yield: 8 servings

Each with: 49 g water; 278 calories (31% from fat, 6% from protein, 63% from carb); 4 g protein; 10 g total fat; 6 g saturated fat; 3 g monounsaturated fat; 1 g polyunsaturated fat; 45 g carb; 3 g fiber; 30 g sugar; 124 mg phosphorus; 108 mg calcium; 1 mg iron; 145 mg sodium; 149 mg potassium; 354 IU vitamin A; 92 mg vitamin E; 2 mg vitamin C; 49 mg cholesterol

Peanut Butter Burritos

These make great snacks for kids, and adults seem to like them too.

6 whole wheat tortillas, 6 inch (15 cm)

¾ cup (195 g) crunchy peanut butter

1 cup (145 g) raisins

1 cup (175 g) chocolate chips

Spread each tortilla with 2 tablespoons peanut butter. Sprinkle with raisins and chocolate chips. Roll up tortillas.

Yield: 6 servings

TIP *Vary the flavor by adding nuts, candies, mini marshmallows, or other flavors of baking chips.*

Each with: 14 g water; 516 calories (45% from fat, 10% from protein, 45% from carb); 13 g protein; 27 g total fat; 7 g saturated fat; 13 g monounsaturated fat; 5 g polyunsaturated fat; 61 g carb; 5 g fiber; 34 g sugar; 226 mg phosphorus; 120 mg calcium; 3 mg iron; 373 mg sodium; 597 mg potassium; 49 IU vitamin A; 13 mg vitamin E; 1 mg vitamin C; 6 mg cholesterol

Creamy Fruit Salad

This is easy to prepare ... and fruit salads are always enjoyed.

14 ounces (397 g) pineapple chunks, in juice

11 ounces (310 g) mandarin oranges, undrained

1 cup (150 g) sliced banana

1 cup (145 g) halved strawberries

¾ cup (113 g) halved seedless green grapes

1 cup (145 g) blueberries, fresh or frozen and thawed

3½ ounces (100 g) instant vanilla pudding mix

½ cup (41 g) granola

Drain chunk pineapple and orange segments, reserving liquid in small bowl. In large bowl, combine banana, strawberries, grapes, and blueberries. Sprinkle pudding mix into reserved liquid; mix until combined and slightly thickened. Fold into fruit until well combined. Spoon into serving dishes. Garnish with granola.

Yield: 8 servings

Each with: 142 g water; 144 calories (4% from fat, 4% from protein, 93% from carb); 1 g protein; 1 g total fat; 0 g saturated fat; 0 g monounsaturated fat; 0 g polyunsaturated fat; 36 g carb; 3 g fiber; 28 g sugar; 121 mg phosphorus; 22 mg calcium; 1 mg iron; 201 mg sodium; 291 mg potassium; 390 IU vitamin A; 0 mg vitamin E; 33 mg vitamin C; 0 mg cholesterol

23

Cooking Terms, Weights and Measurements, and Gadgets

Cooking Terms

Confused about a term I used in one of the recipes? Take a look at the list here and see if there might be an explanation. I've tried to include anything that I thought might raise a question.

Al Dente

To the tooth in Italian—The pasta is cooked just enough to maintain a firm, chewy texture.

Bake

To cook in the oven—Food is cooked slowly with gentle heat, concentrating the flavor.

Baste

To brush or spoon liquid, fat, or juices over meat during roasting to add flavor and to prevent it from drying out

Beat

To smooth a mixture by briskly whipping or stirring it with a spoon, fork, wire whisk, rotary beater, or electric mixer

Blend

To mix or fold two or more ingredients together to obtain equal distribution throughout the mixture

Boil

To cook food in heated water or other liquid that is bubbling vigorously

Braise

A cooking technique that requires browning meat in oil or other fat and then cooking slowly in liquid—The effect of braising is to tenderize the meat.

Bread

To coat the food with crumbs (usually with soft or dry bread crumbs), sometimes seasoned

Broil

To cook food directly under the heat source

Broth or Stock

A flavorful liquid made by gently cooking meat, seafood, or vegetables (and/or their by-products, such as bones and trimming), often with herbs and vegetables, in liquid (usually water)

Brown

A quick sautéing, pan/oven broiling, or grilling done either at the beginning or end of meal preparation, often to enhance flavor, texture, or eye appeal

Brush

Using a pastry brush to coat a food such as meat or bread with melted butter, glaze, or other liquid

Chop

To cut into irregular pieces

Coat

To evenly cover food with flour, crumbs, or a batter

Combine

To blend two or more ingredients into a single mixture

Core

To remove the inedible center of fruits such as pineapples

Cream

To beat butter or margarine, with or without sugar, until light and fluffy—This process traps in air bubbles; later it is used to create height in cookies and cakes.

Cut In

To work butter or margarine into dry ingredients

Dash

A measure approximately equal to $\frac{1}{16}$ teaspoon

Deep-Fry

To completely submerge the food in hot oil—A quick way to cook some food; as a result, this method often seems to seal in the flavors of food better than any other technique.

Dice

To cut into cubes

Direct Heat

Heat waves radiate from a source and travel directly to the item being heated with no conductor between them—Examples are grilling, broiling, and toasting.

Dough

Used primarily for cookies and breads—Dough is a mixture of shortening, flour, liquid, and other ingredients that maintains its shape when placed on a flat surface, although it will change shape once baked through the leavening process.

Dredge

To coat lightly and evenly with sugar or flour

Dumpling

A batter or soft dough that is formed into small mounds that are then steamed, poached, or simmered

Dust

To sprinkle food lightly with spices, sugar, or flour for a light coating

Fold

To cut and mix lightly with a spoon to keep as much air in the mixture as possible

Fritter

Sweet or savory foods coated or mixed into batter, then deep-fried

Fry

To cook food in hot oil, usually until a crisp brown crust forms

Glaze

A liquid that gives an item a shiny surface—Examples are fruit jams that have been heated or chocolate that has been thinned.

Grease

To coat a pan or skillet with a thin layer of oil

Grill

To cook over the heat source (traditionally over wood coals) in the open air

Grind

To mechanically cut a food into small pieces

Hull

To remove the leafy parts of soft fruits such as strawberries or blackberries

Knead

To work dough with the heels of your hands in a pressing and folding motion until it becomes smooth and elastic

Marinate

To combine food with aromatic ingredients to add flavor

Mince

To chop food into tiny irregular pieces

Mix

To beat or stir two or more foods together until they are thoroughly combined

Panfry

To cook in a hot pan with small amount of hot oil, butter, or other fat, turning the food over once or twice

Poach

Simmering in a liquid

Pot Roast

A large piece of meat, usually browned in fat, cooked in a covered pan

Puree

Food that has been mashed or sieved

Reduce

To cook liquids down so that some of the water they contain evaporates

Roast

To cook uncovered in the oven

Sauté

To cook with a small amount of hot oil, butter, or other fat, tossing the food around over high heat

Sear

To brown a food quickly on all sides using high heat to seal in the juices

Shred

To cut into fine strips

Simmer

To cook slowly in a liquid over low heat

Skim

To remove the surface layer (of impurities, scum, or fat) from liquids such as stocks and jams while cooking—This is usually done with a flat slotted spoon.

Smoke

To expose foods to wood smoke to enhance their flavor and help preserve and/or evenly cook them

Steam

To cook in steam by suspending foods over boiling water in a steamer or covered pot

Stew

To cook food in liquid for a long time until tender, usually in a covered pot

Stir

To mix ingredients with a utensil

Stir-fry

To cook quickly over high heat with a small amount of oil by constantly stirring—This technique often employs a wok.

Toss

To mix ingredients lightly by lifting and dropping them with two utensils

Whip

To beat an item to incorporate air, augment volume, and add substance

Zest

The thin, brightly colored outer part of the rind of citrus fruits—It contains volatile oils, used as a flavoring.

Weights and Measurements

First of all, here is a quick refresher on measurements.

3 teaspoons = 1 tablespoon

2 tablespoons = 1 fluid ounce

4 tablespoons = 2 fluid ounces = ¼ cup

5⅓ tablespoons = 16 teaspoons = ⅓ cup

8 tablespoons = 4 fluid ounces = ½ cup

16 tablespoons = 8 fluid ounces = 1 cup

2 cups = 1 pint

4 cups = 2 pints = 1 quart

16 cups = 8 pints = 4 quarts = 1 gallon

Measurements of Liquid Volume

The following measures are approximate but close enough for most, if not all, of the recipes in this book.

1 quart = 1 liter

1 cup = 250 milliliters

¾ cup = 200 milliliters

½ cup = 125 milliliters

⅓ cup = 105 milliliters

¼ cup = 60 milliliters

1 fluid ounce = 30 milliliters

1 tablespoon = 15 milliliters

1 teaspoon = 5 milliliters

Measurements of Weight

Much of the world measures dry ingredients by weight, rather than volume, as is done in the United States. There are several reliable websites, such as www.baking911.com, that make conversions easy. The following basic conversions may also be useful.

1 ounce = 28.4 grams

1 pound = 455 grams (about half a kilo)

Oven Temperatures

Finally, we come to one that is relatively straightforward, the Fahrenheit to Celsius conversion.

100°F = 38°C

150°F = 66°C

200°F = 95°C

225°F = 110°C

250°F = 120°C

275°F = 140°C

300°F = 150°C

325°F = 170°C

350°F = 180°C

375°F = 190°C

400°F = 200°C

425°F = 220°C

450°F = 230°C

475°F = 240°C

500°F = 250°C

Gadgets I Use

The following are some of the tools that I use in cooking. Some are used very often and some very seldom, but they all help make things a little easier or quicker. Why are some things here and others not? No reason except that most of these are things I considered a little less standard than a stove, oven, grill, and mixer.

Blender

Okay, so everyone has a blender. And it's a handy little tool for blending and pureeing things. I don't really think I need to say any more about that.

Bread Machine

When I went on a low-sodium diet I discovered that one of the biggest single changes that you can make to reduce your sodium intake is to make your own bread. Most commercial bread has well over 100 mg per slice. Many rolls and specialty breads are in the 300 to 400 mg range. A bread machine can reduce the amount of effort required to make your own bread to a manageable level. It takes at most 10 minutes to load it and turn it on. You can even set it on a timer to have your house filled with the aroma of fresh bread when you come home. Even if you're not watching your sodium, there is nothing like the smell of bread baking and the taste right out of the "oven."

Canning Kettle

If you are planning on making batches of things like pickles and salsa in volume so you don't have to go through the process every couple of weeks, then you are going to need a way to preserve foods. Most items can be frozen, of course, if that is your preference. But some things just seem to me to work better in jars. What you need is a kettle big enough to make sure the jars can be covered with water when being processed in a boiling water bath. There are also racks to sit the jars in and special tongs to make lifting them in and out of the water easier. I've used a porcelain covered kettle for this for a lot of years, and it also doubled as a stockpot before I got a new one. It's better for canning than for soup because the relatively thin walls allow the water to heat faster (and the soup to burn).

Deep Fryer

Obviously, if you are watching your fat intake, this should not be one of your most often used appliances. I don't use it nearly as often as I used to, but it still occupies a place in the appliance garage in the corner of the kitchen counter. It's a Fry Daddy, big enough to cook a batch of fries or fish for 3 or 4 people at a time.

Food Processor

I'm a real latecomer to the food processor world. It always seemed like a nice thing to have, but something I could easily do without. We bought one to help shred meat and other things for my wife's mother, who was having some difficulty swallowing large chunks of food. I use it now all the time to grind bread into crumbs or chop the peppers and onions that seem to go into at least three meals a week. It's a low-end model that doesn't have the power to grind meat and some of the heavier tasks, but I've discovered it's a real time-saver for a number of things.

Contact Grill

The George Foreman models are the most popular example of this item. My son's girlfriend gave me this for Christmas a few years ago (and he didn't have the good sense to hang on to her . . . but that's a different story). I use it fairly often. When we built our house we included a Jenn-Air cooktop with a built-in grill and for years, that was used regularly. It still is for some things. I much prefer the way it does burgers or steak when it's too cold to grill them outside, but it's difficult to clean and doesn't do nearly as nice a job as the Foreman at things like grilled veggies and fish. And the design allows the fat to drain away, giving you a healthier, lower-fat meal.

Grinder

Many years ago we bought an Oster Kitchen Center. It was one of those all-in-one things that included a stand mixer, blender (the one we still use), food chopper, and a grinder attachment. The grinder was never a big deal that got any use . . . until I started experimenting with sausage recipes. Since then I've discovered that grinding your own meat can save you both money and fat. Buying a beef or pork roast on sale, trimming it of most fat, and grinding it yourself can give you hamburger or sausage meat that is well over 90 percent lean and still less expensive than the fattier stuff you buy at the store. So now the grinder gets fairly regular use.

Hand Chopper

My daughter got this gem at a Wal-Mart in North Carolina while she was in school there. It was from one of those guys with the podium and the auctioneer's delivery and the extra free gifts if you buy it within the next 10 minutes. Neither of us has ever seen one like it since. The food processor has taken over some of its work, but it still does a great job chopping things like onions as fine as you could want without liquefying them.

Pasta Maker

I bought this toy after seeing it on a Sunday morning TV infomercial. It's a genuine Ronco/Popiel "As Seen on TV" special, but try not to hold that against it. Unlike the pasta cutters that merely slice rolled dough into flat noodles, this one mixes the whole mess, then extrudes it through dies with various shaped holes in them. The recipes say you can use any kind of flour, but I've found that buying the semolina flour that is traditionally used for pasta gives you dough that's easier to work with, as well as better texture and flavor. The characterization of it as a "toy" is pretty accurate. There aren't really any nutritional advantages over store-bought pasta. If you buy the semolina, the cost is probably about the same as some of the more expensive imported pasta. But it's fun to play with, makes a great conversation piece, and the pasta tastes good.

Salad Shooter

We seem to end up with a lot of these gadgets, don't we? This is another one that's been around for a while, but it's still my favorite implement for shredding potatoes for hash browns or cabbage for coleslaw.

Sausage Stuffer

This is really an addition to the Kitchen Center grinder. I found it at an online appliance repair site. It is really just a series of different-size tubes that fit on the end of the grinder to stuff your ground meat into casings. I do this occasionally to make link sausage, but most of the time I just make patties or bulk sausage.

Slicer

This was a closeout floor model that I bought years ago. Before going on the low-sodium diet I used to buy deli meat in bulk and slice it myself. Now it's most often used to slice a roast or smoked piece of meat for sandwiches.

Slow Cooker

I've tried to avoid calling it a Crock-Pot, which is a trademark of Rival. Anyway, whatever the brand, no kitchen should be without one.

Smoker

This was another pre-diet purchase that has been used even more since. I started with a Brinkman that originally used charcoal. Then I bought an add-on electric heat source for it that works a lot better in cold weather. Last year the family gave me a fancy MasterChef electric one that seals like an oven and has a thermostat to hold the temperature. Not only do I like the way it does ribs and other traditional smoked foods, but we also use it fairly regularly to smoke a beef or pork roast or turkey breast to use for sandwiches.

Springform Pan

This is a round, straight-sided pan. The sides are formed into a hoop that can be unclasped and detached from its base.

Steamer (Rice Cooker)

I use this primarily for cooking rice, but it's really a Black and Decker Handy Steamer Plus that does a great job steaming vegetables too. It does make excellent rice, perfect every time. So I guess the bottom line is that those of you who have trouble making rice, like me (probably because like me you can't follow the instructions not to peek), should consider getting one of these or one of the Japanese-style rice cookers.

Stockpot

The key here is to spend the extra money to get a heavy-gauge one (another thing I eventually learned from personal experience). The lighter-weight ones not only will dent and not sit level on the stove, but they will also burn just about everything you put in them. Mine also has a heavy glass lid that seals the moisture in well.

Turbocooker

This was another infomercial sale. It is a large, dome-lidded fry pan with racks that fit inside it. You can buy them at many stores too, but mine is the "Plus" model that has two steamer racks and a timer. It really will cook a whole dinner quickly, "steam frying" the main course and steaming one or two more items. The only bad news is most of the recipes involve additions and changes every few minutes, so even if you only take a half hour to make dinner, you spend that whole time at the stove.

Waffle Maker

We don't use this often, but it makes a nice change of pace for breakfast or dinner.

Wok

This is a round-bottomed pan popular in Asian cooking.

Index